Department of Health

Welsh Office

Scottish Office Department of Health

Department of Health and Social
Services, Northen Ireland

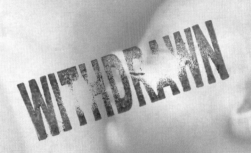

WHY MOTHERS DIE

Report on Confidential Enquiries into Maternal Deaths in the United Kingdom 1994-1996

Director
Gwyneth Lewis   MSc MRCGP MFPHM

Clinical Director
James Drife   MD FRCOG FRCPEd FRCSEd

Other Authors

Beverley Botting	BSc HonMFPHM	Kathryn Sallah	RN RM ADM DipPH
George Gordon	FRCSEd FRCOG	Robert Shaw	MD FRCSEd FRCOG
Ian Greer	MD MRCP MRCOG	Michael de Swiet	MD FRCP
Channi Kumar	MD PhD FRCPsych	William Thompson	MD FRCOG
James Neilson	MD FRCOG	Sheila Willatts	MD FRCA FRCP
Harry Millward-Sadler	FRCPath MHSH		

London: TSO

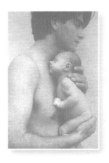

FOREWORD

In the developed world maternal deaths are now, fortunately, extremely rare events. However, the messages that can be gained from this Enquiry, almost 50 years old, are as valid today as when it first started in England and Wales in 1952. Although, sadly, some deaths remain inevitable events, many were associated with a degree of sub-standard care from which valuable lessons may be drawn. Furthermore, these deaths represent the tip of the iceberg of maternal morbidity and by ensuring all women receive optimal care, the recommendations in this Report should help to lessen physical and psychological pain for women and their wider families at a time usually associated with great happiness.

This Report, the fourth combining the United Kingdom as a whole, is the last of this millennium. It is also marked by a change in style and emphasis, which we hope will make it more attractive to read, more widely available and more relevant to general medical, maternity and obstetric practice. Less has been made of the detailed statistical tables of the past, without losing the key messages, and more of the general principles that can be extended into standard maternity care. A new executive summary of the main points and key recommendations for commissioners of services as well as those professional groups who may be involved in caring for pregnant women will be widely circulated among the NHS. The full Report can also be purchased or ordered from any book shop. Through this change we hope that it's findings will be read and implemented by many more people than in the past, including the recommendations, particularly for midwives and GPs, concerning the more public health-centred messages that could be incorporated into routine antenatal clinics. These include understanding the impact of domestic violence in pregnancy, helping identify those women more likely to be at risk of post natal depression, and clear instructions on the correct use of seat belts in pregnancy.

Furthermore, this Report closely follows the publication, in England, of "A First Class Service - Quality in the NHS", in Scotland the White Papers "Designed to Care" and "The Acute Services Review" and in Wales "Quality Care and Clinical Excellence". A similar paper will shortly be published in Northern Ireland. Many of the recommendations in this Report, particularly those for the use and audit of evidence based guidelines, are in tune with this new approach. It is an example of an area in which health professionals have been willing, for many years, to undertake a critical clinical audit in all cases of maternal death. This is evidenced by the very high reporting rate (95%) of maternal deaths. In the future, such reporting and participation will become a requirement of clinical practice, and we congratulate all staff who have been involved in such cases for willingly and freely giving of their time and expertise and showing how such a comprehensive Confidential Enquiry can be achieved.

REPORT ON CONFIDENTIAL ENQUIRIES INTO MATERNAL DEATHS IN THE UNITED KINGDOM

i

Finally, a Report such as this would not be possible without the continuing valuable support of the Royal Colleges of Obstetricians and Gynaecologists (RCOG), Midwives, General Practitioners, Psychiatrists, Pathologists, and Anaesthetists. As a result of previous Reports many Colleges have developed evidence-based guidelines for clinical practice which are included or referenced in this book. We are also indebted to the RCOG audit unit for reauditing the availability of such guidelines: the thought-provoking results are contained in Chapter 18. Furthermore, we must thank all the authors, local and central Assessors, Directors of Public Health and the professionals involved in each case for their dedicated work which has helped produce this Report only 18 months after the end of the triennium; a further full year ahead of the old schedule. We particularly congratulate the new Chairman of the Clinical Sub-group, Professor James Drife, for his hard work, dedication and vitality, and Dr Gwyneth Lewis, who has co-ordinated the Enquiries for the past four years and who has shown imagination and perseverance in setting the new schedule and steering the Report to publication.

This century has seen momentous changes in the safety of pregnancy for women and their babies. It is right to look back with gratitude to those who began this Enquiry and to recognise the part it has played in reducing the risks in childbirth. Complacency, however, would be a mistake. We look forward to the implementation of this Report's recommendations and to further improvements, especially in the health of underprivileged women.

CMO England	Professor Liam Donaldson
CMO Scotland	Sir David Carter
CMO Wales	Dr Ruth Hall
CMO Northern Ireland	Dr Henrietta Campbell

References

The Department of Health. *A First Class Service- Quality in the new NHS*. The Department of Health. London; 1998.

The Scottish Office Department of Health White Paper. *Designed to Care - Renewing the National Health Service in Scotland.* SODH; 1997.

The Scottish Office Department of Health. *Acute Services Review Report.* The SODH. TSO; 1998.

Welsh Office. *Quality Care and Clinical Excellence.* Cardiff. Welsh Office. 1998.

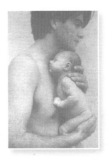

WHY MOTHERS DIE
CONTENTS

REPORT ON CONFIDENTIAL ENQUIRIES INTO MATERNAL DEATHS IN THE UNITED KINGDOM

Special issues

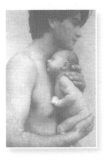

PREFACE

The "Maternal Mortality Reports" have been appearing throughout the working lifetime of all NHS staff. Indeed, the current system of Confidential Enquiries was started in 1952, only four years after the NHS was founded, and maternal deaths had been reported to the "Ministry" on an ad hoc basis for many years before that. The Enquiries have earned the respect of clinicians over the years and the findings and recommendations of successive Reports have underpinned a large part of obstetric practice.

This places a considerable responsibility on those who are now responsible for the Enquiries. It also brings disadvantages. Familiarity may dull the impact of these triennial publications and messages may be repeated from Report to Report without action being taken. Hence the new look of this Report. It differs from its predecessors not only in appearance but also in content, with new Chapters on Psychiatric disorders and on the role of the Midwife.

Some aspects of the Enquiries, however, have not changed. They are still a self-audit conducted by professionals - the longest-running example of such audit in the world. At a time of increasing pressures about imposing external audit on medicine, these Enquiries are a leading example of how doctors can review their own work and bring about dramatic improvements in health care. The involvement of midwives in this process is particularly welcome.

Looking back at the first Report, which covered 1952-54, it is easy to assume that the remarkable changes have resulted from a general improvement in the health of the population over the last four decades. This is far from true. Deaths from abortion, for example, have fallen from 153 in 1952-54 to one in 1994-96 because abortion has become legal. Deaths from haemorrhage have fallen from 188 to nine because of several measures, including routine oxytocic injections, ultrasound diagnosis of placenta praevia, and improved intensive care. Even deaths from thromboembolism, now the leading cause of *Direct* deaths, have fallen from 138 in 1952-54 to 46 in 1994-96, partly because women no longer take prolonged bed rest after a normal delivery.

The task now is to improve results that are already very good. This is not easy but it can be done. An example is provided by the anaesthetists, who have year by year reduced mortality. In 1952-54 anaesthesia caused 49 deaths; in 1982-84 it caused 18 deaths; and in 1994-96 only one death was due to anaesthesia. This reduction has been achieved by painstaking attention to detail and a refusal to compromise standards. The recommendations in this Report show how lives can still be saved in other areas.

We have to make these improvements while continuing to ensure that for the majority of women pregnancy and childbirth remain as natural and enjoyable as possible. Maximum safety does not mean unnecessary medicalisation. The increasing role of evidence-based practice should help to ensure that only effective interventions are used but when it comes to rare catastrophes, scientific data may be lacking. This Report therefore represents a blend of clinical experience and evidence-based recommendations. We hope it will help professionals and the women for whom they care.

James Drife
Gwyneth Lewis

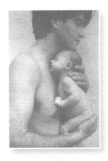

AIMS OF THE ENQUIRY AND DEFINITIONS OF MATERNAL MORTALITY

Aims and objectives of the Enquiry

These are:

- to assess the main causes of, and trends in, maternal deaths; to identify any avoidable or substandard factors; to promulgate these findings to all relevant health care professionals,

- to reduce maternal mortality and morbidity rates still further, as well as the proportion of cases due to substandard care,

- to make recommendations concerning the improvement of clinical care and service provision, including local audit, to purchasers of obstetric services and professionals involved in caring for pregnant women,

- to suggest directions for future areas for research and audit at a local and national level, and

- to produce a triennial Report for the four Chief Medical Officers of the United Kingdom.

Definitions of maternal mortality

The International Classification of Diseases, Injuries and Causes of Death - ninth revision (ICD9) defines a maternal death as "the death of a woman while pregnant or within 42 days of termination of pregnancy, from any cause related to or aggravated by the pregnancy or its management, but not from accidental or incidental causes". These are subdivided into *Direct*, *Indirect* and *Fortuitous*, but only *Direct* and *Indirect* deaths are counted for statistical purposes. In addition, the latest revision, ICD10, recognises that some women die as a consequence of *Direct* or *Indirect* obstetric causes after this period and has introduced a category for *Late* maternal deaths defined as "those deaths occurring between 42 days and one year after abortion, miscarriage or delivery that are due to *Direct* or *Indirect* maternal causes". The previous Report included all *Late* deaths occurring up to one year after delivery or abortion, as does this. The precise definitions for these are given in Table 1.

For the period covered by this Report the Office for National Statistics (ONS) continued to use ICD9 coding on death certificates, for the purposes of internal consistency, but this does not affect the number of deaths described in this Report in any way.

Table 1

Definitions of maternal deaths.	
Maternal deaths*	Deaths of women while pregnant or within 42 days of termination of pregnancy, from any cause related to or aggravated by the pregnancy or its management, but not from accidental or incidental causes.
Direct*	Deaths resulting from obstetric complications of the pregnant state (pregnancy, labour and puerperium), from interventions, omissions, incorrect treatment, or from a chain of events resulting from any of the above.
Indirect*	Deaths resulting from previous existing disease, or disease that developed during pregnancy and which was not due to direct obstetric causes, but which was aggravated by the physiological effects of pregnancy.
Late**	Deaths occurring between 42 days and one year after abortion, miscarriage, or delivery that are due to Direct or Indirect maternal causes.
Fortuitous*	Deaths from unrelated causes which happen to occur in pregnancy or the puerperium.

* ICD9

** ICD10

Denominator data used for calculating mortality rates

There are a number of statistical definitions and denominators that can be used to enable comparison of data collected through the Enquiry with data collected by the Registrars General, described below and shown in Table 2. They also enable comparision of trends in maternal mortality over time.

Maternities

Maternities are the number of pregnancies that result in a live birth at any gestation or a stillbirth occurring at or after 24 completed weeks' gestation and are required to be registrable by law. However, it is impossible to know the exact number of pregnancies which occurred during this, or any preceding, triennium since not all pregnancies result in a registrable live or still birth. Because of the unreliability of these data, due to the lack of appropriate denominators, the most common denominator used throughout this, and the previous, Report is the number of maternities (mothers delivered of live or stillborn infants) rather than the total number of pregnancies. The total number of maternities for the United Kingdom in 1994-96 was 2,197,640.

Estimated pregnancies

This denominator is used for calculating the rate of early pregnancy deaths. It is a combination of the number of maternities, together with legal terminations, hospital admissions for spontaneous abortions (at less than 24 weeks' gestation) and ectopic pregnancies, with an adjustment to allow for the period of gestation and maternal age at conception. The estimate for the United Kingdom 1994-96 was 2,914,600. However, the resulting total is still an underestimate of the actual number of pregnancies since these figures do not include other pregnancies which miscarry early, those where the woman is not admitted to hospital, or indeed those where the woman herself may not even know she is pregnant. Further details are available in Appendix 1.

Deaths from obstetric causes per million women aged 15-44

This denominator assumes that all women of childbearing age are at risk of becoming pregnant. It lacks the rigour of confining the rate calculated to women who actually were pregnant but has the advantage of enabling comparison with other causes of women's deaths.

Table 2

Maternal mortality definitions used in this Report.	
Maternal mortality definitions	**Reason for use**
Deaths from obstetric causes per million women aged 15-44.	This enables comparison with the other causes of death in this age group.
Deaths from obstetric causes per 100,000 maternities.	Maternities are the number of mothers delivered of registrable live births at any gestation or stillbirths of 24 weeks or later, i.e. these are the majority of women at risk of death from obstetric causes.
Deaths from obstetric causes per 100,000 estimated pregnancies.	Because the data for spontaneous abortions and ectopic pregnancies are unreliable this denominator is only used when calculating rates of death in early pregnancy.

Precise details of these, together with background figures and tables for the United Kingdom 1994-96, can be found in Appendix 1; Trends in Reproductive Epidemiology and Women's Health.

SUMMARY OF KEY RECOMMENDATIONS

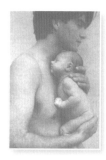

SUMMARY OF KEY RECOMMENDATIONS

Reporting maternal deaths and assisting with the Enquiry

Any health care professional who is aware of the death, from any cause, of a woman who is either pregnant or within one year following delivery, termination of pregnancy, ectopic pregnancy, or miscarriage is required to report it to their Director of Public Health or the Enquiry direct. The contact point for the Enquiry in England is Dr Gwyneth Lewis on 0171 972 4345.

"A First Class Service - Quality in the new NHS[1] " states: "All relevant hospital doctors and other health professionals will be required to participate in the work of the Confidential Enquiries". Full case notes must be made available to the Enquiry Assessors, and are treated in strict confidence. All professional staff who cared for the woman must provide information on request. Reports must be completed within nine months of the death.

Each trust should nominate a maternal death liaison officer to draw up local protocols for keeping the notes, assisting the Assessors and disseminating the recommendations. Guidelines for this are contained in Appendix 3.

Commissioning for maternal health

It is clear that some women who died had felt inhibited about seeking help. The socially excluded, the very young, or those from some minority ethnic groups did not always appear to have their specific concerns understood. Commissioners and trusts should provide those least likely to use services with the opportunity to gain acceptable professional and social support during their pregnancies.

The guidelines for the management of specific conditions set out here should be regularly reviewed and audited. Their implementation through local health care contracts, care and audit plans has the potential to reduce maternal deaths or severe morbidity.

Childbearing women suffering from psychiatric disorders, including postnatal depression, require a multi-professional approach. Commissioners should identify a clinician in each district to be responsible for managing a perinatal mental health service. This would provide continuity of care as a mentally ill woman and her baby pass through maternity and paediatric services and back into the community.

With regard to domestic violence, local trusts and community teams should develop inter-agency guidelines for the identification of vulnerable women and the provision of support for them and their families.

Auditable standards for maternity care

Each unit should identify a lead professional to develop and regularly update local multidisciplinary guidelines for the management of obstetric problems. Guidelines should be provided for the following:

- The management of pre-eclampsia and eclampsia
- The management of obstetric haemorrhage
- The use of thromboprophylaxis
- The use of antibiotics for caesarean section
- The management of women who decline blood products
- The identification and management of ectopic pregnancy

Guidelines should be prominently placed in all antenatal and postnatal wards, the delivery suite and in Accident and Emergency Departments, and given to all new members of staff.

The implementation of the guidelines should be subject to regular audit.

Each maternal death or case of severe morbidity should be discussed at multidisciplinary audit meetings.

Units should organise regular "fire drills" for cases of massive haemorrhage so that when these emergencies occur all members of staff - including the blood bank - know exactly what to do to ensure that large quantities of cross-matched blood can be delivered to the labour ward without delay.

A register of all cases of suspected or proven amniotic fluid embolism, whether the woman survived or not, is to be established for the United Kingdom. Details are available in Chapter 5.

Professional training

All staff should become familiar with the contents of this Report. Staff training, particularly in relation to audit and local guidelines, should be organised on a regular basis. This Report identified the need for training in the recognition of domestic violence, the early identification and management of postnatal depression and the correct use of car seat belts.

Specific recommendations for all health professionals providing maternal care

Antenatal care

Routine enquiries

Early identification of women at risk of postnatal mental illness or self harm should become part of routine practice. At booking, brief details should be taken about the presence or history of maternal psychiatric disorder, alcohol and substance abuse, severe social problems and previous self harm. Mechanisms should be in place to ensure effective psychiatric liason as well as to provide appropriate support

A sensitive enquiry about domestic violence should be routinely included when taking a social history. Ideally this information should be sought in the absence of the woman's partner. Advice or information about local sources of help should be available.

Routine information

Women should receive advice and support on healthy lifestyles, including diet and exercise, smoking and substance misuse and safety in the home and workplace.

Women should be educated about the correct use of seat belts during pregnancy. Three-point seat belts should be worn, with the lap strap placed as low as possible beneath the "bump" lying across the thighs with the diagonal shoulder strap above the bump lying between the breasts. Diagrams and further information are contained in Chapters 13 and 15.

All women should be made aware of the symptoms associated with pre-eclampsia, their importance and the need to obtain urgent professional advice.

Women with known epilepsy

Epilepsy is a potentially fatal disease. GPs and midwives should check with relatives that they know what to do in the case of a fit and should provide instruction, particularly on the need to place the patient in the recovery position once the fit is over. Pregnant women who are at risk of fits should be advised not to bathe alone, or to use a shower instead.

Pulmonary embolism

Even in the first trimester, pregnancy carries an increased risk of thrombosis. Additional risk factors such as bed rest may indicate thromboprophylaxis, as should a family history or known thrombophilia. Specialist advice should be sought if a thrombophilia screen is positive.

Close attention should be paid to any pregnant woman with chest or leg symptoms to exclude the presence of deep vein thrombosis or pulmonary embolism by Duplex ultrasound and ventilation/perfusion lung scanning respectively. Neither of these procedures carries any significant risk to mother or fetus.

Pre-eclampsia and eclampsia

A single senior clinician should have responsibility for the overall management for each case, and in particular for fluid balance. There should also be a clear system in place for transferring these women, if necessary, to a more specialised centre at an appropriate stage.

Medical problems in pregnancy

Minor signs or symptoms may have considerable significance in pregnancy and any pregnant woman seen in an Accident and Emergency Department, apart from those with minor injuries, should be discussed with the duty obstetrician. It should not be left to Accident and Emergency nurses or junior medical staff to decide whether or not there is an obstetric problem.

Chest X-ray is safe in pregnancy and is a simple screening test for dissection of the aorta. It should **always** be performed in unwell pregnant women with chest pain.

Patients with severe medical conditions or those taking anticoagulants require management in co-ordination with specialist centres. Obstetricians and midwives should liaise early with other health care professionals when patients have non-obstetric illness, including diabetes or epilepsy.

Ectopic pregnancy

It is essential that GPs and other clinicians including staff in Accident and Emergency Departments, consider the diagnosis of ectopic pregnancy in any woman of reproductive age who complains of abdominal pain. The clinical presentation is often not "classical". Gastrointestinal symptoms, notably diarrhoea and painful defaecation, may be prominent in ectopic pregnancy.

β-human chorionic gonadotrophin testing should be considered in any woman with unexplained abdominal pain whether or not she has missed a period or had abnormal vaginal bleeding.

When ectopic pregnancy is suspected, or when a woman with a predisposing history complains of severe abdominal pain, rapid referral and assessment are vital.

Laparoscopic surgery rather than open surgery should only be undertaken by an operator experienced in the technique.

Women in haemorrhagic shock following rupture of ectopic pregnancy need to be transferred promptly to the operating theatre. Transfer must not be delayed by attempts to try to re-establish a normal circulating plasma volume.

The Royal College of Obstetricians and Gynaecologists will shortly be producing further guidelines on the management of ectopic pregnancy, and the summary of these should be made available to all local GPs and staff in Accident and Emergency Departments.

Delivery

All women undergoing caesarean section should be assessed for prophylaxis against thromboembolism. If multiple risk factors are present the most effective method of prophylaxis, heparin at appropriate doses, should be used.

There is clear evidence from controlled trials showing the benefit of prophylactic antibiotics for caesarean section.

Care is required in using prostaglandins for induction of labour because of the risk of hyperstimulation and uterine rupture.

Placenta praevia, particularly in patients with a previous uterine scar, may be associated with uncontrollable uterine haemorrhage at delivery and caesarean hysterectomy may be necessary. At caesarean section, a very experienced operator is essential and a consultant must be immediately available.

When infection develops and the patient is systemically ill, urgent and repeated bacteriological specimens, including blood cultures, must be obtained. In serious cases doctors should be prepared to give parenteral antibiotics before the diagnosis can be confirmed.

Postnatal care

Midwives, GPs and other medical staff should give particular attention to women in the puerperium with chest or leg symptoms after vaginal or caesarean delivery to exclude the presence of deep vein thrombosis or a pulmonary embolism.

Puerperal sepsis is not a disease of the past. GPs and midwives must be aware of the signs and be prepared for the immediate treatment and referral of any recently delivered woman with a fever and/or offensive vaginal discharge.

Women who have a history of psychiatric disorder, substance abuse, or self harm should be carefully followed up for signs of postnatal recurrence or exacerbation of their problem.

A woman's weight may remain raised after pregnancy and account should be taken of this when considering oral contraception. Puerperal cardiomyopathy is a known risk factor for cerebral thrombosis and women with this condition should not be prescribed oral contraception.

Termination of pregnancy and spontaneous abortion

Ideally, all women should undergo ultrasound examination before termination of pregnancy to establish gestational age, viability and site.

Laparoscopy, and/or laparotomy, is essential if perforation of the uterus occurs during suction termination of pregnancy, because of the risk of bowel damage and life-threatening sequelae.

In cases of septic abortion, evacuation of the uterus should be performed by experienced surgeons, optimally around one hour after intravenous antibiotics.

References

1.   The Department of Health. *A First Class Service - Quality in the new NHS.* London: The Department of Health; 1998.

2.   The Scottish Office Department of Health White Paper. *Designed to Care - Renewing the National Health Service in Scotland.* Edinburgh: SODH; 1997.

3.   The Scottish Office Department of Health. *Acute Services Review Report.* Edinburgh: SODH; 1998.

4.   Welsh Office. *Quality Care and Clinical Excellence.* Cardiff: Welsh Office; 1998.

1

INTRODUCTION AND KEY FINDINGS

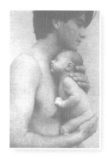

CHAPTER 1
INTRODUCTION AND KEY FINDINGS

Background

This Report, the fourth covering the United Kingdom as a whole, continues the unbroken series of Confidential Enquiries into Maternal Deaths which started in 1952 for England and Wales, 1956 for Northern Ireland and 1965 for Scotland. Not only is this the last Report to be published in this millennium, but also it sets new standards for case ascertainment. Furthermore, it has widened its scope to include important public health messages concerning advice to and care of pregnant or recently delivered women. These are derived from a more detailed assessment of *Fortuitous* deaths and those occurring as a result of psychiatric illness or substance abuse.

Appendix 1 to this Report gives details of the general trends in reproductive epidemiology. Details of the method of enquiry can be found in Appendix 2.

Overall maternal mortality rates

These can be calculated in two ways:

- through official death certification to the Registrars General (the Office for National Statistics (ONS) and its equivalents), or

- through deaths known to this Enquiry. The overall maternal death rate is calculated from the number of *Direct* and *Indirect* deaths. The preceding section on Aims and Definitions gives a fuller explanation of this terminology.

The number of *Direct* and *Indirect* deaths identified by the Enquiry always exceeds those officially reported. This is because ONS data are based on death certificates where the cause of death is directly or secondarily coded for a pregnancy-related condition such as postpartum haemorrhage, eclampsia etc. A large proportion of women known to the Enquiry die of conditions indirectly influenced by their pregnant state, for example cardiac disorders and epilepsy, but these are excluded from the official statistics. The same applies to those women who require long-term intensive care and whose cause of death is registered as a non-pregnancy condition such as multiple organ failure although the precipitating cause was an obstetric event. Conversely, the maternal deaths known to the Registrars General may include *Late* deaths as it is not possible to identify from the death certificate when the delivery or termination occurred.

In terms of international comparison, it is important to note two points. The first is that the criteria used by the UK Assessors for *Indirect* deaths are more inclusive than those used in other countries. The second is that case ascertainment is lower in the vast majority of other countries because they do not undertake such comprehensive enquiries. For example in this Enquiry all cases of cardiac disease, asthma and epilepsy are coded as *Indirect,* as are cases of suicide unless obviously occurring in women with a long standing previous psychiatric history.

An important note on improved case ascertainment for the 1994-96 Enquiry

Until recently it has not proved possible to estimate, with any degree of certainty, the degree of under-reporting of cases to this Enquiry. However, for the first time in the history of these Enquiries it is now possible for the Office of National Statistics (ONS) to run a computer program to identify deaths that previously would have passed unrecognised. Before 1993, only the underlying cause of death was coded for computer record. For deaths occurring from 1993 onwards, computer programs, originally developed in the USA and adapted by ONS, have been used to code cause of death automatically. As a result, all conditions given anywhere on the certificate are now coded and held on the computer record and ONS have been able to undertake a more extensive search of death draft entry information to identify all conditions listed in 1994-96 which suggest a maternal death. This has led to the identification of 67 deaths not otherwise known to the Enquiry; 10 *Direct* (nine cases of pulmonary embolism and one of amniotic fluid embolism), 40 *Indirect* and 17 *Late* deaths. These have increased the numbers known to the Enquiry, and hence the overall and specific maternal mortality rates compared to the last triennium. It is not possible to know whether or not similar numbers remained undetected in previous triennia, but it is probable that such a degree of under-reporting existed in earlier years. Furthermore, efforts have also been made to increase the profile of the Enquiry and more health care professionals, in particular Local Supervising Authority (LSA) responsible midwifery officers, have been reporting maternal deaths. As a result **it is not always possible to draw meaningful comparisons between the figures for this triennium and those which preceded it. This Report's figures will therefore act as a new baseline against which future rates will be judged.**

Maternal death rates derived from the 1994-96 Enquiry: the effect of the additional cases

Table 1.1 shows the maternal mortality rates derived from the Enquiry with and without improved case ascertainment as compared to the rates for 1991-93. As can be seen, due to the small numbers involved, the rates for 1994-96 change significantly with the inclusion of the extra cases. The overall rate (*Direct* and *Indirect* deaths) for the Enquiry, should these have not been included, is calculated to be 9.9 per 100,000 maternities, the same as the revised figure for the last Report. Table 1.3 at the end of this Chapter gives the total number of maternities for this, and the previous three triennia broken down by age group.

Table 1.1

Maternal death rates per 100,000 maternities showing the effect of improved case ascertainment; United Kingdom 1994-96.						
Type of death	1991-93		1994-96 Without extra cases*		1994-96 With extra cases*	
	No.	Rate	No.	Rate	No.	Rate
Direct	128	5.6	124	5.6	134	6.1
Indirect	100	4.3	94	4.3	134	6.1
Total	228	9.9	218	9.9	268	12.2

* see text

Deaths known to the Registrars General

Table 1.2 shows that the maternal mortality rate derived from death certificate notifications has risen to 7.4 from 6.4 per 100,000 maternities for 1991-93. The rates for previous triennia were 7.2 per 100,000 in 1988-90 and 7.7 per 100,000 maternities in 1985-87. The overall rates for this Enquiry are shown for comparison although it is important to note the shaded column giving the 1994-96 figures which reflect the introduction of improved case ascertainment.

There has also been a small rise in the percentage of deaths due to obstetric causes in women aged 15-44 as shown in Table 1.3, although the percentage of such deaths in this population remains the same as for the four previous triennia.

Table 1.2

Maternal deaths and mortality rates per 100,000 maternities reported to the Registrars General and the Enquiries; United Kingdom 1985-96.				
	1985-87	1988-90	1991-93	1994-96
Total maternities	2,268,766	2,360,309	2,315,204	2,197,640
Maternal deaths known to the Registrars General				
Number	174	171	149	163
Rate	7.7	7.2	6.4*	7.4
Direct maternal deaths known to the Enquiry				
Number	137	145	128	134
Rate	6.0	6.1	5.6	6.1
Indirect deaths known to the Enquiry				
Number	86	93	100	134
Rate	3.8	3.9	4.3	6.1
Total *Direct* and *Indirect* deaths known to the Enquiry				
Number	223	238	228	268
Rate	9.9	10.1	9.9	12.2

* final ONS revised figures for 1991-93. The rate available in time for the publication of the previous Report was 6.0

Source: England and Wales Mortality Statistics Cause Series DH2
    Birth Statistics Series FM1
    Scotland - Registrar General Annual Report 1985-96
    Northern Ireland - Registrar General Annual Report 1985-96

Table 1.3

Mortality rates per million female population aged 15-44 years. All causes and maternal deaths; United Kingdom 1979-96.			
Triennium	All Causes	Maternal deaths	% deaths in age group due to maternal causes
1979-81	697.2	6.6	1.0
1982-84	641.7	4.7	0.7
1985-87	622.5	4.2	0.7
1988-90	625.9	4.1	0.7
1991-93	608.1	4.0	0.7
1994-96	610.3	4.3	0.7

ICD 9th revision 1978-96, ICD 630-676
Source: 1979-96 Mortality Statistics, cause. Series DH Table 2
1979-96 The Registrar General's Annual Report, Scotland
1979-96 The Registrar General's Annual Report, Northern Ireland.

Summary of cases known to the Enquiry: 1994-96

During this triennium 376 deaths were reported to or identified by the Enquiry. There were 323 such cases in 1991-93. Taking into account the number of cases identified by the new ONS search, the numbers that would have expected to have been reported without improved case ascertainment may have been roughly comparable.

Regrettably, and despite repeated requests, either no forms or only the death certificate were available in 40 cases. However, it was still possible to code the deaths according to type. Of the 376 there were 134 *Direct* and 134 *Indirect* deaths, each representing 36% of reported cases. Thirty-six (9%) were classified as *Fortuitous* and 72 (19%) as *Late*. In this triennium the total number of *Direct* and *Indirect* maternal deaths reported to the Enquiry, 268, is higher than the 229 reported in the previous triennium, but as explained before, 50 of these are *Direct* and *Indirect* deaths identified through the new case ascertainment system. Comparison with the previous Report (40% *Direct* and 31% *Indirect*) shows proportionately fewer *Direct* and slightly more *Indirect* deaths in this triennium although these differences must be interpreted with caution.

The number of deaths by underlying cause, and the Chapter to which they have been allocated, are shown in Table 1.4. Rates by cause of death, per million maternities, compared to previous triennia are shown in Table 1.5.

Table 1.4

Chapter	Cause	Number of cases
Direct deaths		
2	Thrombosis and thromboembolism	48
3	Hypertensive disease of pregnancy	20
4	Haemorrhage	12
5	Amniotic fluid embolism	17
6	Early pregnancy deaths*	15
	Ectopic*	12
	Spontaneous miscarriage	2
	Legal termination	1
7	Sepsis	14
8	Other _Direct_	7
	Genital tract trauma	5
	Other	2
9	Anaesthetic	1
	Total number of _Direct_ deaths	**134**
Indirect deaths		
10	Cardiac	39
11	Psychiatric	9
12	Other Indirect	86
	Total number of _Indirect_ deaths	**134**
Fortuitous deaths		
13		**36**
Late deaths **		
14	_Direct_	4
	Indirect	32
	Fortuitous	36
	Total number of _Late_ deaths	**72**

Number of maternal deaths by cause; United Kingdom 1994-96.

*   includes one ruptured abdominal pregnancy
** _Late_ deaths classified as _Direct_ or _Indirect_ according to ICD(10) are not counted for statistical purposes.

Table 1.5

Chapter	Cause	Rate 1985-87	Rate 1988-90	Rate 1991-93	Rate 1994-6
	Death rates by major cause of death per million maternities; United Kingdom 1985-96. The shaded column for 1994-96 reflects the new system of case ascertainment.				
2	Thromboembolism	14.6	14.0	15.1	21.8*
3	Pregnancy-induced hypertension	11.9	11.4	8.6	9.1
4	Haemorrhage	4.4	9.3	6.5	5.5
5	Amniotic fluid embolism	4.0	4.7	4.3	7.7
6	Early pregnancy	10.6	10.2	7.8	6.8
7	Sepsis	2.6	3.0	3.9	6.4
8	Total uterine trauma/other *Direct***	11.8	7.2	6.0	3.2
	Uterine trauma	2.6	1.3	1.7	2.3
	Other *Direct*	9.2	5.9	4.3	0.9
9	Anaesthetic	2.6	1.7	3.5	0.5
10	Cardiac *Indirect*	10.1	8.9	16.0	17.7
11	Other *Indirect*	27.0	30.5	27.2	39.1
12	Psychiatric *Indirect****	-	-	-	4.1
2-12	Total *Direct* and *Indirect*	99.6	100.9	98.9	121.9
13	*Fortuitous*****	11.3	16.5	19.9	16.4
14	*Late*****	N/A	20.3	19.9	32.8

*   includes 9 cases found under new ascertainment system
**   new composite Chapter
***   new Chapter; previously counted in other *Indirect*
**** these are excluded, by International definition, from maternal mortality statistical calculations
N/A   not available for the 1985-87 Enquiry

Summary of key findings 1994-96

These are:

● An increase in overall maternal mortality rates (*Direct* and *Indirect* deaths) known both to the Registrars General and to this Enquiry,

● an increase in *Direct* and *Indirect* maternal mortality rates,

Specific causes of death

Direct

Thrombosis and thromboembolism remain the major direct cause of maternal death and the rates have risen substantially to 21.8 per million maternities in this triennium compared to 15.1 in the last. They account for almost 36% of all *Direct* maternal deaths. Hypertensive disease of pregnancy is the second leading cause of death, closely followed by amniotic fluid embolism, early pregnancy and sepsis. Together these five categories account for 85% of all *Direct* maternal deaths.

Increase in rates

- A striking increase has occurred in the number of deaths associated with thromboembolism, in particular pulmonary thromboembolism, of which 18 cases (38%) occurred before 24 weeks' gestation. The rate for pulmonary Thromboembolism has increased from 13 per million maternities (30 cases) in the last triennium to 20.9 (46 cases) for this, but this includes nine extra cases found under the new case ascertainment system. If these had been excluded, the rate would have increased to 17.7 per million maternities.

- An increase was seen in the rate of death from amniotic fluid embolism to 7.7 compared to 4.3 per million maternities in the last Report.

- An increase was seen in the rates of death from sepsis to 6.4 from 3.9 per million maternities in the last triennium. The majority of these were cases of puerperal sepsis, and only two women had had a caesarean section.

- A small increase in the rate of death from uterine rupture: 2.3 compared to 1.7 per million maternities in the last Report.

- A slight increase in the rates of death from pregnancy-induced hypertension: 9.1 compared to 8.6 per million maternities in the last triennium. However, the rate is still lower than for the previous two triennia.

Decrease in rates

- Deaths directly associated with anaesthesia have fallen from 3.5 per million maternities in the last Report to 0.5 in this Report. There was only one death directly due to an anaesthetic in this triennium.

- Haemorrhage, too, has caused fewer deaths, the rate being 5.5 compared to 6.5 per million maternities reported in the last triennium.

- Other *Direct* causes of death have fallen to 0.9 compared to 4.3 per million maternities for 1991-93.

REPORT ON CONFIDENTIAL ENQUIRIES INTO MATERNAL DEATHS IN THE UNITED KINGDOM

- There has been a small decrease in deaths in early pregnancy, which are mainly due to ectopic pregnancies and spontaneous miscarriage. The rates are 6.8 per million maternities for this triennium compared to 7.8 in the last Report. There was only one death as a result of a termination of pregnancy.

- There were four *Late Direct* deaths in this triennium, compared to 10 in the last Report.

Indirect

There has been a small increase in *Indirect* deaths, probably due to increased case ascertainment. The number of *Late Indirect* deaths is 31 compared to 23 in the last Report.

Substandard Care

Substandard care has been very difficult to evaluate in many of the cases in this Report due to the lack of key records and case notes. Whilst it is clear that many of the cases received less then optimum care it has not always been possible to quantify these with certainty. Cases where major substandard care clearly occurred, in which different management would probably have changed the outcome, are described in the relevant Chapter. Lessons to be drawn from these cases are highlighted, and reflected in the recommendations. Without direct access to the case notes it will never be possible adequately to establish the number of deaths due to substandard care, and it is for this reason **this Report recommends that the full case notes be made available to the CEMD Assessors in future.**

However, it is possible to establish the main causes of substandard care, which, again, are due to:

- failure of junior staff or GPs to diagnose or refer the case to a senior colleague or to hospital,

- failure of consultants to attend, and inappropriate delegation of responsibility,

- in some units, the continuing lack of a clear policy for the prevention or treatment of conditions such as pulmonary embolism, eclampsia or massive haemorrhage,

- lack of team work, and

- failure of the lead professional to identify diseases or conditions which do not commonly occur in their own speciality, or to seek early advice.

Ethnic origin

A breakdown of major causes of death in each Chapter by ethnic origin is shown in Table 1.6. Due to the small numbers involved, for ease of calculation, and because specific coding was sometimes incomplete, the ONS codes for Black African, Black Caribbean, Black Other and Black Mixed have been grouped together, as have Indian, Bangladeshi and Pakistani. The very small numbers occurring in other groups are also grouped together.

Table 1.6

Major causes of death where ethnic group was known: *Direct* and *Indirect* deaths; United Kingdom 1994-96.						
Cause of death	White	Black	Indian/ Pakistani/ Bangladeshi	Other*	Not stated	Total
Thromboembolism	33	3	1	2	9	48
Pregnancy-induced hypertension	14	5			1	20
Haemorrhage	10	1			1	12
Amniotic fluid embolism	11	2	1	1	2	17
Ectopic pregnancy	8	2	2			12
Spontaneous miscarriage	2					2
Termination of pregnancy		1				1
Uterine trauma	2	3				5
Other *Direct*	1		1			2
Sepsis	12	1			1	14
Anaesthetic	1					1
Cardiac *Indirect*	23	6	3	1	6	39
Other Indirect	68	8	4		6	86
Psychiatric *Indirect*	9					9
Total	**194**	**32**	**12**	**4**	**26**	**268**

* Middle Eastern 3, Chinese 1.

ONS do not collect data by the ethnic group of the mother apart from country of birth. Therefore it is not possible to calculate directly maternal death rates by ethnic group as many mothers will be second, third or more generations born in the UK. Ethnic group information is now being collected as part of the Hospital Episode Statistics (HES) System for England, but is not complete for the years covered by this Report. There was 35% coverage in 1995-96 and 54% coverage in 1996-97. The ethnic distribution was similar in both years. Using the 1996-97 distribution by ethnic group as a best estimate for the period covered by this Report leads to the estimates of maternal death rates by ethnic group for **England** shown in Table 1.7. From this it appears that Black women (a composite of Black African, Black Caribbean, Black Mixed and Black Other) have a three times greater risk of maternal mortality. But it should be noted that due to the very small numbers it takes only small differences in the estimated proportions of a particular ethnic group to make a large difference in the maternal death rates.

There was no evidence of any excess in substandard care for these women. In some cases the care they received was of an exceptionally high standard. Some women were recently arrived immigrants pregnant on arrival in the UK, and others were poor attenders at antenatal clinics, or did not speak English. Several moved addresses during their pregnancy, making community follow up difficult. This important aspect of the Enquiry will be greatly expanded in the next Report when specific data should be available. This, combined with more data on substandard care, may point to inequalities in accessing the maternity services, or the need for further support for women from specific sections of the community. However, it is stressed again that these results require caution in their interpretation because of the many possible confounding factors, and the play of chance when dealing with small numbers.

Table 1.7

Numbers of *Direct* and *Indirect* maternal deaths by ethnic group and **estimated** rate per 100,000 maternities; **England** 1994-96.		
Ethnic group	Total *Direct* and *Indirect* maternal deaths	Estimated rate per 100,000 maternities
White	194	11
Black African/Caribbean/ Mixed/Other	32	31
Indian/Bangladeshi/Pakistani	12	8
Other	4	4
Total (for which ethnic data were available)	242	11

Age and parity

Maternal mortality is closely related to both maternal age and parity, as shown by the data presented in Tables 1.8 and 1.9. Maternal death rates rose with age, as shown in Table 1.8. The mortality rate for women over 40 is now higher than the rate for "grande multiparous" women.

Published all-cause mortality data for women also show increasing rates throughout the age group 16-45, but the contribution of maternal causes peaked for ages 25-34, being lowest for women aged under 20 or 40 and over.

There was a different pattern of maternal mortality with parity shown in Table 1.9, with rates for *Direct* deaths being lowest for women in their second pregnancy.

Table 1.8

Total number of *Direct* and *Indirect* deaths by maternal age, United Kingdom 1985-96 and rate per 100,000 maternities. (Table 1.13 at the end of this Chapter gives actual numbers of maternities by age.)										
Age	1985-87		1988-90		1991-93		1994-96		Total 1985-96	
	No.	Rate	No.	Rate	No.	Rate	No.	Rate	No.	Rate
<20	15	7.8	17	8.8	7	4.2	15	10.2	54	7.6
20-24	47	7.3	38	6.0	30	5.5	40	9.0	155	7.0
25-29	53	6.8	74	8.8	87	10.6	71	9.6	285	9.0
30-34	60	13.7	57	11.4	61	10.9	70	11.5	248	11.8
35-39	35	23.0	31	18.5	35	19.1	53	24.1	155	15.7
40+	13	41.3	18	57.2	7	20.6	11	29.1	49	30.3
Not stated			3		1		8		9	
Total and overall rate	223	9.8	238	10.1	228	9.9	268	12.2	955	10.5

Table 1.9

Number of *Direct* and *Indirect* maternal deaths by estimated parity of the mother; United Kingdom 1985-96 and rate per 100,000 maternities.								
Parity	1985-87		1988-90		1991-93		1994-96	
	No.	Rate	No.	Rate*	No.	Rate	No.	Rate
0	87	9.3	57	N/A	76	8.0	94	10.6
1	50	6.8	44	N/A	58	7.4	55	7.5
2	30	8.8	10	N/A	51	13.0	37	9.7
3	27	21.1	5	N/A	17	12.2	21	16.4
4+	26	29.6	13	N/A	18	25.6	7	10.8
NS	3		109		8		54	
Total and overall rate	223	9.8	238	10.1	228	9.8	268	12.2

* Note: due to the large number of cases for the 1988-90 triennium where parity was not stated it is not possible to calculate meaningful rates.

Marital status

Sixty-two per cent of the women who had a *Direct* or *Indirect* maternal death in 1994-96 were known to be married at the time of death, which is consistent with the 65% of live births born inside marriage in 1996 in the United Kingdom. This suggests that being unmarried is not in itself a risk factor for maternal mortality overall. Therefore, marital status will not be considered in the later chapters of this Report.

Geographical distribution

There was no over or under representation among English Regions, Scotland, Wales, or Northern Ireland, or by individual provider unit, other than that which could have been expected by chance.

Type of antenatal care

Table 1.10 shows the type of antenatal care received by women who had either *Direct* or *Indirect* deaths and who had reached at least 24 completed weeks' gestation. In 121 cases care was shared between midwives and/ or GPs and the hospital. In 20 cases the care was mainly shared between the midwife and GP, with one hospital visit, and in eighteen cases the women were cared for solely in the community until delivery. In 23 cases the woman attended the consultant unit only, in most instances due to underlying or pre-existing disease. In three cases the woman was cared for solely by midwives throughout the antenatal period but none of these deaths was due to any failings of the care provided by the midwife or the fact that the woman had not been seen by a doctor. Three women had private antenatal care from an obstetrician, but only one delivered in a private hospital. Two women had concealed pregnancies and another two did not know they were pregnant. Ten were poor attenders or sought no care at all.

During the period covered by this Report some trusts and health authorities introduced changes to antenatal care, increasing the proportion of care provided in the community by midwives and GPs. There is no indication that these changes led to an increase in maternal deaths associated with substandard care.

Table 1.10

Antenatal care in pregnancies >24 completed weeks' gestation, *Direct* and *Indirect* deaths; United Kingdom 1994-96.			
Type of antenatal care	*Direct*	*Indirect*	Total
Consultant-led unit only	6	17	23
Traditional shared care	60	61	121
Midwife/GP mainly	12	8	20
Midwife/GP only	12	6	18
Midwife only	1	2	3
Private obstetrician	2	1	3
Concealed pregnancy	2		2
Unaware she was pregnant	1	1	2
Very late in booking (34 weeks' +)	5	5	10
Total	101	101	202

Place of delivery

Table 1.11 shows the place of delivery. Most deliveries occurred in a consultant unit. There were two planned home births and in one of these cases care was substandard in that warning signs of puerperal sepsis appear to have been missed. This is discussed in Chapter 7. Three births occurred in a GP-or midwife-led unit, but only one was associated with substandard care. Sixteen caesarean sections were performed in Accident and Emergency (A&E) Departments, seven being post-mortem sections on women certified dead on arrival (DOA) and six peri-mortem caesarean sections while the woman was still undergoing cardio-pulmonary resuscitation. One live birth and another early neonatal death were associated with the latter. Three unplanned emergency caesarean sections also took place in A&E with one live birth.

Table 1.11

Place of delivery by type of death; United Kingdom 1994-96.						
Type of death	Consultant Unit	GP/ midwife unit	A&E	ICU	Home	Total
Direct	79	1	6	1	2	89
Indirect	73		6	1		80
Fortuitous	11		4	1		16
Late	65	2			1	68
Total	228	3	16	3	3	253

Type of delivery

Previous Reports have included a Chapter on deaths after caesarean section. It has, however, become increasingly difficult to draw useful conclusions by considering all caesarean sections together, because of the diverse indications for the operation. The Chapter on caesarean section (Chapter 13 of the last Report) has therefore been discontinued and the data are discussed here.

Table 1.12 shows the type of delivery, where known, for *Direct* and *Indirect* deaths occurring after 24 completed weeks' gestation. A total of 93 women had caesarean sections. All the caesarean sections, including 17 elective operations, were carried out for obstetric indications, or because of underlying or pre-existing disease. No elective caesarean section was performed at the request of the woman herself and only one was performed because of a previous caesarean section. In many cases of elective caesarean section the woman had significant underlying medical problems, such as primary pulmonary hypertension, or other cardiac disease. In other cases there were underlying conditions, such as polyhydramnios or multiple previous uterine scars.

Emergency caesarean sections have been grouped into "planned", where some little time was available to prepare the woman adequately for theatre, and "unplanned" where the operation had to be performed immediately as soon as the underlying problem became apparent. Peri- and post-mortem sections have been described in the preceding section on place of delivery as these were all carried out in A&E Departments on women moribund on arrival.

As in the previous Report, a fatality rate per thousand caesarean sections cannot be given because of inaccuracies in known denominator data. The clinical usefulness of such an overall rate is questionable, as most of the women had significant impairment to their health before operation. The specific causes are discussed in the appropriate Chapters.

Compared with the previous Report, there was a reduction in the total number of deaths after caesarean section (93 compared to 103 for 1991-93). due to a reduction in the "planned" category (45 compared to 57 in 1991-93). Otherwise the figures are similar to those in the last Report: deaths after elective section were 17 compared to 15 in the last Report, and after "unplanned" caesarean section were 18 compared to 19 in the last Report. There were eight peri-mortem caesarean sections (compared to nine in 1991-93) and the number of post-mortem caesarean sections was unchanged.

Table 1.12

Number of cases by type of delivery: *Direct* and *Indirect* deaths; United Kingdom 1994-96.			
Type of delivery	*Direct*	*Indirect*	Total
Spontaneous Vaginal	28	30	58
Forceps	3	4	7
Ventouse	5	3	8
Vaginal breech	2	-	2
Laparotomy*	1	-	1
Caesarean section			
Elective	9	8	17
Planned emergency	26	19	45
Unplanned emergency	10	8	18
Peri-mortem	4	4	8
Post-mortem	1	4	5
Caesarean section total	50	43	93
Total delivered	**89**	**80**	**169**
Total undelivered at more than 24 weeks' gestation	12	21	33
Total died before 24 weeks' gestation	33	33	66
Total	**134**	**134**	**268**

* for extra-uterine pregnancy

Table 1.13

Number of maternities (in thousands) by age band: United Kingdom 1985-96.					
Age group	1985-87	1988-90	1991-93	1994-96	Total 1985-96
Under 25	837,8	825,0	714,9	590,4	2,968,100
25-29	777,7	836,4	819,8	738,4	3,172,300
30-34	437,6	499,9	558,4	610,7	2,106,600
35-39	152,1	167,5	188,0	220,0	727,700
40+	26,6	31,5	34,0	37,8	129,900
Total	**2,231,800**	**2,360,300**	**2,315,100**	**2,197,300**	**9,104,500**

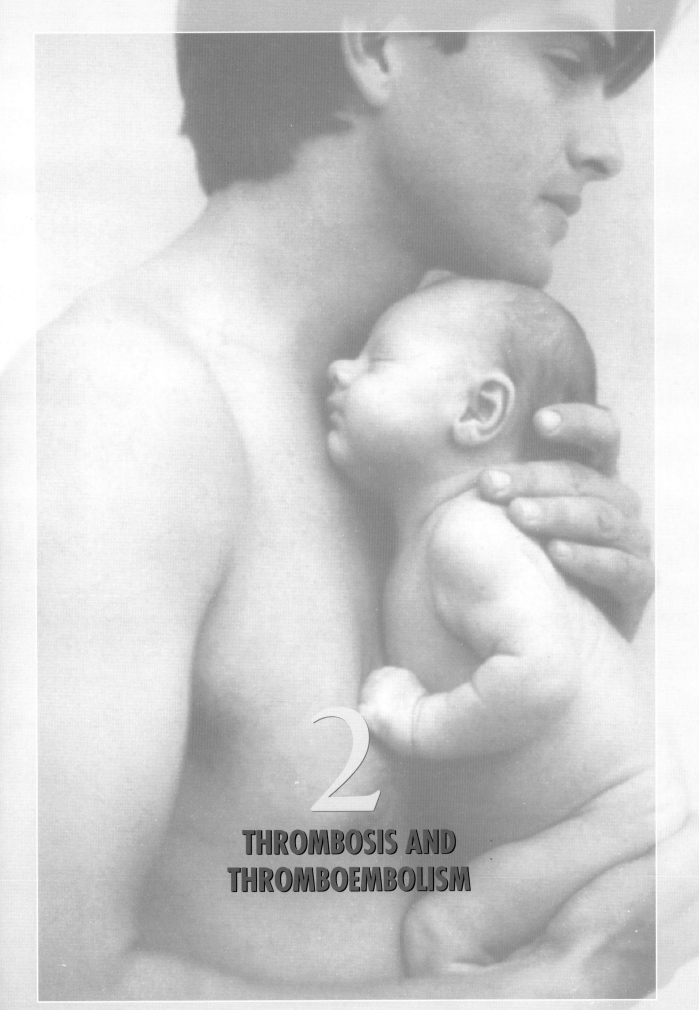

2

THROMBOSIS AND
THROMBOEMBOLISM

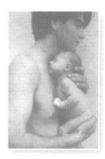

CHAPTER 2
THROMBOSIS AND THROMBOEMBOLISM

Summary

Forty-eight deaths from thrombosis or thromboembolism are counted in this Chapter. Forty-six were from pulmonary embolism and two from cerebral thrombosis secondary to a deep vein thrombosis (DVT). In addition there were two *Late* deaths from pulmonary embolism which are counted in Chapter 14.

Of the 46 deaths from pulmonary embolism, three occurred after operative procedures in early pregnancy. There were 15 other antenatal deaths, mainly in the first trimester of pregnancy. Of the 25 postpartum deaths, 15 occurred after caesarean section and 10 followed vaginal delivery. In three cases the only information available was from the death certificate, and the mode of delivery was not stated.

The total of 46 deaths from pulmonary embolism represents a significant increase from the 30 cases in 1991-93. There were increases in all categories, the largest increases being in deaths after vaginal delivery and after ectopic pregnancy or abortion. Although part of this increase could be due to increased case ascertainment, this would only account for 9 of the extra 16 cases by comparison with 1991-93.

Substandard care was present in many cases, although it is impossible to quantify this with accuracy due to the incomplete details available on some report forms. Often there was a failure to appreciate the importance of risk factors such as obesity, or of symptoms such as calf pain. There is a need to educate all doctors, not just obstetricians, that the risk of thromboembolism is increased from early pregnancy until the late puerperium.

There were at most four deaths because of failure of treatment. Once patients are treated for venous thromboembolism in pregnancy they usually survive. The problems are failure of diagnosis and, in particular, failure even to consider the possibility of venous thromboembolism and failure to give adequate prophylaxsis.

Wider use of thromboprophylaxis (not only after caesarean section) and better investigation of classic symptoms (particularly in high-risk women) are urgently recommended.

Thrombosis and thromboembolism: key recommendations

Wider use of thromboprophylaxis (not only after caesarean section) and better investigation of classic symptoms (particularly in high risk women) are urgently recommended.

Obstetricians and gynaecologists are reminded that even in the first trimester, pregnancy carries a risk of thrombosis and additional risk factors such as bed rest and dehydration may indicate thromboprophylaxis, as should a family history or known thrombophilia. Both unfractionated heparin and low molecular weight heparins are safe in early pregnancy as they do not cross the placenta.

Close attention should be paid to any pregnant woman with chest or leg symptoms to exclude the presence of DVT or PE by Duplex ultrasound and ventilation/perfusion lung scanning respectively, both of which do not carry any significant risk to mother or fetus.

All women undergoing caesarean section should be assessed for prophylaxis against VTE. Multiple risk factors are often present and in these cases the most effective method of prophylaxis, heparin at appropriate doses, should be used.

Midwives, general practitioners and other medical staff should take particular attention of women in the puerperium with chest or leg symptoms after vaginal delivery, to exclude the presence of DVT or potential PE.

Women with risk factors for DVT (bed rest, pre-eclampsia, other medical disorders, family history) should be carefully screened and consideration given to thromboprophylaxis.

Pulmonary embolism

Pulmonary embolism (PE) remains the single major direct cause of maternal death in the United Kingdom. The total of 46 deaths (excluding *Late* deaths) equates to a rate of 2.1 per 100,000 maternities compared to 1.3 in the previous Report. The comparison with previous triennia is shown in Table 2.1.

Table 2.1

	Total	Deaths after abortion/ ectopic	Antepartum deaths	Deaths in labour	Deaths after caesarean section	Deaths after vaginal delivery	Rate per 100,000 maternities
Deaths from Pulmonary Embolism (excluding *Late* deaths) and rates per 100,000 maternities; United Kingdom 1985-96.							
1985-87	30	1	16	0	7	6	1.3
1988-90	24	3	10	0	8	3	1.2
1991-93	30	0	12	1	13	4	1.3
1994-96	46*	3	15	0	15	10	2.1

* includes three deaths for which details are not available

There are increases in all categories, though the increase in those after vaginal delivery is particularly striking.

Many of the women had risk factors for venous thromboembolism (VTE) and appropriate prophylaxis might have altered the outcome. There is still a lack of awareness about the importance of risk factors and the need for thromboprophylaxis. Although prophylactic measures against VTE can result in complications, these need to be balanced against their potential to prevent fatalities. The recommendations of the RCOG Working Party on Prophylaxis against Thromboembolism in Gynaecology and Obstetrics [1] were published in March 1995 and we have not yet had a full triennium in which their effect on PE after caesarean section can be assessed.

Age

Age has been identified in previous Reports as a risk factor for VTE. In this triennium, for those cases where there are sufficient data, one of the women was a teenager, 32 were aged 20-34 and 13 were aged 35 or over. Using the table of maternities by age band in Annex 1 to Chapter 1 the maternal mortality from pulmonary embolism for women under 35 years of age is 2.3 per 100,000 maternities in that age group, but rises to 5.0 per 100,000 for women aged 35 or older.

Antepartum deaths

Three deaths occurred after operative procedures in early pregnancy. Two were after terminations of pregnancy and one followed an operation for an ectopic pregnancy. There were no features of substandard care in these cases.

A total of 15 other patients died from PE during the antenatal period. Summaries are given in Table 2.2. The gestations were as follows:

Up to 12 weeks,   10;
13 to 24 weeks,   3;
24 weeks to term,   2.

Table 2.2

Antepartum Deaths from Pulmonary Embolism; United Kingdom 1994-96.			
Age	Gestation in Weeks	Risk Factors	Features
< 20	6	Past history and symptoms.	Past history of DVT on O/C. Rx Warfarin. Presented at A&E with calf pain. Sent home Dx muscle strain. Died of PE next day.
20-29	11	None apparent.	Admitted by physicians at 11/40 with chest pain. Diagnosed PE and treated but died few days later.
	20	None apparent.	Collapsed and admitted. Spontaneous abortion and failed to recover consciousness. Died shortly afterwards. Autopsy showed PE, not diagnosed prior to death.
30-34	6	Bed rest.	In-patient for psychiatric problems. Collapsed and died. Autopsy showed PE.
	8	Bed rest.	In-patient for hyperemesis. Collapsed. Autopsy showed PE.
	8	Symptoms suggestive of PE.	Saw GP with chest pain. Treated for sore throat. Collapsed and died. Autopsy showed PE.
	8	Past history.	Had previous PE on O/C. Died at home. Pregnancy not booked.
	11	None apparent.	Collapsed and died at home. Autopsy showed PE.
	18	Symptoms suggestive of PE.	Presented to A&E with chest pain. Dx anxiety. Collapsed and died a few days later.

Table 2.2 (continued)

Antepartum Deaths from Pulmonary Embolism; United Kingdom 1994-96.			
Age	Gestation in Weeks	Risk Factors	Features
35-40	10	Age. Symptoms suggestive of PE.	Complained of shortness of breath. A&E Dx panic attack. Collapsed and died a few days later. Autopsy showed PE.
	12	Age.	Collapsed, Dx PE. Anticoagulants started but died same day.
	13	Age. Classic symptoms.	Seen by GP for leg pain on two successive days. DVT considered unlikely. Chest pain some days later. Admitted to medical ward with clinical picture of DVT. Medical registrar held off heparin as did not believe blood gas results. Died next day of PE.
	22	Age. Obese.	Collapsed during induction for IUD. Autopsy showed PE.
	24	Age.	Collapsed and died at home. Autopsy showed PE.
	26	Age. Obese. Suggestive symptoms.	Admitted by physicians for shortness of breath. Dx Chest infection. One week bed rest. Died after discharge of PE.

Two-thirds of the antepartum deaths were in the first trimester. **Obstetricians and gynaecologists are reminded that even in the first trimester pregnancy carries a risk of thrombosis and additional risk factors, such as bed rest and dehydration, may indicate thromboprophylaxis, as should a family history or known thrombophilia.** Both unfractionated heparin and low molecular weight heparins are safe in early pregnancy as they do not cross the placenta.

Many of these women, however, were not under the direct care of an obstetrician at the time of their death although several had seen other specialists as outpatients and some were even inpatients at the time. Details of the cases are summarised in Table 2.2 but one case is described in more detail here:

An older multiparous woman was seen by her GP with leg pain on two consecutive days at 12 weeks of pregnancy. DVT was considered but thought unlikely. Five days later she presented with chest pain and was admitted to a general medical ward in hospital. She was seen by junior medical staff who recognised the clinical picture of DVT but did not start treatment. Her blood gases worsened but the results were thought to be an error. The next day she collapsed and died. Autopsy showed a pulmonary embolus.

There was substandard care in this case. The GP should have arranged admission for investigation when DVT was considered. The hospital medical staff should have arranged prompt investigation and treatment.

Other risk factors in addition to pregnancy were often present, and there were sometimes multiple factors in one individual. These included obesity (weight >80 kg at booking), bed rest, dehydration and in two instances a known past history of pulmonary embolus. Combinations of risk factors - such as age and operative delivery - can lead to an increase in risk greater than the additive effect of the two factors [2].

The thromboprophylactic method chosen will depend on the patient, but heparin is the most effective technique presently available. Low molecular weight heparins have not yet been proven to be more effective than unfractionated heparin in pregnancy but they have fewer side effects and only need to be given once a day.

A past history of PE and/or DVT is a high risk factor for recurrence in pregnancy. Many women, particularly those with a family history, will have underlying thrombophilia, which can be found in about 50% of patients with VTE in pregnancy. Knowledge of this condition is rapidly evolving and patients with thrombophilia should be seen by specialists with particular expertise in this area. In this triennium, two women with past histories of VTE developed problems in very early pregnancy before formal booking. Previous investigation (e.g. in relation to contraception) and a warning to contact an obstetrician as soon as pregnancy is suspected would be prudent, but might not have prevented these two deaths.

It is of particular concern that five women had presented to GPs or casualty departments with symptoms of chest pain, shortness of breath or calf pain but had been discharged home. More complete investigation might have led to treatment which could have prevented the fatal PE which occurred a few days later. Most diagnoses can now be made using Duplex ultrasound scanning, which is now available in virtually all major hospitals. Its use is recommended in any case where there is suspicion, as clinical diagnosis is notoriously unreliable. Women and indeed doctors need to be reassured that nowadays only very low radiation doses are required for ventilation perfusion scanning, chest X-ray and even X-ray venography.

Close attention should be paid to any pregnant woman with chest or leg symptoms to exclude the presence of DVT or PE by Duplex ultrasound and ventilation/perfusion lung scanning respectively, neither of which carry any significant risk to mother or fetus.

Deaths after caesarean section

Caesarean section, like other major surgical procedures, remains a risk factor for VTE. Fifteen deaths occurred after caesarean section in this triennium. Complete details are available for 13 of these cases, as summarised in Table 2.3, but in the other two the details and timing of death are unknown. One case is described in more detail here:

> A primigravid woman had a normal pregnancy until pregnancy-induced hypertension developed near term. Labour was induced but caesarean section was carried out because of breech presentation combined with placental abruption. A live baby was delivered. The woman was anaemic after delivery and received a blood transfusion but she received no thromboprophylaxis. She went home a few days after delivery but collapsed and died on the ninth day. Autopsy confirmed PE.

Care was substandard. As well as the risk factors of caesarean section and a low haemoglobin, the woman was a cigarette smoker. She was not seen by a consultant. When acute complications of pregnancy, such as abruption, are successfully treated, the importance of thromboprophylaxis must not be overlooked.

Table 2.3

Deaths from Pulmonary Embolism following caesarean section; United Kingdom 1994-96.			
Age Group	Days after Delivery	Risk Factors	Features
25-29	4	Bed rest. Pre-eclampsia.	In-patient bed rest for APH and PIH. Had C/S, PPH and blood transfusion. TED stockings only. Collapsed and died a few days post C/S.
	9	C/S. Anaemic, smoker.	Labour induced for PIH, breech and abruption. Eventual C/S. No consultant involvement or prophylaxis.
	12	Bed rest. Grossly obese (BMI >35). Symptoms suggestive of PE.	Severe PIH and bed rest. C/S. Had prophylaxis for 5 days then home. Complained of calf pain day 6 - seen by midwife and GP. Treated for respiratory tract infection day 8 when complaining of shortness of breath. Collapsed and died 4 days later.
	23	Symptoms suggestive of PE.	C/S. Home day 6. No prophylaxis. Seen two weeks after delivery with chest pain and haemoptysis - treated as chest infection. On day 23 admitted with PE but died shortly afterwards.

Table 2.3 (continued)

Age Group	Days after Delivery	Risk Factors	Features
	26	Grossly obese (BMI > 35). Bed rest.	Bed rest for premature rupture of membranes. C/S at 35 weeks. Had TED and was anticoagulated.
30-34	2	Grossly obese. Bed rest.	One week bed rest for PIH. C/S for failed induction. Anticoagulated but collapsed a day later and transferred to ICU but died.
	10	Prolonged bed rest. Laparotomy.	Inpatient for 6 weeks with extra-uterine pregnancy. Laparotomy to deliver dead fetus. Had prophylaxis post-op for five days. Died at home. Perhaps pre-delivery prophylaxis might have helped.
	22	Bed rest and paraplegia.	Paraplegic. Admitted with PIH. Three weeks bed rest then C/S. No prophylaxis.
	42	Bed rest. Smoker.	C/S for PIH. No prophylaxis other than TED stockings.
35-42	21	Age. Diabetic. Bed rest. Wound infection.	In hospital for two weeks post C/S. Wound infection. On low dose heparin. ? higher dose required.
	24	Age.	Collapsed after ARM ? AFE. Survived and had C/S. No prophylaxis given. Home a week later. Collapsed and died three weeks later ? earlier episode PE.
Not Known	3	Past history.	PE in earlier pregnancy. Admitted at 30 weeks' with PE. Umbrella filter to vena cava. Further PE - emergency C/S. Died shortly afterwards.

The table title: Deaths from Pulmonary Embolism following caesarean section; United Kingdom 1994-96.

Only two of the 13 deaths for which full details were available occurred in women aged 35 or over. Guidelines currently emphasise that such women should receive thromboprophylaxis and the relatively low number of deaths in this age group might suggest that such prophylaxis is effective. Eight of the 13 women received some form of prophylaxis - five subcutaneous heparin, and three TED stockings alone. According to the RCOG Guidelines, however, most of these cases would be classified as high risk, with three or more moderate risk factors (see the Annex to this Chapter). In such cases, the Guidelines recommend both heparin prophylaxis and leg stockings.

However, the dose of herapin recommended by the RCOG for caesarean section is relatively low. In practice it might be better to give high risk patients higher dose prophylaxsis such as unfractionated herapin 7,500 units 12 hourly, enoxaparin 40mg 24 hourly, dalteparin 5,000 units 24 hourly or other low molecular weight herapin in equivalent dose. Such doses of herapin are recommended by the RCOG for thromboprophylaxsis in the antenatal period in those at risk because of previous thromboembolism.

The timing of the PE after caesarean section shows a change from 1991-93. Most deaths occurred between 15 and 42 days, mainly in the 21-28 day interval (see Table 2.5).This represents a shift to later presentation and may reflect the effects of some form of PTE prophylaxis delaying but not fully preventing the formation of thrombus. In patients with significant risk factors, such as very obese women, consideration should be given to prolonged thromboprophylaxis, for example for six weeks after delivery.

All women undergoing caesarean section should be assessed for prophylaxis against VTE. Multiple risk factors are often present and in such cases the most effective method of prophylaxis, heparin at appropriate doses, should be used.

Deaths after vaginal delivery

There were ten deaths from PE after vaginal delivery, a marked increase on the four in 1991-93. The details of these cases are summarised in Table 2.4. No deaths from PE occurred in the first week after vaginal delivery, and most occurred between days 15 and 28 as shown in Table 2.5.

Table 2.4

Deaths from Pulmonary Embolism following vaginal delivery: United Kingdom 1994-96.			
Age Group	Days after Delivery	Risk Factors	Features
18-25	10	Obese. Cardio-myopathy. Bed rest.	Shortness of breath at 38 weeks. Cardiomyopathy diagnosed and anticoagulation started. Labour induced. Post-delivery on ICU then cardiac ward but died of PE despite treatment.
	12	Obese. Symptoms of DVT.	SVD post-term. Leg pain day 5. Seen by GP day 10 and admitted for venogram. NAD and discharged home but died of PE two days later.

Table 2.4 (continued)

Age Group	Risk Factors	Days after Delivery	Features
	32	? Oral contraception early puerperium.	Induced delivery. Early discharge home and prescribed oral contraception at 14 days. Not clear if started.
26-30	17	Bed rest for PIH.	Patient with HbSc and severe PIH. Induced for IUD, Several days on ICU. Home after 2 weeks. Three days later died in A&E of PE.
	21	Obese. Bed rest. Multiple symptoms suggestive of PE.	PIH - bed rest 7 days. Induced for IUD. Home day 3. Two days later saw midwife with leg pain, and GP on day 8. Dx phlebitis and Rx antibiotics. Day 15 had chest pain and referred to A&E. CXR and ECG normal and discharged home. Day 21 collapsed and died.
31-35	23	Obese. Family history. Symptoms suggestive of PE.	SVD. Seen by GP postnatally with shortness of breath, but not investigated. Collapsed a day later and admitted with PE. Anticoagulation started but died the next day.
	29	Obese. Bed rest. Symptoms suggestive of PE. Family history.	SVD. Immobile with long stay in hospital for respiratory tract infection. After discharge saw GP with pleuritic pain, infection diagnosed. Collapsed and died.
	40	None.	SVD, but PPH and blood transfusion. Collapsed at home five weeks later.
36-40	14	None.	Induced for post term. Uneventful postpartum. Sudden collapse and died on day 14.
	30	Chest symptoms.	Normal pregnancy and delivery. Seen by GP for ? respiratory tract infection a few days before death from PE. R iliac vein thrombosis at autopsy.

REPORT ON CONFIDENTIAL ENQUIRIES INTO MATERNAL DEATHS IN THE UNITED KINGDOM

Table 2.5

Interval between delivery and Pulmonary Embolism; United Kingdom 1994-96.						
Days post-partum	0-7	8-14	15-28	29-42	Not known	TOTAL
Vaginal delivery	0	3	3	4		10
Caesarean section	3	3	6	1	2	15
TOTAL	3	6	9	5	2	25

In half the cases the patients were obese (>80kg) and most of these women weighed more than 100kg. Several had had bed rest before delivery (because of hypertension or other medical problems), or after delivery, on an ICU or in the postnatal ward. Some of the patients had complained to midwifery or medical staff of chest symptoms, shortness of breath or leg/calf pain - symptoms suggestive of developing or actual PE or DVT.

In two cases there was a family history of DVT or PE as well as signs and symptoms. These women may have had an underlying thrombophilia. This emphasises the need to take a family history at booking and to seek specialist guidance when this is positive.

Most of the deaths after vaginal delivery occurred after spontaneous, not instrumental, delivery. There is a need for the development of guidelines on thromboprophylaxis after normal delivery. The RCOG Guideline focuses largely on caesarean section. Many maternity units have now drawn up their own guidelines for vaginal delivery, whereby women, such as those over 35 and the obese, receive thromboprophylaxis.

Two deaths were probably unavoidable - one in a patient already fully anticoagulated, with a cardiomyopathy, and the other in a woman who had been fully investigated with a negative venogram two days prior to death from PE.

Midwives, GPs and other medical staff should take particular attention of women with chest or leg symptoms after vaginal delivery, to exclude the presence of DVT or potential PE.

Women with risk factors for DVT (bed rest, pre-eclampsia, other medical disorders, family history) should be carefully screened and consideration given to thromboprophylaxis.

Late deaths

Two *Late* deaths related directly to PE are recorded in this triennium. They are described here but counted in Chapter 14:

A young obese, parous woman had in a previous pregnancy developed a DVT antenatally. She booked late in this pregnancy and was prescribed low-dose aspirin for prophylaxis. She had a normal delivery at term. After delivery superficial thrombophlebitis was diagnosed and she was given TED stockings. Heparin was prescribed but it was cancelled. Four months later she was investigated by the physicians for recurrent breathlessness and diagnosed as hyperthyroid. She died a few days later of massive PE. Autopsy revealed recurrent pulmonary emboli and pulmonary hypertension.

A teenager had a caesarean section for a failed induction with pre-eclampsia. She had prolonged bed rest and wore TED stockings after delivery. She was admitted two months after delivery with a stroke and hemiplegia, recovered and was sent home. She was readmitted two weeks later with chest pain and a PE. She was anticoagulated and was readmitted four weeks later and died. Autopsy revealed a dilated cardiomyopathy with systemic and pulmonary emboli.

Cerebral thrombosis

There were only two cases of cerebral thrombosis in this triennium. One woman had a past history of DVT and PE and the second was anticoagulated for a DVT in her current pregnancy:

A young woman who had had a DVT and PE in her late teens was admitted to hospital in mid-pregnancy, disorientated. She then became unconscious. A cerebral vein thrombosis was diagnosed. She was anticoagulated but remained unconscious on a ventilator. At 28 weeks' gestation a caesarean section was performed and the ventilator was switched off because of irreversible brain damage.

A parous woman in her thirties developed a DVT a few weeks before term. She was anticoagulated and had a spontaneous vaginal delivery at term. Twelve hours later she became disorientated then unconscious. She was transferred to specialist neurological care but died a few days later from a sagittal sinus thrombosis and massive intracerebral haemorrhage.

There was a strong family history of DVT in close relatives subsequently shown to be due to Antithrombin III deficiency. This emphasises the need for adequate screening, in particular thrombophilia screening, and specialist advice in such cases.

Comments

Once again, the major cause of direct maternal deaths is pulmonary embolism. Although some antenatal deaths, and some deaths after vaginal delivery, occurred without warning and without apparent risk factors, many patients in these categories - and the majority after caesarean sections - had multiple risk factors or symptoms suggestive of PE and/or DVT.

The risk of VTE after any operation is further increased when surgery is performed in pregnancy. This was highlighted in the 1995 RCOG Report [1], which included a risk assessment chart shown in the Annex to this Chapter. The full effect of these RCOG guidelines is yet to be seen. It should be noted, however, that these guidelines highlight the need for more effective prophylaxis when multiple risk factors are present. Multiple factors were present in many of the deaths in this triennium. Such women need subcutaneous heparin as the preferred option at appropriate doses and for appropriate duration.

REPORT ON CONFIDENTIAL ENQUIRIES INTO MATERNAL DEATHS IN THE UNITED KINGDOM

As noted above, the risk of VTE is increased by surgery in pregnancy and this includes the first trimester. The deaths in this triennium also indicate the need for considering thromboprophylaxis in such cases.

Each unit should be advised to develop its own guideline, based on existing national guidelines, which can be applied within the requirements of their own unit.

Implementation of such guidelines in local health care contracts, care and audit plans has the potential to reduce significantly deaths from PE in the next triennium.

A recurrent finding in many cases was of a past personal or family history of VTE. There seems to be a lack of awareness of potential thrombophilia in such cases. A strong family history or personal history of VTE should be recognised as risk factors and properly investigated. Specialist advice should be sought if a thrombophilia screen is positive.

Prolonged bed rest antenatally or after delivery should prompt the use of TED stockings as a simple measure to try and reduce VTE. In this triennium there was a failure to appreciate the risk of thromboembolism after vaginal delivery in patients with multiple risk factors. Prolonged thromboprophylaxis may be advisable in patients with ongoing risk factors. Specific notice must be taken of any symptoms of breathlessness, chest or leg pain which might well herald the development of VTE.

There was also a failure to appreciate the risk of VTE in early pregnancy. Awareness of this risk needs to be increased among all doctors, not just obstetricians and gynaecologists.

References

1. Royal College of Obstetricians and Gynaecologists. *Report of a Working Party on Prophylaxis against Thromboembolism in Gynaecology and Obstetrics*. London: RCOG, 1995.

2. Greer I (ed). Thrombo-embolic disease in obstetrics and gynaecology. *Bailliere's Clinical Obstetrics and Gynaecology* 1997; **11**: 403-615.

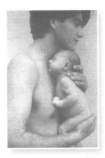

ANNEX TO CHAPTER 2
PROPHYLAXIS AGAINST THROMBOEMBOLISM IN CAESAREAN SECTION

The following recommendations, taken from the RCOG Working Party Report on Prophylaxis against Thromboembolism, are of relevance to patients requiring caesarean section.

A risk assessment of all patients undergoing elective or emergency caesarean section should be performed and prophylaxis instituted as appropriate. See box below.

Risk Assessment Profile for Thromboembolism in Caesarean Section

LOW-RISK - Early mobilisation and hydration

Elective caesarean section - uncomplicated pregnancy and no other risk factors

MODERATE RISK - Consider one of a variety of prophylactic measures

- Age >35 years
- Obesity (>80 kg)
- Para 4 or more
- Gross varicose veins
- Current infection
- Pre-eclampsia
- Immobility prior to surgery (>4 days)
- Major current illness, e.g. heart or lung disease, cancer, inflammatory bowel disease, nephrotic syndrome
- Emergency caesarean section in labour

HIGH RISK - Heparin prophylaxis +/- leg stockings

- A patient with three or more moderate risk factors from above
- Extended major pelvic or abdominal surgery, e.g. caesarean hysterectomy
- Patients with a personal or family history of deep vein thrombosis, pulmonary embolism or thrombophilia; paralysis of lower limbs
- Patients with antiphospholipid antibody (cardiolipin antibody or lupus anti-coagulant)

Management of different risk groups

Low-risk patients

Patients undergoing elective caesarean section with uncomplicated pregnancy and no other risk factors require only early mobilisation and attention to hydration.

Moderate risk patients

Patients assessed as of moderate risk should receive subcutaneous heparin (doses are higher during pregnancy) or mechanical methods. Dextran 70 is not recommended until **after** delivery of the fetus and is probably best avoided in pregnant women.

High-risk patients

Patients assessed as high risk should receive heparin prophylaxis and, in addition, leg stockings would be beneficial.

Prophylaxis until the 5th postoperative day is advised (or until fully mobilised if longer).

The use of subcutaneous heparin as prophylaxis in patients with an epidural or spinal block remains contentious. Evidence from general and orthopaedic surgery does not point to an increased risk of spinal haematoma.

Prophylaxis against thromboembolism in pregnancy

The RCOG Working Party also made recommendations for prophylaxis against thromboembolism in pregnancy, which are summarised in the box below.

> ### Prophylaxis against thromboembolism in pregnancy
>
> Patients with a previous history of venous thromboembolism in pregnancy or the puerperium and no other thrombotic risk factor should receive thromboprophylaxis for up to 6 weeks post partum (subcutaneous heparin and then oral warfarin if desired).
>
> Patients at higher risk, e.g. those having had multiple episodes of thromboembolism, may require heparin throughout the pregnancy.

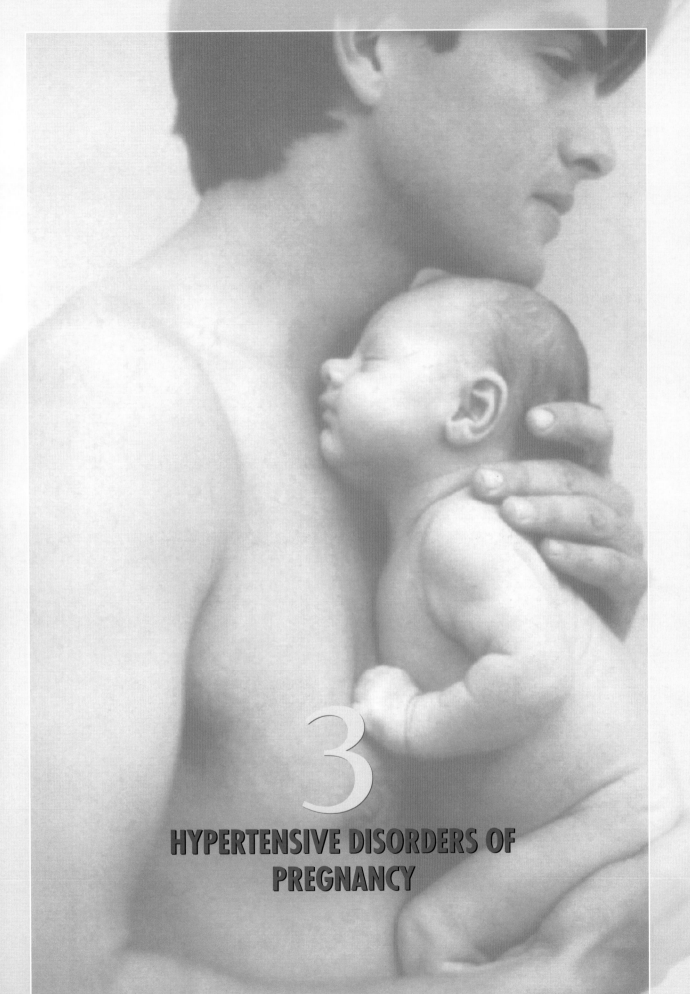

3

HYPERTENSIVE DISORDERS OF PREGNANCY

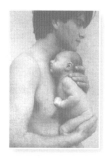

CHAPTER 3
HYPERTENSIVE DISORDERS OF PREGNANCY

Summary

There were 20 *Direct* deaths due to hypertensive disorders of pregnancy in the United Kingdom during this triennium, the same number as in the last Report. In addition there was one *Late Direct* death counted in Chapter 14 but discussed here, again the same as in the last triennium. In only one case was there evidence of pre-existing hypertension. There were eight cases of eclampsia. In three cases death certificate details were the only information available.

Substandard care, despite early consultant involvement in some cases, was evident in 10 of the 17 *Direct* deaths where sufficient details were available to make an assessment. This amounts to 59% of the cases, compared with 80% in each of the previous two triennia. Underlying factors remain similar to those in previous Reports, including inadequate consultant involvement and failure to take prompt action, to appreciate the severity of the disorder, to monitor the problem appropriately, to refer or transfer appropriately, and to treat appropriately, particularly with regard to fluid balance.

The Assessors recommend that an obstetrician-led special interest team of appropriate size and composition should be set up in each unit to formulate and update pre-eclampsia and eclampsia protocols and to advise in difficult cases. In addition a system should be in place where a single senior clinician has responsibility for overall management, in particular for fluid balance. Very few of the cases in the present series had appropriate laboratory tests performed despite serious and often deteriorating disease. The importance of adequate monitoring of renal, hepatic, haematological and coagulation parameters must be emphasised to staff caring for women with hypertensive disorders.

Many cases develop rapidly and can progress to a severe form within days of antenatal assessment. Routine antenatal education should make women aware of the type of symptoms associated with pre-eclampsia and the need to obtain further advice. As cases do occur between 26 and 33 weeks' gestation, it is important to continue to have formal antenatal reviews during this time. As several cases were associated with a failure of medical and midwifery staff to appreciate the severity or presence of the problem, there is a continuing need to alert all those providing antenatal care to the importance of screening for pre-eclampsia and appropriately assessing its severity.

Pregnancy-induced hypertension: key recommendations

An obstetrician-led special interest team of appropriate size and composition should be set up in each unit to formulate and update pre-eclampsia and eclampsia protocols and to advise in difficult cases. They should also co-ordinate regular staff training.

As in the previous Report, the need is emphasised for appropriate protocols to prevent junior staff being exposed to potentially dangerous clinical situations of which they have little experience.

A single senior clinician should have responsibility for the overall management of each case, in particular for fluid balance. There should also be a clear system in place with regard to transfer of these patients at an appropriate stage, if necessary.

All women should receive antenatal education so that they are aware of the symptoms associated with pre-eclampsia, its importance and the need to obtain urgent professional advice.

There is need for continued education of medical and midwifery staff, particularly in the community, with regard to the implications of pre-eclampsia and the need for accurate diagnosis, assessment and prompt referral when required.

Pre-eclampsia and eclampsia were the sole underlying causes of death in 19 cases in whom the blood pressure was normal in early pregnancy. One woman had evidence of pre-existing hypertension but her blood pressure was normal in early pregnancy. In three women, the only information available was from the death certificate, thus limiting investigation. Seven of the women were parous.

Cases counted in other Chapters

In eight other cases, severe pre-eclampsia was a significant factor but the deaths were considered by Assessors to have been directly due to other causes and are, therefore, counted in the relevant Chapters. The causes of death were berry aneurysm, respiratory arrest, cardiac disease, three cases of pulmonary embolism, and two of postpartum haemorrhage, one of which is described below:

> A woman who died of post-partum haemorrhage, whose case is considered more fully in Chapter 4, had been admitted with presumed pre-eclampsia and severe thrombocythaemia. This was considered to be HELLP syndrome although key diagnostic features were absent. She was delivered by caesarean section in a small district general hospital.

Care was considered substandard as a patient with a problem of such severity should have been delivered in a tertiary centre with better haematological support.

The details of one *Late Direct* death, counted in Chapter 14 are:

> A woman was admitted with moderate hypertension without proteinuria at 37 weeks' gestation. She had an uneventful vaginal delivery after labour induction and was discharged on the third postpartum day on antihypertensive agents with adequate blood pressure control. She was subsequently admitted under the care of the physicians with headache and a neurological deficit due to a subarachnoid haemorrhage from a berry aneurysm. Despite treatment, she entered a persistent vegetative state and died approximately six months later.

Table 3.1 shows the number and rates per million maternities of deaths from pre-eclampsia and eclampsia in the United Kingdom 1985-96.

Table 3.1

The number of women who died from hypertensive disorders of pregnancy and the death rate per million maternities; United Kingdom 1985-96.						
	Pre-eclampsia		Eclampsia		Total	
	Number	Rate	Number	Rate	Number	Rate
Triennium						
1985-87	15	6.7	12	5.4	27	12.1
1988-90	12	5.1	14	5.9	27	11.0
1991-93	12	5.3	8	3.4	20	9.0
1994-96	12*	5.4	8	3.6	20	9.0

* - In 3 of these deaths only death certificate information is available, and there is no record of eclampsia. .

A comparison of the ages of the women who died of hypertensive disorders of pregnancy in the United Kingdom from 1988 to 1996 is given in Table 3.2. It is striking that in 1994-96 five women who died were aged 20 or under, giving a death rate of 34.2 per million maternities in this age group. Two of these young women had concealed their pregnancies. This highlights firstly the requirement to communicate the importance of antenatal care to young women, secondly the fact that young women are at particular risk of pre-eclampsia - an established risk factor which is often overlooked - and thirdly the need to make it possible for young women to seek medical help.

Table 3.2

Number of maternal deaths and the death rates per million maternities from hypertensive disorders by age; United Kingdom 1985-1996.										
	1985-87		1988-90		1991-93		1994-96		1985 -96	
Age	Number	Rate	Number	Rate	Number	Rate	Number	Rate	Number	Rate
<25	10	11.9	8	9.6	3	4.4	11	18.6	32	10.8
25-29	5	6.4	5	5.6	11	13.4	2	2.7	23	7.3
30-34	7	16.0	8	16.0	4	7.2	4	6.5	25	11.9
35-39	3	19.7	4	23.8	2	10.6	2	9.1	11	15.1
40+	2	75.1	2	63.5	-	-	-	-	4	24.7
N S							1		1	
All ages	27	12.1	27	11.4	20	8.6	20	9.1	96	10.5

NS - not stated

REPORT ON CONFIDENTIAL ENQUIRIES INTO MATERNAL DEATHS IN THE UNITED KINGDOM

The duration of pregnancy at delivery is shown in Table 3.3

Table 3.3

Duration of pregnancy in delivered women; United Kingdom 1994-96.			
Duration of pregnancy (weeks)	Pre-Eclampsia	Eclampsia	Total
Up to 28	2	2	4
29-32	2	3	5
33-37	3	1	4
38 +	1	0	1
Total	8	6	14

Three patients died undelivered between 29 and 37 weeks' gestation. All delivered patients reached 26 weeks' gestation or more. Nine of the deaths following delivery occurred before 33 weeks' gestation, four due to pre-eclampsia and five due to eclampsia. Further data was not available for three cases.

Mode of delivery

Amongst the 14 women known to have been delivered 11 had caesarean sections. There were no twin pregnancies. There was one assisted breech delivery in which the baby was stillborn. There were one spontaneous and one ventouse vaginal delivery.

Eclamptic fits

Eclampsia occurred in eight patients. All but two of these had received no treatment by the time of their first fit, six having suffered a convulsion outside hospital. Two of these 8 were without a previous diagnosis of pre-eclampsia. One case had a seizure in hospital, after a caesarean section for pre-eclampsia at term, and appeared to be making a good recovery but was found collapsed and pulseless after being left unattended in a bath on the fourth day after delivery. The other woman had severe pre-eclampsia with backache, epigastric pain and nausea and was initially managed conservatively at 28 weeks' gestation before transfer to the local perinatal centre after her seizure. Only one was known to have had more than a single fit.

Immediate cause of death

The immediate causes of death in all cases are shown in Table 3.4. As in the last triennium, there was a continued reduction in deaths from cerebral haemorrhage, with only one death ascribed to subarachnoid haemorrhage, although the *Late* death was initiated by a subarachnoid haemorrhage. The two deaths classified under "other causes" were due to drowning in the bath at home (presumed following an eclamptic fit), and septicaemia, the origin of which is unclear. Acute Respiratory Distress Syndrome (ARDS) was the commonest mode of death, and in all cases, the pre-eclampsia was complicated by other problems.

One woman died from ARDS precipitated by Mendelson's syndrome after aspiration during an eclamptic fit at home, one woman had an underlying HELLP syndrome (haemolysis, elevated liver enzymes and low platelets, a form a severe pre-eclampsia involving the liver), one had septicaemia and two had pulmonary oedema with or without DIC. Another had ARDS precipitated by rapid transfusion for anaemia during labour. The woman who died from bronchopneumonia had underlying HELLP syndrome. Poor control of fluid balance with circulatory overload was evident in three cases in this Report.

Table 3.4

Cause of death due to eclampsia and pre-eclampsia; United Kingdom 1985-96.				
Cause of death	1985-87	1988-90	1991-93	1994-96
Cerebral				
Intracerebral haemorrhage	11	10	5	3
Subarachnoid	-	2	-	1
Infarct	-	2	-	-
Oedema	-	-	-	3
Total	**11**	**14**	**5**	**7**
Pulmonary				
ARDS	9	9	8	6
Oedema	1	1	3	2
Haemorrhage	1	0	-	-
Pneumonia	1	0	-	1
Total	**12**	**10**	**11**	**9**
Hepatic				
Necrosis	1	1	-	-
Ruptured liver	-	-	-	2
Liver failure	-	-	-	1
Other	3	2	4	1
Total	**4**	**3**	**4**	**4**
Overall Total	**27**	**27**	**20**	**20**

Substandard care

In 15 of the 17 deaths for which care could be evaluated, there was evidence of substandard care. In five cases, however, this was minor and is unlikely to have altered the outcome. The 10 cases with a major deficiency of care, which is likely to have altered the outcome, will be discussed further.

Women who did not seek antenatal care

In the following cases, antenatal care may well have altered the outcome of the pregnancy:

> A schoolgirl felt unable to tell anyone she was pregnant. After a convulsion at home, she was admitted to a medical ward. After a further convulsion the pregnancy was identified. Obstetric referral diagnosed eclampsia which was treated appropriately. She had a caesarean section and was transferred to the ICU but subsequently died from septicaemia, the cause of which is unclear. The lack of antenatal care is likely to have contributed to her death.

> In another case the woman, apparently through fear of hospitals, failed to attend for antenatal care and presented in labour with severe iron-deficiency anaemia and severe pre-eclampsia. Over-transfusion led to pulmonary oedema and later she developed ARDS which is likely to have been precipitated by transfusion-related lung injury and pre-eclampsia.

If she had been able to attend antenatal care it is likely that the anaemia would have been diagnosed and treated at an earlier stage and thus one of the main problems from which she suffered may have been avoided. Similarly, it is possible that the pre-eclampsia could have been identified at an earlier stage.

Failure of communication

> A woman referred for termination of pregnancy after a failure of depot progestogen contraception was found to be 22 weeks pregnant and termination was declined by a hospital clinic. The GP failed to organize antenatal care as he understood that the hospital was arranging this. The patient did not attend for any care. At 32 weeks' gestation, she was found convulsing and hypertensive. She underwent a caesarean section and was admitted to the ICU where she subsequently died from multi-organ failure.

There was a degree of substandard care in that no adequate arrangements were made for antenatal care following the refusal of termination of pregnancy.

General Practitioner (GP) and Community Midwife care

Care was substandard in the following cases:

> A woman at 31 weeks' gestation developed +++ proteinuria, but her blood pressure was normal. One week later, she was found dead at home, having attended her GP's surgery the previous day for a repeat prescription for antacid, possibly because of epigastric pain associated with fulminating pre-eclampsia. When last seen by a family member before her death, she was complaining of feeling unwell and had a swollen face. The autopsy was compatible with underlying eclampsia.

Care was substandard in that the midwife did not refer her to the GP or obstetrician when +++ proteinuria was found, but rather, sent a mid stream specimen of urine, which showed no evidence of infection. The GP failed to make any assessment of the patient when she requested a repeat prescription for antacid.

REPORT ON CONFIDENTIAL ENQUIRIES INTO MATERNAL DEATHS IN THE UNITED KINGDOM

In another case, the GP failed to act on + + + proteinuria at 28 weeks' gestation and failed to recognize and act on a fundal height measurement which was clearly small-for-dates. At 30 weeks' gestation the GP reviewed her and found her to have hypertension and proteinuria indicative of fulminating pre-eclampsia. The GP arranged admission urgently but left her to wait in the street for the ambulance. On admission she had HELLP syndrome and intrauterine death was diagnosed. Labour was induced and she delivered a growth-restricted stillborn infant. She died 18 days later from respiratory complications.

In a further case the woman did not receive an antenatal check two weeks after her last visit, due to poor communication between the hospital and the GP. At 33 weeks' gestation she referred herself to a maternity unit while on holiday as she felt unwell. Blood pressure and urinalysis were unremarkable and she was advised to keep her next GP review appointment. Twenty days after this assessment, she was found convulsing at home and she died from the convulsion despite attempts at resuscitation. It is noteworthy that she had a history of chronic hypertension, although blood pressure in early pregnancy was satisfactory.

Consultant unit responsibility

In six of the cases where there was substandard hospital care, a consultant obstetric unit was involved. In these cases, four principal factors were evident:
- failure to take prompt action,
- delay in delivery,
- delay in transfer to an ICU, appropriate high dependency area or Regional referral unit, and
- inadequate consultant involvement.

Inadequate consultant involvement included:
- failure to inform consultants,
- failure of consultants to attend,
- inadequate consultant management.
- failure to appreciate severity of the condition, and
- failure in fluid management leading to circulatory overload.

In most cases there were combinations of these inter-related factors.

In two cases, there were critical delays of 48 hours or more before delivery or transfer. The Assessors considered that these delays may have adversely affected the outcome:

In the first, delay was caused by a shortage of neonatal intensive care facilities. The patient's condition had rapidly deteriorated with severe pre-eclampsia. She was a primigravida whose uterus was found to be small-for-dates although she had an apparently normal blood pressure at 27 weeks' gestation. Her GP referred her to hospital. On admission, she had a blood pressure of 140/100 mmHg with + + + proteinuria. HELLP syndrome was diagnosed and she was transferred to another unit as the Neonatal Unit in the initial hospital was closed. The fetus was dead when she arrived at the hospital. During attempted induction of labour, fluid imbalance was associated with developing pulmonary oedema. Positive pressure ventilation was required to improve her oxygenation before caesarean section. She subsequently developed ARDS and DIC which progressed to multi-organ failure and death. The fetal death had been precipitated by placental abruption, which may have contributed to the coagulopathy.

Care was substandard in the initial hospital, where there was a failure to appreciate the severity and rapid deterioration of the pre-eclampsia and delay in referring to a second hospital for delivery, particularly when no neonatal beds had been available in the first hospital for more than 24 hours before transfer. In the second hospital, there may have been inappropriate fluid balance during the attempted induction of labour, and this could have contributed to the pulmonary oedema. There was also a delay in involving the senior anaesthetist.

In the second case, delay in delivery also occurred, due to efforts to gain fetal maturity. The woman was admitted at 28 weeks' gestation, complaining of upper abdominal pain which was unrelieved by antacid. She had hypertension and +++ proteinuria. She was admitted to hospital and steroids were initiated to enhance fetal lung maturity. Three days after admission, she complained of backache, epigastric pain and nausea. Her blood pressure was subsequently recorded at 200/120 mmHg. She was found in a postictal state. She was stabilised and transferred by ambulance to the regional perinatal centre which was 10 minutes away. Intrauterine fetal death occurred, labour was induced and uncontrollable intraperitoneal haemorrhage occurred. Laparotomy, subcapsular haematoma and liver rupture were present and results of liver function tests taken earlier that day showed grossly elevated liver enzymes.

Care was substandard in that there was a failure to appreciate the severity of her condition and to arrange earlier transfer and intensive management.

Failure to inform consultants and failure of consultants to attend

In a number of cases the consultant, either anaesthetic or obstetric and sometimes both, should have been informed earlier. One has been considered above because delay in transfer also occurred. Other examples are:

A patient at 34 weeks' gestation was admitted with chest pain and found to have a blood pressure of 180/110 mmHg along with +++ proteinuria. Senior staff were involved and management was appropriate before caesarean section, which was performed promptly. Immediate post-caesarean section management was in the ICU. She was transferred back to the postnatal ward after approximately 24 hours. One day later, she developed pulmonary oedema. Subsequent cardiac arrest occurred and resuscitation, although carried out promptly, failed.

Care was substandard in that after delivery she was discharged from the ICU prematurely and there was a delay in recognising the severity and implications of her pulmonary oedema in the postnatal ward. This may have been due to lack of consultant involvement after delivery and illustrates the need for continued high levels of care in the puerperium by experienced senior staff.

One of the women already described as having no antenatal care was admitted at 37 weeks' gestation. She had severe pre-eclampsia with +++ proteinuria and her blood pressure was

180/100 mmHg. She also had a microcytic anaemia with a haemoglobin of 5 g%. Four units of blood were transfused rapidly, the baby was delivered by ventouse, blood pressure was controlled with hydralazine and phenytoin was given. She developed severe pulmonary oedema, was transferred to the ICU, subsequently developed ARDS and died a month after delivery from its complications.

Care was substandard with regard to the obstetric management. Pulmonary oedema followed on from the rapid transfusion of four units of blood during labour and immediately after delivery, precipitating a transfusion-associated lung injury which, in combination with pre-eclampsia, led to her death. There was lack of consultant involvement and consultation in the management of the case which presented difficulties with the combination of severe anaemia and severe pre-eclampsia in labour. The patient's inability to seek antenatal care is also likely to have contributed to the degree of anaemia and to late identification of severe pre-eclampsia, and has been discussed above.

Inappropriate consultant management

A woman was apparently being treated for infertility with a progestogen challenge test and clomiphene. Three days after this treatment had been commenced in a consultant unit, she was admitted, collapsed, as an emergency to the A&E Department of another hospital. Pregnancy and eclampsia were diagnosed and emergency caesarean section performed at 32-34 weeks' gestation. She died 48 hours later, secondary to eclampsia.

There was substandard care in that the infertility specialist had failed to recognise pregnancy and signs of pre-eclampsia. The GP was not aware of the pregnancy until her admission to hospital. The GP attended immediately before her admission to hospital because of seizures (subsequently found to be due to eclampsia) and the outcome may have been altered if a Flying Squad had attended at home.

In three deaths, circulatory overload occurred, followed by pulmonary oedema and/or ARDS. This is a recurrent theme in these Reports and is caused by a failure to appreciate the reduced intravascular compartment in pre-eclampsia, together with poor control of fluid balance. Sometimes the fluids were ordered separately by the obstetrician, the anaesthetist and even the haematologist, each independently using fluid as a vehicle for their particular aspect of therapy, without co-ordination. There is also a failure to appreciate that oliguria is a common feature after delivery in severe pre-eclampsia. Fluid management can be extremely difficult in these cases and requires the involvement of experienced senior staff and optimal assessment of fluid balance and circulatory status. Of particular importance is assessment for possible pulmonary oedema. One member of staff should have responsibility for the overall fluid management to allow optimal control.

Comments

The number of deaths from the hypertensive disorders of pregnancy is the same as in the previous triennium. There appears, however, to have been a reduction in cases where there was a major degree of substandard care, 55% in the present Report, compared to 80% in the previous one. While this is a welcome improvement, there remains no room for complacency and several areas need to be addressed.

There was no clear pattern to the timing of antenatal visits in relation to the development of pre-eclampsia. Many cases develop rapidly and can progress to a severe form within days of a satisfactory antenatal assessment. The median time between the last antenatal attendance and severe pre-eclampsia, or eclampsia, was 6 days (range 0-28 days) in those attending for care. The median gestation was 32 weeks' (range 26-40 weeks). Because some cases occurred between 26 and 33 weeks' gestation, it is important to continue formal antenatal reviews during this time. However, in view of the rapid development of some cases, even with such regular assessment, **routine antenatal education should make women aware of the symptoms associated with pre-eclampsia, its importance and the need to obtain formal assessment. Suitable educational material is produced by APEC (Action on Pre-eclampsia). Such information should be available to women from a variety of sources including GPs, midwives and hospital antenatal clinics.**

In two cases, after an increase in blood pressure or significant proteinuria had been found, there was no follow up arranged for two weeks, indicating failure of staff to appreciate the implications of possible pre-eclampsia. **There is therefore a need for continued education of medical and midwifery staff, particularly in the community, with regard to the implications of pre-eclampsia and the need for accurate diagnosis, assessment and prompt referral when required.**

As in the last Report, there were failures of adequate assessment of severity and progression of the disorder in terms of biochemistry, including uric acid and liver function, and haematological parameters, including platelet count and coagulation status. Such investigations play a key role in the assessment and management of patients with pre-eclampsia. Appropriate assessment and follow up of patients, particularly those with proteinuria, are emphasised, especially in view of the rapid deterioration of many cases. Optimal management depends on local geography, but may include day care facilities, short stay wards and domiciliary midwife and GP assessment. Such assessment should not be restricted to patients with hypertension and proteinuria occurring together, but is indicated in any patient with either significant proteinuria or hypertension alone.

With regard to treatment of hypertension, there has been an improvement from previous Reports, with better control of blood pressure. This apparent improvement in management of hypertension may also have played a role in the continued reduction in deaths from intracerebral haemorrhage, and this is a welcome development.

There was also increasing use of anticonvulsants and it is likely that greater use of magnesium sulphate will be seen in future after the publication by the Eclampsia Trial Collaborative Group[1] demonstrating the superiority of magnesium sulphate over diazepam and phenytoin for the secondary prevention of eclampsia. However, as eclampsia remains a relatively rare condition, most obstetricians will see only the occasional case, and will therefore have limited experience of the use of magnesium sulphate, which itself carries significant side effects and hazards when used inappropriately. **Each unit should therefore develop its own protocol with regard to the use of magnesium sulphate for prophylaxis of seizures.** Increasingly, consideration is being given to prophylactic anticonvulsants in the treatment of pre-eclampsia although obstetricians vary in the anticonvulsant they use[2]. The value of such treatment is uncertain[3] and is currently the subject of a large clinical trial with magnesium sulphate (the MAGPIE trial).

The most frequent mode of death from hypertensive disorders in pregnancy is the development of ARDS. This condition rarely complicates pre-eclampsia unless other problems develop, such as disseminated intravascular coagulation, pulmonary oedema, fluid overload or over-transfusion[4,5] as noted in several cases in the present Report. Pulmonary oedema can easily arise due to fluid overload in pre-eclampsia, particularly as there is already increased vascular permeability due to endothelial damage. If good attention is given to fluid balance, pulmonary oedema may be prevented with, in turn, less risk of lung injury and subsequent ARDS. The implications of ARDS must be appreciated and prompt referral to specialist help is essential. As in previous Reports, **it is a mandatory requirement that strict attention be paid to fluid balance** in light of the failures documented in this Report and the frequent occurrence of ARDS with many cases related to inappropriate fluid balance. Often too many persons become involved in treatment without appropriate co-ordination, leading to inadvertent fluid overload and the serious problems noted above.

Problems can be compounded by junior medical staff being expected, or asked, to carry out executive clinical responsibilities. As in the previous Report, **the need is emphasised for appropriate protocols to prevent junior staff being exposed to potentially dangerous clinical situations of which they have little experience.**

Each unit must identify a lead obstetric consultant to develop a system for the management of patients with pre-eclampsia and eclampsia. This will include protocol development and updating, and appropriate staff training. There should also be a clear system in place with regard to transfer of these patients at an appropriate stage.

References

1.   Eclampsia Trial Collaborative Group. Which anticonvulsant for women with eclampsia? Evidence from the collaborative eclampsia trial. *Lancet* 1995; **345**: 1455-63.

2.   Gülmezoglu, A.M. & Duley, L. Use of anticonvulsants in eclampsia and pre-eclampsia: survey of obstetricians in the United Kingdom and Republic of Ireland. *British Medical Journal;* 1998; **316**; 975-6.

3.   Duley, L., Gulmezoglu, A.M. & Henderson-Smart, D. Anticonvulsants for women with preeclampsia (Cochrane review). In: *The Cochrane Library*. Issue 1 1998 Oxford: Update Software.

4.   Mabie, W.C., Barton, J.R. & Sibai, B.M. Adult Respiratory Distress Syndrome in pregnancy. *American Journal of Obstetrics & Gynecology* 1992; **167**: 950-7.

5.   Catanzarite, V.A. & Willms D. Adult respiratory distress syndrome in pregnancy: report of three cases and review of the literature. *Obstetrical and Gynecological Survey* 1997; **52**, 381-92.

APEC Address:

Action on Pre-eclampsia,

31 - 33 College Road,

Harrow,

Middlesex,

HA1 1EJ

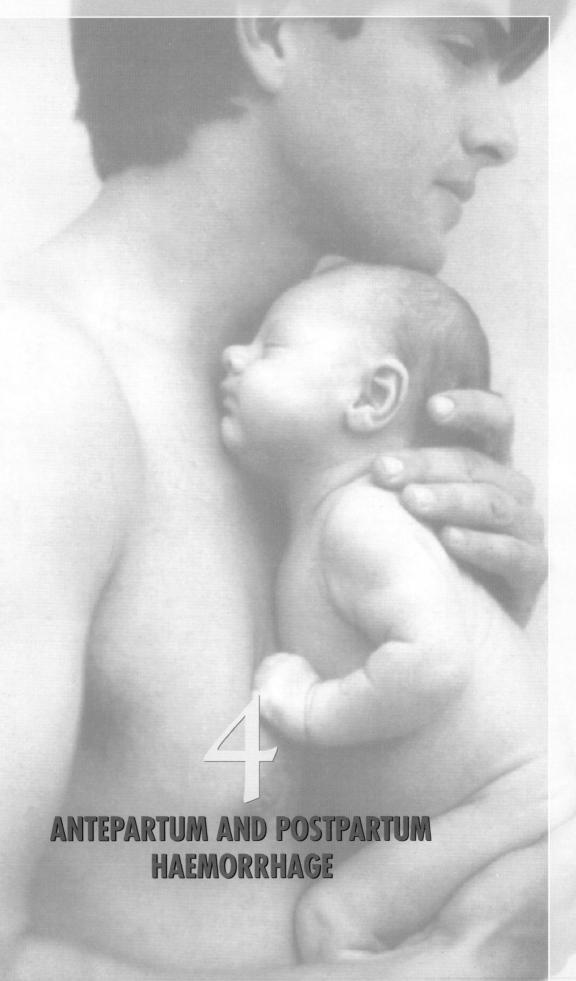

4

ANTEPARTUM AND POSTPARTUM HAEMORRHAGE

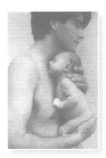

CHAPTER 4
ANTEPARTUM AND POSTPARTUM HAEMORRHAGE

Summary

Of the 12 deaths directly due to ante-partum and post-partum haemorrhage, three were due to placenta praevia, four to placental abruption and five to post-partum haemorrhage. There were no *Late* deaths. In eight cases care was substandard: reasons included poor communication between the labour ward and the blood bank, and failure to take appropriate action when predisposing factors were recognised. The number of *Direct* deaths from haemorrhage has again fallen compared with 1988-90 and 1991-93, but is still higher than in 1985-87.

Obstetric haemorrhage: key recommendations

Placenta praevia, particularly in patients with a previous uterine scar, may be associated with uncontrollable uterine haemorrhage at delivery and caesarean hysterectomy may be necessary. A very experienced operator is essential and a consultant must be readily available.

Minor signs or symptoms may have considerable significance in pregnancy and any pregnant woman admitted to an Accident and Emergency department should be discussed with the duty obstetrician. Accident and Emergency nurses should not be asked to decide whether or not there is an obstetric problem.

Obstetric or maternity units should organise regular "fire drills" so that when these emergencies occur all members of staff - including the blood bank - know exactly what to do to ensure that large quantities of cross-matched blood can be delivered to the labour ward without delay.

The speed with which obstetric haemorrhage can become life-threatening also emphasises the need for good communication between the labour ward and the blood bank. Ideally both should be on the same site.

Every unit must have a protocol for the management of massive haemorrhage.

Only deaths due to haemorrhage from the genital tract are included in this Chapter. Deaths due to haemorrhage from other sites (including ectopic pregnancy) are considered in the appropriate Chapters.

In 1994-96 there were 12 *Direct* deaths from haemorrhage with a mortality rate of 5.5 per million maternities, compared with 6.4 per million in 1991-93. There were no *Late* deaths. Of the 12 *Direct* deaths five were caused by post-partum haemorrhage, three by placenta praevia and four by placental abruption. All but two of the twelve women were of caucasian ethnic origin. Care was considered substandard in eight cases (66%), compared with 11 of the 15 deaths (73%) in 1991-93 and 14 of the 22 deaths (64%) in 1988-90.

Table 4.1 shows the number of *Direct* deaths from haemorrhage by cause and the death rate per million maternities in the four triennia, 1985-96, in the United Kingdom.

Table 4.1

Number and cause of deaths from haemorrhage and rates per million maternities; United Kingdom 1985-96.					
Triennium	Placental abruption	Placenta praevia	Postpartum haemorrhage	Total	Rate per million maternities
1985-87	4	0	6	10	4.5
1988-90	6	5	11	22	9.2
1991-93	3	4	8	15	6.4
1994-96	4	3	5	12	5.5

Previous Reports have drawn attention to the increased risk with age, particularly for those age 35 and over. This trend is still seen in the present triennium, as shown in Table 4.2.

Table 4.2

The number of deaths from haemorrhage, and death rates per million maternities by age from haemorrhage; United Kingdom 1988-96. (Numbers of maternities are shown in Table 1.13)								
	1988-90		1991-93		1994-96		Total 1988-96	
Age group	No.	Rate	No.	Rate	No.	Rate	No.	Rate
<25	2	3.1	1	6.0	2	3.2	5	2.3
25-29	6	7.2	7	8.5	3	4.1	16	6.7
30-34	8	16.2	5	26.5	2	3.3	15	9.0
35-39	4	23.9	1	5.3	4	18.7	9	15.6
40+	2	63.9	1	29.4	1	26.4	4	29.6
All ages	22	9.2	15	6.4	12	5.5	49	7.1

Placenta praevia

Three deaths were associated with placenta praevia. Two involved placenta percreta in association with a lower uterine scar:

> A woman who had a twin pregnancy and a previous caesarean section experienced antepartum haemorrhage. Placenta praevia was diagnosed by ultrasound. Near term, further bleeding occurred and emergency caesarean section was performed by a Specialist Registrar. Placenta percreta was diagnosed and there was massive bleeding after delivery of the second twin. A consultant attended promptly. Coagulopathy quickly developed. Treatment included subtotal hysterectomy, internal iliac artery ligation and aortic clamping. Transfer to the intensive care unit (ICU) was being arranged when cardiac arrest occurred, seven hours after delivery.

Although consultant support was readily available, the fact that this operation was undertaken by a Specialist Registrar represents substandard care. Bleeding from placenta praevia can be sudden and torrential, as shown by two cases in this Report. Subtotal hysterectomy was carried out rather than total hysterectomy, which would have been preferable but was very difficult because the placenta was invading through the lower segment into the bladder. Massive blood transfusion was required and there were some communication difficulties between the operating theatre and the blood bank. These can be difficult to avoid in a life-threatening emergency:

> A woman who had one previous caesarean section experienced several episodes of haematuria during pregnancy and a minor antepartum haemorrhage at term. Ultrasound scans in mid-pregnancy had shown that the placenta was low lying but later scans seemed to exclude placenta praevia. During labour (which was induced by amniotomy) further bleeding occurred. After forceps delivery, haemorrhage began and she became hypotensive before delivery of the placenta. Despite transfusion and subtotal hysterectomy by a consultant, she died less than four hours after delivery. The measured blood loss was over 15 litres.

Placenta praevia percreta can be difficult to diagnose on ultrasound, as shown by this case and a case in the 1991-93 Report. With hindsight there were warning signs in the form of haematuria in pregnancy, minor antepartum haemorrhage and bleeding in labour, but an ultrasound scan appeared to exclude placenta praevia. Care was substandard because the maternity hospital was several miles away from the main hospital and the blood bank, and difficulties in communication contributed to delay in obtaining blood for transfusion.

The problems of placenta praevia when associated with a lower uterine scar have repeatedly been emphasised in these Reports. Placenta praevia percreta is a very difficult condition to treat, and even with the best care it may be impossible to prevent death in such cases. Nevertheless these two cases emphasise the need for, and the importance of, excellent communication between labour ward and blood bank. The second case illustrates the dangers of their being on separate sites, in view of the speed with which exsanguination can occur in obstetric haemorrhage.

The third death also illustrates the fact that diagnosis of placenta praevia is not always straightforward:

> At 20 weeks' gestation an ultrasound scan on a parous woman showed a posterior placenta in the lower segment, apparently clear of the cervical os. On a scan in the third trimester the placenta appeared extensive, anterior and posterior to the os. A third scan showed that the presenting part was below the placenta. At 36 weeks the woman was found unconscious at home with severe bleeding. Despite resuscitation, rapid transport to hospital and prompt caesarean section the baby was stillborn and the woman died later in intensive care.

The blood loss, although severe, does not satisfactorily account for the sudden loss of consciousness but no other cause was found so the death is counted in this Chapter. Care has to be regarded as substandard because a patient with placenta praevia should be admitted to hospital as the pregnancy approaches term. Nevertheless this case illustrates the fact that placental localisation can be very difficult even when good ultrasound facilities are available.

Placental Abruption

There were four cases of placental abruption. Two occurred in the middle trimester of pregnancy:

> A woman was admitted at 25 weeks' gestation with abdominal pain and mild hypertension. Preterm labour was diagnosed and she was treated with dexamethasone and ritodrine, which was later discontinued. About 18 hours after admission she complained of further pain and vaginal bleeding and an ultrasound scan showed that the fetus had died. Placental abruption was diagnosed. A coagulation screen was normal, as was the haemoglobin level. An attempt was made to induce labour with prostaglandin pessaries. After another 10 hours she complained of epigastric pain and became shocked with a haemoglobin of 6.6 g%. Concealed haemorrhage was diagnosed. Treatment included amniotomy, oxytocin, antibiotics and a central venous line. She remained shocked and the cervix remained unfavourable. Another prostaglandin pessary was inserted and Willetts' forceps were attached. Hysterotomy was undertaken more than 36 hours after admission. There was a couvelaire uterus and the blood loss was 4 litres. She was transferred to the ICU. On day five, her condition deteriorated and she received a liver transplant. Two days later she collapsed, and she died while undergoing re-exploration of the abdomen. Autopsy confirmed placental abruption.

Placental abruption characteristically occurs in the third trimester of pregnancy, when it is usually followed by labour and vaginal delivery. Before 28 weeks' gestation, however, as this case demonstrates, labour may not occur and induction of labour may be difficult, allowing time for coagulopathy to develop. With hindsight, hysterotomy should have been carried out more promptly, when it became clear that induction of labour was not succeeding. Nevertheless the management of this unusual case was not considered substandard.

> A parous woman with no previous caesarean sections experienced two episodes of vaginal bleeding in the middle trimester of pregnancy. At 22 weeks' gestation she collapsed with abdominal pain and died less than 90 minutes later. Autopsy showed partial placental abruption and congestion of the lungs but no sign of amniotic fluid embolism.

Placental abruption does not normally lead to maternal death so quickly. There remains some doubt about the cause of death in this case. Care was not substandard.

The other two cases of placental abruption occurred in the third trimester. In one of these cases, death also occurred quickly:

> A parous woman in the third trimester was admitted to an Accident and Emergency Department at night because she was feeling unwell. She was noted to be pale and clammy but she was not in pain and her pulse and blood pressure were normal. She was placed in a cubicle and was thought to be asleep. When a doctor saw her, just over two hours after admission, she was dead. Her haemoglobin was 3.0g%. At emergency caesarean section the uterus contained two litres of blood.

An immediate obstetric opinion should have been obtained when this woman was admitted after midnight, "pale and clammy" in late pregnancy. Failure to do so amounts to substandard care. Severe internal bleeding is not always accompanied by pain, as shown by this case and some deaths from ectopic pregnancy (see Chapter 6). The rule in this Accident and Emergency Department was that "any patient who is 20 weeks pregnant or more should be discussed with the obstetric ward if it is felt that there is any obstetric problem". This is inadequate. Accident and Emergency nurses should not be asked to decide whether or not there is an obstetric problem. Minor signs or symptoms may have considerable significance in pregnancy and any pregnant woman admitted to an Accident and Emergency department should be discussed with the duty obstetrician.

Inadequate details are available of the fourth case of placental abruption:

> A young woman with sickle cell trait was admitted at 36 weeks' gestation with abdominal pain and hypotension. At emergency caesarean section there was only a small abruption but she developed coagulopathy and multiple organ failure and died later in intensive care.

If worthwhile lessons are to be learned from such tragedies it is essential that full details are available to the Assessors. Public opinion repeatedly reminds us that if we cannot prevent a death we should do all we can to avoid the same thing happening to someone else.

Primary postpartum haemorrhage

Five deaths were due to postpartum haemorrhage. Four of these deaths were associated with caesarean section and in two of those cases the woman had undergone previous caesarean sections. One death occurred after vacuum extraction. No death from postpartum haemorrhage occurred after normal delivery.

One death was due to difficulty with haemostasis at operation:

> A woman who had undergone two previous caesarean sections was booked for elective caesarean section at 38 weeks' gestation. She was admitted in spontaneous labour two days before that date and caesarean section was performed by a registrar. "Some bleeding" was noted from the angle of the uterine incision. Twenty-one hours after the operation she collapsed on the postnatal ward. Laparotomy revealed a retroperitoneal haematoma. Hysterectomy was performed by two consultants and she was transferred to an ICU in another hospital. At a further laparotomy a 2mm tear in the common iliac vein and a 1cm laceration in the liver were repaired. She was returned to the ICU but died the next day.

Care was substandard. A third caesarean section can be difficult and a registrar should seek help from a consultant. When blood loss at caesarean section is excessive this must be acknowledged and the patient must be carefully monitored afterwards, with regard to pulse and blood pressure. Collapse can occur without revealed bleeding. It should also be remembered that a young woman may maintain a normal blood pressure until sudden and catastrophic decompensation occurs.

Two patients died of haemorrhage due to platelet dysfunction which was present before caesarean section:

> A woman had an inherited congenital abnormality of the platelets. Antenatal care was given by a consultant. At 37 weeks' gestation she received a platelet transfusion and underwent elective caesarean section and sterilisation. She was transferred to the postnatal ward but became hypotensive. Laparotomy revealed generalised bleeding. She received massive platelet transfusions in the ICU but died seven days after delivery with acute respiratory distress syndrome (ARDS).

This patient had repeated transfusions and had been admitted to an ICU after her previous caesarean section. Care was substandard because she should have been transferred electively to an ICU after her caesarean section. Pre-operative plasmapheresis might have been considered.

> A young woman developed hypertension in the third trimester of her first pregnancy. Her platelet levels fell and HELLP syndrome was diagnosed. She was treated with steroids under the supervision of a haematologist and underwent caesarean section in a small district general hospital. Severe haemorrhage occurred and was treated with transfusion and hysterectomy but she died within two hours of the operation.

Although consultant obstetric, anaesthetic and haematological care was given, care was substandard because caesarean section for severe thrombocytopenia was undertaken in a small district general hospital. More support might have been available at a tertiary centre.

The fourth death after caesarean section was a case of secondary haemorrhage in a woman in poor health:

> A woman whose previous children all had fetal alcohol syndrome was admitted at 34 weeks' gestation with ruptured membranes. Caesarean section was carried out because of fetal distress. Afterwards she developed delirium tremens, a severe wound infection and wound dehiscence, which was repaired. Three weeks after delivery severe vaginal bleeding occurred. At laparotomy dense bowel adhesions were found and subtotal hysterectomy was performed. Further bleeding occurred and vaginal packing was required. Her condition deteriorated and she died a week later in an ICU.

The woman's general health was poor and her total circulating protein concentration was low. The tissues at operation were very friable. There was no apparent substandard care, though it is not known whether prophylactic antibiotics were given at caesarean section.

One woman bled after assisted delivery:

> An older primigravid woman with a fear of hospitals went into labour at home at 39 weeks' gestation after normal antenatal care. She was transferred to hospital because of delay in the second stage and vacuum extraction was performed because of fetal distress. One hour after delivery her temperature was 38.2°C. At two hours she felt unwell and at three hours she collapsed with massive atonic postpartum haemorrhage. The platelet count was 36,000. She was anaesthetised and underwent laparotomy two hours later. There was "offensive" free fluid in the peritoneal cavity. She died some hours after delivery.

The reason for the atonic postpartum haemorrhage is unclear, and it is possible that sepsis was an underlying cause. There was delay in carrying out the laparotomy. Care was substandard. One unit of incompatible blood was given during resuscitation, but this probably did not affect the outcome.

Substandard care

Care was substandard in eight cases. In one of the cases of placenta praevia caesarean section was undertaken by a Specialist Registrar. In another case of placenta praevia the diagnosis was missed on ultrasound scan and there was delay in obtaining blood for transfusion because of the distance between the labour ward and the blood bank. In the third case of placenta praevia there was doubt about the diagnosis on scan.

In one case of placental abruption, the Accident and Emergency Department failed to seek an immediate obstetric opinion. In two cases of postpartum haemorrhage, predisposing factors - platelet dysfunction or intraoperative haemorrhage - were recognised but were inadequately treated. In another case of postpartum haemorrhage, inadequate precautions were taken after difficulty with haemostasis at caesarean section, and in another case, one unit of incompatible blood was given and there was delay in carrying out laparotomy.

Comment

It is gratifying that there has been a further fall in the number of deaths from haemorrhage in this triennium compared to 1991-93 and 1988-90. Studies from other countries[1] and "near-miss" investigations[2] suggest that life-threatening haemorrhage occurs in 1 in 1000 deliveries, which means there are 600 cases of life-threatening obstetric haemorrhage in the UK every year. The low numbers of deaths indicate that in general this condition is being well treated.

Nevertheless the number of deaths from this cause in the present triennium remains higher than in 1985-87 and there are lessons to be drawn from the deaths that have occurred. One is the frightening speed with which death can occur from obstetric haemorrhage, particularly in cases of placenta praevia. This is the reason for a recommendation that has been repeatedly made in these Reports:

Placenta praevia, particularly in patients with a previous uterine scar, may be associated with uncontrollable uterine haemorrhage at delivery and caesarean hysterectomy may be necessary. A very experienced operator is essential and a consultant must be readily available.

This advice is now even more important than it was in the past, as changes in the patterns of training have led to the loss of some Specialist Registrar posts. Trainees in future may be less experienced than "traditional" Senior Registrars. The treatment of severe haemorrhage may require not only the technical ability to carry out caesarean hysterectomy but the ability to decide quickly that this operation is necessary.

Accident and Emergency nurses should not be asked to decide whether or not there is an obstetric problem. Minor signs or symptoms may have considerable significance in pregnancy and any pregnant woman admitted to an Accident and Emergency department should be discussed with the duty obstetrician.

The speed with which obstetric haemorrhage can become life-threatening also emphasises the need for good communication between the labour ward and the blood bank. Both should be on the same site. Every unit must have a protocol for the management of massive haemorrhage.

Although postpartum haemorrhage is relatively common (occurring after about 1% of deliveries[i]), life-threatening haemorrhage requiring immediate treatment affects only 1 in 1000 deliveries, as mentioned above. It will therefore occur about four times a year in a large maternity hospital. This is infrequent enough to make practice drills necessary. The recommendation in previous Reports is repeated: **units should organise regular "fire drills" so that when these emergencies occur all members of staff - including the blood bank - know exactly what to do to ensure that large quantities of cross-matched blood can be delivered to the labour ward without delay.**

With obstetric haemorrhage in particular, vigilance is necessary to ensure that past lessons are not forgotten. Recommendations from previous Reports are therefore summarised again. In addition to the recommendations printed in bold type above, previous Reports have emphasised:

- accurate estimation of blood loss,
- prompt recognition and treatment of clotting disorders,
- early involvement of a consultant haematologist,
- involvement of a consultant anaesthetist in resuscitation,
- the use of adequately sized intravenous cannulae, and
- the importance of monitoring central venous pressure.

References

1. Drife, J. Management of primary postpartum haemorrhage. *British Journal of Obstetrics and Gynaecology* 1997; **104**: 275-7.

2. Mantel, G., Buchmann, E., Rees, H. & Pattinson, R. C. Severe acute maternal morbidity: a pilot study of a definition for a "near miss". *British Journal of Obstetrics and Gynaecology* 1998; **105**: 985-90.

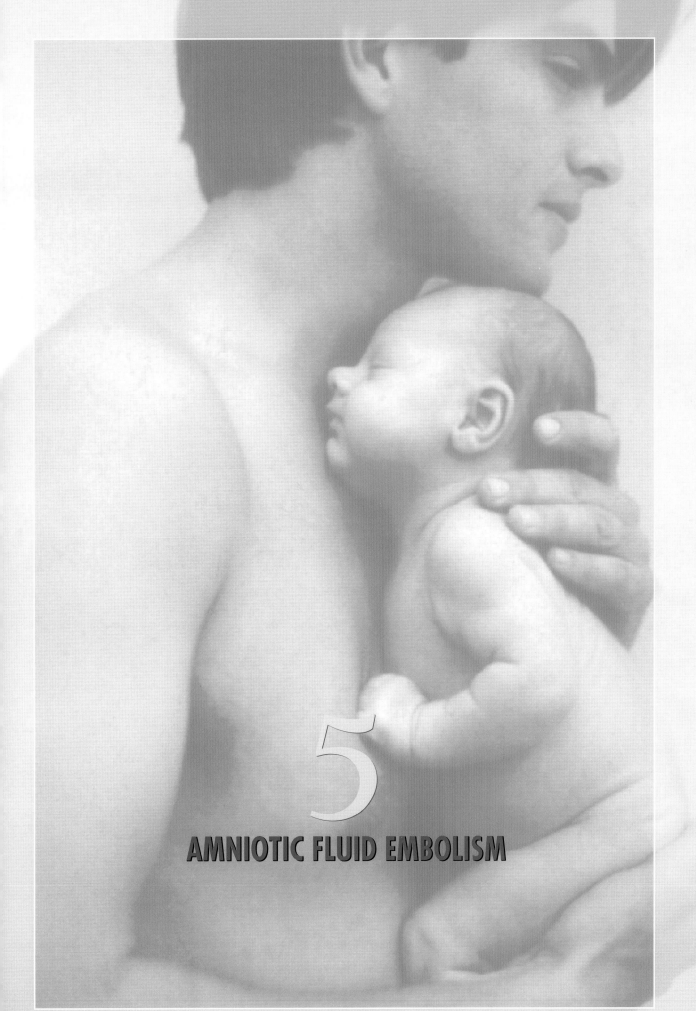

5

AMNIOTIC FLUID EMBOLISM

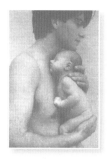

CHAPTER 5
AMNIOTIC FLUID EMBOLISM

Summary

There were 17 deaths due to amniotic fluid embolism in the United Kingdom in 1994-96, compared with 10 in 1991-93, 11 proven and one diagnosed on clinical grounds in 1988-90 and nine in 1985-87. All but one of the women were aged over 25, and 12 were over 30. Two women were nulliparous and three were of high parity (para 4 or more). Seven had received prostaglandin or oxytocin and two had had amniotomy. Fourteen were delivered by forceps or caesarean section, the indication in eleven of these cases being maternal collapse. In eight cases the interval between collapse and death was short, in two cases this information was not available and in the other seven cases the interval was greater than six hours.

Amniotic fluid embolism

Seventeen *Direct* deaths were attributed to amniotic fluid embolism (AFE). In 10 cases the diagnosis was confirmed by the finding of squames or hair in the lungs on histological examination. There were four deaths in which a clinical diagnosis of AFE was made without confirmation of the diagnosis at autopsy. In the remaining three cases inadequate information was available to the Assessors. The acceptance of a clinical diagnosis of AFE began with the last Report: prior to 1991-93 the Reports accepted only deaths in which autopsy provided histological evidence of squames in the lungs.

Clinically diagnosed cases

An asthmatic woman who weighed over 100kg had a history of a previous caesarean section followed by a "collapsed lung" requiring intensive care. She developed polyhydramnios and required blood transfusion for anaemia. Elective caesarean section was carried out at 36 weeks. Just after delivery of the placenta, cardiac arrest occurred. At autopsy the lungs showed anaphylactoid reaction but no squames were seen. The heart was dilated and flabby, weighing 500g, compared to a normal weight of around 300g. This case is also discussed in Chapter 16 on Pathology.

A primigravid woman went into spontaneous labour at term. Labour was augmented by syntocinon and lasted less than eight hours. She felt unwell in the last two hours of labour. There was very little liquor in labour and thick meconium was noted in the second stage. Instrumental delivery was performed, syntometrine was given and the placenta was delivered. She became suddenly cyanosed while the episiotomy was being repaired. She was transferred to an intensive care unit (ICU) where pulmonary oedema was diagnosed but she died a few hours later. No autopsy was carried out.

Care was not substandard in this case. Although cyanosis and sudden collapse are suggestive of AFE, it is not typical for collapse to occur after the placenta has been delivered.

A parous woman underwent amniocentesis because of her age. She had undergone previous instrumental deliveries because of large babies but was persuaded to attempt a vaginal delivery. Several days after term, induction of labour was begun with 1mg of prostaglandin gel followed six hours later by 2mg. About three hours later a strong contraction was noted. An epidural was set up. Fetal distress was diagnosed, and a trial of forceps was planned but caesarean section was carried out. The baby was stillborn and was heavier than her previous babies. Severe haemorrhage occurred at operation. After some delay hysterectomy was carried out. The patient was transferred to an ICU but died three days later.

The clinical picture of a sustained strong uterine contraction followed by fetal distress, stillbirth and severe haemorrhage is strongly suggestive of amniotic fluid embolism. There was delay in carrying out hysterectomy and this was considered substandard care.

The fourth clinically diagnosed case is described below, in the section on substandard care.

Age

Table 5.1 shows how the risk of the condition increases with age. In the previous two triennia no case of amniotic fluid embolism occurred in a woman under the age of 25. In this triennium only one of the patients was under 25.

Table 5.1

	1988-90		1991-93		1994-96		Total 1988-96	
	Number of maternal deaths and the death rates per million maternities from amniotic fluid embolism by age; United Kingdom 1988-96. (Numbers of maternities are shown in Table 1.13)							
Age	No.	Rate	No.	Rate	No.	Rate	No.	Rate
<25	0	0	0	0	1	1.6	1	0.4
25-29	6*	7.2	4	4.9	3	4.0	13	5.4
30-34	4	8.0	4	7.2	6	9.8	14	9.3
35-39	0	0	2	10.6	4	18.1	6	10.4
40+	2	63.3	0	0	3	79.3	5	37.0
Total	12	4.7	10	4.3	17	7.7	39	5.6

* One not histologically confirmed

Precise figures by age are not available for 1985-87.

Parity

Amniotic fluid embolism has been thought to be associated with high parity, though in 1991-93 none of the deaths was associated with high parity. In 1994-96, of the 14 women for whom parity information was available, two were primigravid, three had one previous delivery, five had two previous deliveries, and four had three or more previous deliveries.

Antenatal complications

Antenatal complications were present in about half the cases. Two women had undergone amniocentesis. Another two had developed polyhydramnios, one of whom had an intrauterine death. One woman had placenta praevia, one had fibroids, and one had a cervical suture inserted.

Induction or augmentation of labour

Amniotic fluid embolism has been thought to be associated with induction of labour and the use of oxytocic drugs, but in this triennium four of the women collapsed before labour began and another four went into labour spontaneously.

Six women had labour induced: five with prostaglandins (gel in two cases and tablets in three cases) and one with amniotomy and oxytocin. One woman received oxytocin in labour and another underwent amniotomy in labour.

Mode of delivery

Two woman died undelivered and one miscarried after collapsing at 22 weeks' gestation. Nine women were delivered by caesarean section and four by forceps. Information was not available about one case. In most cases of operative delivery the indication was maternal collapse.

In three of the cases of forceps delivery, instrumental delivery was undertaken after the signs of AFE had occurred. In the fourth case, signs of AFE occurred after delivery, though the woman had felt unwell during the last two hours of her labour.

In two of the caesarean sections, symptoms of AFE appeared after the operation had been started. The other seven caesarean sections were undertaken after symptoms of AFE had occurred. One of these was a post-mortem caesarean section:

> A parous woman underwent amniocentesis because of her age. In late pregnancy she developed hypertension and proteinuria. Labour was induced with prostaglandin 1mg, repeated twice. A few hours after the third pessary she collapsed, cyanosed and foaming at the mouth. A live baby was delivered by caesarean section but the woman could not be resuscitated. At autopsy histological examination of the lungs confirmed the presence of fetal squames.

Although this case shows an association between amniocentesis, induction of labour and amniotic fluid embolism, there was no substandard care in this case. This was one of the few occasions in these Reports when peri-mortem caesarean section resulted in the birth of a live baby.

Speed of collapse

In nine cases the collapse was sudden and resuscitation proved impossible. In seven of these cases the diagnosis was histologically confirmed.

In seven cases the interval between death and collapse was longer, varying between six hours and three days. Three of these cases were histologically confirmed.

Substandard care

Care was substandard in five cases. In one (summarised above) this was because there was delay in carrying out hysterectomy to treat severe haemorrhage. In the others there were deficiencies in the midwifery or anaesthetic care:

> A "grande multipara" was admitted in early labour at term after a normal pregnancy (apart from anaemia in the third trimester). She remained in hesitant labour for 24 hours. Amniotomy was carried out when the cervix was 9cm dilated. When vaginal examination was repeated over 3 hours later she collapsed. The baby, which was large, was delivered by forceps and survived. The mother died shortly after delivery and histological examination confirmed the presence of squames in the lungs.

Care was substandard in this case. Hesitant labour is unusual in a "grande multipara" and once the cervix reaches 9cm dilatation it is very worrying if more than three hours elapse before the second stage of labour begins. Persistent strong contractions at the end of the first stage may have contributed to the outcome in this case. As fewer "grande multiparous" women are seen, staff may lose their ability to recognise danger signs in such labours.

> A woman with a history of a cone biopsy, recurrent miscarriages, preterm deliveries and a caesarean section had a cervical suture inserted and had several admissions with abdominal pain. She went into preterm labour, was treated with ritodrine and developed supraventricular tachycardia. The cervical suture was removed and amniotomy was carried out. Fetal bradycardia led to caesarean section. She became cyanosed before the baby was delivered. Cardiac arrest occurred. She was resuscitated and transferred to the ICU but died soon afterwards. Histological examination confirmed the presence of squames in the lungs.

Although she had been seen by a consultant physician because of her supraventricular tachycardia, the anaesthetic was given by a senior house officer. Care was therefore substandard, though this probably did not affect the outcome. In view of the poor obstetric history, it is also disappointing that the caesarean section was not performed by a consultant obstetrician.

> A parous woman developed polyhydramnios at 37 weeks' gestation. Glucose tolerance was normal. At 38 weeks she noticed diminished fetal movements and intrauterine fetal death was diagnosed four days later. Labour was induced with a cervagem pessary followed by another about two hours later "because of failure to progress". After a labour lasting just over two hours she collapsed with shortness of breath. The baby was quickly delivered by forceps, after which postpartum haemorrhage occurred. She was declared dead less than six hours after the insertion of the first pessary. AFE was confirmed histologically.

Cervagem pessaries contain 1mg Gemeprost. When they are used to induce abortion in cases of intrauterine fetal death in the second trimester, the manufacturer recommends insertion into the posterior fornix at 3-hourly intervals up to a maximum of five administrations. The manufacturer recommends that "they should not be used for the induction of labour or cervical softening at term as fetal effects have not been ascertained". The listed indications for Gemeprost do not include intrauterine death at term, and other forms of prostaglandin are generally used in such cases. A two-hour interval between pessaries, particularly in an older parous woman, was felt to represent substandard care.

> A parous woman with uterine fibroids had labour induced at 38 weeks' gestation because of a history of "slight shoulder dystocia" and patient request. One 3mg prostin pessary was inserted, followed by another 3mg prostin pessary. One hour after the second pessary, contractions began and two hours later there was fetal bradycardia. The cervix was 2cm dilated and caesarean section was carried out. The baby was acidotic and the uterus was "slightly lax". Two and a half hours after operation the patient became dyspnoeic and shocked and had a convulsion. Coagulopathy developed and haemorrhage was treated by hysterectomy. She died five days later in ICU after a repeat laparotomy for bleeding.

Amniotic fluid embolus was not confirmed histologically but this did not rule out the diagnosis in view of the length of time between collapse and autopsy. Care was substandard because a lower dose of prostin should have been used and the indications for induction of labour were in any case weak. Particular caution should be exercised in inducing labour in an older parous woman with any uterine abnormality.

Comment

The number of deaths from amniotic fluid embolism has risen from 10 in 1991-93 to 17 in 1994-96. This is the highest total in any of the last four Reports. Only the present Report and the previous one have accepted cases diagnosed on clinical grounds: in 1991-93 there were two such cases and in the present triennium there were four (and another three cases in which information was inadequate). If these seven cases are excluded the number of histologically confirmed deaths has varied little over the last four Reports - from nine in 1985-87 to 10 in 1994-96.

The Reports have shown consistently that age is a risk factor for amniotic fluid embolism. One woman in the present triennium was aged under 25 (and obese), three were in their late twenties and the rest were 30 or over. The average age of childbearing in the UK continues to rise and this is a possible reason for an increase in the numbers of cases of amniotic fluid embolism.

No single obstetric intervention was identified as a risk factor for amniotic fluid embolism, but it should also be noted that in only one case did the condition complicate an entirely straightforward pregnancy in a woman of low parity. Antenatal complications included amniocentesis, polyhydramnios, placenta increta, fibroids, cervical suture and intrauterine fetal death.

The use of oxytocic drugs has been thought to be a risk factor for amniotic fluid embolism, but nine of the women in this triennium received neither prostaglandin nor oxytocin. Nevertheless, two of the nine underwent amniotomy and another two were women of high parity, in whom normal uterine contractions can be expected to be particularly strong.

The death rate from amniotic fluid embolism could be reduced by avoiding uterine over-stimulation and by prompt diagnosis of obstructed labour. This, however, applies only to a small number of cases. The previous Report suggested that a more promising strategy for reducing deaths was better treatment of women who survive long enough to be transferred to intensive care. In the present triennium there were seven such cases but only one of these had substandard care after delivery. Examination of the other cases has not suggested how the intensive care of this condition can be improved.

Amniotic fluid embolism remains a frustrating challenge and only general recommendations can be made. Rates of obstetric intervention in the form of amniocentesis and induction and augmentation of labour should be kept as low as possible, and research into the condition is still necessary.

The UK amniotic fluid embolism register

A confidential register of all cases of AFE is to be established for the United Kingdom. The aim is to identify any differences or common factors between survivors and fatalities, which may help to reduce maternal deaths from this condition.

The entry criteria are:

- Acute hypotension or cardiac arrest
- Acute hypoxia (dyspnoea, cyanosis or respiratory arrest)
- Coagulopathy (laboratory evidence of intravascular coagulation or severe haemorrhage)
- Onset of all of the above during labour, caesarean section or within 30 minutes of delivery
- No other clinical condition or potential explanation for the symptoms and signs.

All cases of suspected or proven AFE, whether they survived or not, should be reported to:

Mr Derek Tuffnell, Consultant Obstetrician,
Bradford Royal Infirmary,
Duckworth Lane
Bradford,
BD9 6RJ
West Yorkshire.

Tel   01274 364520
Fax 01274 366690

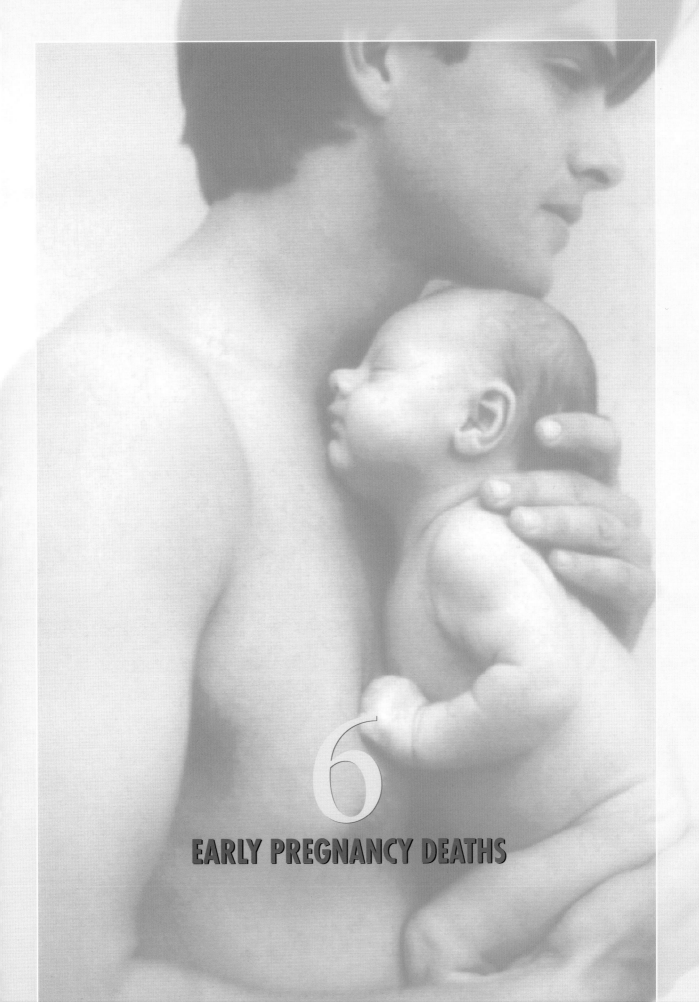

6

EARLY PREGNANCY DEATHS

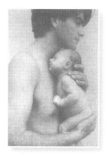

CHAPTER 6
EARLY PREGNANCY DEATHS

Summary

This Chapter considers all deaths from ectopic pregnancy, spontaneous abortion, or termination of pregnancy, before 24 weeks' gestation. Corresponding Chapters in previous Reports included deaths before 20 weeks. Since all such deaths reported in 1994-96 occurred before 20 weeks, direct comparison with previous triennia is possible. Other deaths in early pregnancy are counted in the relevant Chapters of this Report.

There were 12 deaths from ectopic pregnancy (compared to eight in 1991-93), two following spontaneous miscarriage (compared to three in 1991-93) and one as a direct consequence of a legal termination of pregnancy (compared to five in 1991-93). These figures are also shown in Table 6.1.

In addition, there were 15 *Direct* deaths from pulmonary embolism in pregnancies before 24 weeks' gestation (which are discussed and counted in Chapter 2), and one *Indirect* death from myocardial infarction following termination of pregnancy (counted in Chapter 10).

It is gratifying to identify a decrease in deaths associated with termination of pregnancy. Nevertheless many of the early pregnancy deaths showed features of substandard care and, in some cases, deviation from guidelines published in previous Reports. Excluding two cases with insufficient details the proportion of deaths from ectopic pregnancies associated with substandard care was 80%, as in the previous Report. Both cases of spontaneous miscarriage, and the one death following a termination of pregnancy were also associated with substandard care.

Early pregnancy: key recommendations

Ectopic pregnancy

It is essential that GPs and other clinicians, including staff in Accident and Emergency Departments, consider the diagnosis of ectopic pregnancy in any woman of reproductive age who complains of abdominal pain. It is important to recognise that the clinical presentation is often not "classical". β-hCG testing should be considered in any young woman with unexplained abdominal pain whether or not she has missed a period or had abnormal vaginal bleeding.

Gastrointestinal symptoms may be prominent in ectopic pregnancy, notably diarrhoea and painful defaecation.

An ultrasonically "empty" uterus in a woman who presents with vaginal bleeding in pregnancy may indicate an ectopic pregnancy.

When ectopic pregnancy is suspected, or when a young woman with a predisposing history complains of severe abdominal pain, rapid referral and assessment are vital.

The decision to treat ectopic pregnancy by laparoscopic rather than open surgery should be based on the experience and expertise of the operator and a judgement about the suitability of the procedure for the individual woman.

Women in haemorrhagic shock following rupture of ectopic pregnancy need to be transferred promptly to the operating theatre. Transfer must not be delayed by attempts to try to re-establish a normal circulating plasma volume.

Several of the women who died were socially disadvantaged, and included recent immigrants, women with little English, and those with itinerant occupations or previous substance abuse. Such factors may make assessment or communication difficult or lead to a delay in seeking help.

An RCOG guideline on treatment of ectopic pregnancy, including laparoscopic treatment, is being prepared and should be available during 1999.

Spontaneous abortion

When there is evidence of serious clinical decline postoperatively, or in association with miscarriage, and especially when sepsis is suspected, it is vital that there is direct and rapid involvement of senior obstetric staff and other relevant specialists including intensive care doctors.

In cases of septic abortion, evacuation of the uterus should be performed by experienced surgeons, optimally around one hour after intravenous antibiotics.

Termination of pregnancy

Ideally, all women should undergo ultrasound examination before termination of pregnancy to establish gestational age, viability, and site.

Failure to obtain tissue at suction termination of what appears, ultrasonically, to be an intrauterine pregnancy suggests an abnormal site of implantation, including cornual pregnancy.

Laparoscopy, and/or laparotomy, is essential if perforation of the uterus occurs during suction termination of pregnancy, because of the risk of bowel damage and life-threatening sequelae.

There remain questions as to whether dilatation and evacuation is a safe and appropriate method of terminating second trimester pregnancies when effective medical alternatives exist.

As previously discussed in the section on Definitions, the denominator used for early pregnancy deaths is the number of "estimated pregnancies". This is a combination of the number of maternities, together with legal terminations, hospital admissions for spontaneous miscarriages (at less than 24 weeks' gestation) and ectopic pregnancies, with an adjustment to allow for the period of gestation and maternal age at conception. It is the preferred denominator for deaths in early pregnancy. The estimate for the United Kingdom 1994-96 was 2,914,600. However, this is still an underestimate of the actual number of pregnancies since the figure does not include other pregnancies which miscarry early, those where the woman is not admitted to hospital, or those where the woman herself may not even know she is pregnant. Further details are available in Appendix 1 to this Report.

Table 6.1 shows the number of women dying from ectopic pregnancy and rates per thousand estimated pregnancies for 1987-96. Table 6.2 shows the rates, per 100,000 estimated pregnancies, for deaths following spontaneous abortion and legal termination of pregnancy.

Table 6.1

Deaths from ectopic pregnancies and rates per 1,000 estimated pregnancies; England and Wales 1988-90 and United Kingdom 1991-96.					
	Total estimated pregnancies in thousands	Total estimated ectopic pregnancies	Ectopic pregnancies per 1,000 pregnancies	Deaths from ectopic pregnancies	Death rate per 1,000 estimated ectopic pregnancies
England and Wales 1988-90	2,886.9	24775	9.6	15	0.5
United Kingdom 1991-93 1994-96	3,137,4 2,914,6	30160 33550	9.6 11.5	9* 12	0.3 0.4

NB Comparative figures for 1985-87 not available
Sources:
    1982-90 England HIPE/Hospital Episode Statistics (HES)
    Wales Hospital Activity Analysis (HAA)
    1991-96 England HES, Wales HAA
    Scottish Morbidity Records (SMR) 1 Inpatients and Daycases Acute
    Scottish Morbidity Records (SMR) 2 Inpatients and Daycase Maternity
    DHSS Northern Ireland
    And see Table A.1 in Appendix 1

Table 6.2

	Spontaneous	Legal	Illegal	Total	Rate per million maternities	Rate per million estimated pregnancies
1985-87	5[1]	1[2]	0	6	2.7	N/A
1988-90	6	3	0	9	4.0	N/A
1991-93	3	5	0	8	3.5	2.5
1994-96	2	1	0	3	1.4	1.0

Direct abortion deaths by type of abortion, rates per million maternities and estimated pregnancies; United Kingdom 1985-96.

[1] Includes one death from missed abortion.

[2] Does not include one unexplained death associated with legal abortion.

N/A - Data not available on/numbers of estimated pregnancies for these years.

Ectopic pregnancy

Of the 12 deaths from ectopic pregnancy, eight were considered to be associated with substandard care. This resulted from delayed diagnosis and inappropriate investigation and treatment. In two other cases insufficient information was made available for the Assessors to make a judgement as to whether care was acceptable or not. In the two remaining cases, collapse was so sudden that there was little scope for any effective medical intervention.

Ectopic pregnancy is often difficult to diagnose. It is essential that GPs, and other clinicians, always consider the possibility of ectopic pregnancy in a woman of reproductive age who complains of abdominal pain. The clinical presentation may not be "classical" and, in particular, that there may be no history of a missed period. Gastrointestinal symptoms were prominent in some of the cases described here, notably diarrhoea and painful defaecation. Several of the women also showed features of social exclusion, including immigrant status, little English, itinerant occupation, or previous substance abuse. As in previous Reports, deaths occurred despite clear clinical pointers to the diagnosis of ectopic pregnancy and, in some cases, despite repeated consultations with medical staff.

> A patient underwent an ultrasound scan because of vaginal bleeding at eight weeks of pregnancy. This showed no evidence of intrauterine pregnancy and a diagnosis of probable complete miscarriage was made by the ultrasonographer. Subsequent attendances to general practitioners and A&E departments with acute abdominal pain, vaginal bleeding, fainting episodes, and pallor produced diagnoses of pelvic inflammatory disease and constipation which preceded her final collapse and death from ruptured ectopic pregnancy.

Previous Reports have emphasised the fact that an ultrasonically empty uterus in a woman who presents with vaginal bleeding in pregnancy may indicate an ectopic pregnancy. Further investigation should be based on suggestive symptoms, clinical signs and β-hCG estimation, which is readily available. In this case insufficient attention was paid to symptoms and signs.

Ultrasound can also be misleading in the diagnosis of cornual pregnancy (see later) and of more advanced extrauterine pregnancies, as in the next case. This also applies to another woman who died of a pulmonary embolus and is counted and discussed in Chapter 2:

> A fetus was thought to be small for gestational age on ultrasound examination prompted by a raised serum alpha-fetoprotein result. Detailed examination was undertaken by an experienced sonographer who confirmed this impression and also noted an echogenic mass in the lower abdomen. Fetal karyotyping was performed. Less than two weeks later, the patient re-presented to hospital with abdominal pain and tenderness and tachycardia, and was admitted. A junior doctor prescribed repeated doses of opiate analgesia for increasing pain without apparently making a diagnosis. The patient was found dead in bed the following morning. Autopsy showed an "abrupted" abdominal pregnancy.

With hindsight, the pelvic mass seen on ultrasonography was presumably the empty uterus. Although advanced extrauterine pregnancy can be a very difficult diagnosis to make by ultrasound, it is regrettable that it was not apparently considered here. Junior doctors should not prescribe regular doses of opiate without making a diagnosis or asking a more senior colleague to assess the patient.

> A young woman complained repeatedly of intermittent abdominal pain and episodes of faintness. She was amenorrhoeic and had a positive pregnancy test at six weeks' gestation. She was noted to be pale by one of several GPs that she consulted. A month later she was visited twice in one day by her GP, because of abdominal pain and diarrhoea. The gastrointestinal symptoms masked the clear diagnosis of ectopic pregnancy. No referral was made to a specialist and no ultrasound examination was requested. The patient collapsed at home the next day and was found to be asystolic by the attending paramedics. Cardiorespiratory resuscitation was effected during transfer to the local A&E Department where resuscitation continued. Eventual ultrasound examination identified free fluid in the peritoneal cavity, and the gynaecological team was called. Despite rapid laparotomy and salpingectomy for a ruptured ectopic pregnancy, the patient died shortly afterwards in the ICU.

This case illustrates how presentation to different doctors, together with some atypical symptoms, can lead to failure to consider the diagnosis of ectopic pregnancy despite strong clinical indicators. It is also vital that staff in A&E departments consider the diagnosis in women of reproductive age who present with hypovolaemic shock. Ultrasound examination in such circumstances merely delays definitive surgical intervention; the presence of intraperitoneal blood can be demonstrated much more rapidly by paracentesis.

> A young woman with a history of pregnancy terminations complained of severe abdominal pain one evening. Her GP gave advice over the telephone but later visited because the pain had worsened. There was no history of a missed period and because the patient complained of nausea, it was assumed that the problem was gastrointestinal in origin. Less than an hour later, the woman had a cardiac arrest in the presence of the GP, who had been re-called. Cardio-

pulmonary resuscitation was initiated, and continued until arrival at hospital. Attempts were then made to resuscitate the patient by infusion through multiple intravenous cannulae, with minimal success, before laparotomy was undertaken. This showed a ruptured ectopic pregnancy and three litres of blood in the peritoneal cavity. The patient died in theatre.

In this case the delay in diagnosis was again caused by the presence of gastrointestinal symptoms. It was compounded by futile attempts at resuscitation before laparotomy. It is important to re-emphasise the traditional teaching that women in haemorrhagic shock following rupture of ectopic pregnancy need to be transferred promptly to the operating theatre without delays to try to re-establish a normal circulating plasma volume.

When ectopic pregnancy is suspected, or when a young woman with a predisposing history complains of severe abdominal pain, rapid medical attendance and assessment are vital:

> Another young woman with a history of previous terminations of pregnancy was seen, at home, by a locum doctor during the night because of severe abdominal pain. A further call to the Practice the following day was made by a neighbour because the patient appeared unwell and continued to complain of pain. The GP arrived three hours later to find the woman dead. Autopsy showed her to have a ruptured ectopic pregnancy.

Delay in diagnosis may result from communication problems. Two women for whom English was not their first language died from ruptured ectopic pregnancies:

> One had oligomenorrhoea following medical treatment of endometriosis and had attended her GP for another reason two weeks before emergency admission to an A&E Department, shocked from a ruptured ectopic pregnancy. Despite rapid resuscitation and surgery, death occurred subsequently from adult respiratory distress syndrome. Whether the outcome would have been different if the patient had been able to speak English, or had access to a clinician with knowledge of her language, remains speculative.

> The other woman was admitted in asystole to an A&E Department; it is not known what, if any, prior symptoms she might have had.

There has been a trend in recent years towards less use of laparoscopy for diagnostic purposes in suspected ectopic pregnancy, with greater reliance on ultrasound and quantitative β-hCG estimation. At the same time there has been more use of laparoscopy for surgical treatment of confirmed ectopic pregnancy. Ultrasound examination, however, can be especially misleading in the diagnosis of advanced extrauterine pregnancy, as mentioned above, and of cornual pregnancy:

> A woman had a termination of pregnancy in a private clinic at eight weeks' gestation. A suction curettage was performed and apparently appropriate tissue noted in the cannula during the procedure. A week later, however, she was re-referred because she still felt pregnant and her pregnancy test remained positive. An ultrasound scan was reported as showing a nine-week intrauterine pregnancy. A repeat suction curettage was performed but no tissue was obtained. Consideration was given in theatre to performing a laparoscopy, but this was not done because a pregnancy test in theatre was negative. She was discharged home but, in light of a subsequently

reported high serum β-hCG result, an appointment was made for her to re-attend the clinic. In the meantime, she attended an A&E Department with acute abdominal pain and a diagnosis of probable urinary tract infection was made. Later the same day, she returned to the same A&E Department and had a cardiac arrest. Resuscitation was attempted but failed. At autopsy, there were 3.5 litres of blood in the peritoneal cavity and a ruptured cornual pregnancy in an otherwise normal uterus.

Although cornual pregnancy is difficult to diagnose by ultrasound, it should have been obvious after the second unsuccessful attempt at suction termination that the pregnancy was abnormally sited. An ultrasound scan or laparoscopy should have been performed in theatre to clarify the site of implantation. The patient should not have been discharged home without knowledge of the β-hCG result. The fact that this took place in the private sector, where there may not have been "on site" laboratory services, may be relevant. When she attended the A&E Department with abdominal pain, the previous history should have alerted the staff to the serious nature of her complaint. The management of this woman was sub-standard in many respects.

"Minimal access" surgical treatment of ectopic pregnancy has become more popular but may be associated with hazards:

> A parous woman with an intrauterine contraceptive device presented with acute lower abdominal pain and vaginal bleeding two weeks after what was thought to be a delayed period. There was marked pelvic tenderness and a diagnosis of pelvic inflammatory disease was made despite hypotension and absence of pyrexia. The diagnosis of ectopic pregnancy was made after β-hCG testing and ultrasonography. Although two litres of blood were present in the peritoneal cavity, salpingostomy was performed via the laparoscope, by a non-consultant member of staff. The patient required laparotomy later the same day because of further intra-abdominal bleeding by which time a further two litres of blood had accumulated (from the ovarian vein). Salpingo-oophorectomy was performed. She died subsequently from ARDS despite intensive care, including ECMO.

In this case, the consequences of delay in diagnosis, despite the classical features of ectopic pregnancy, were compounded by ill-judged surgical treatment in a woman with major haemoperitoneum and a normal, contralateral fallopian tube. A similar case was reported during the previous triennium. An RCOG guideline on treatment of ectopic pregnancy, including laparoscopic treatment, is being prepared and should be available during 1999.

> Another woman died after diagnostic laparoscopy for presumed ectopic pregnancy. She had positive β-hCG results but no pregnancy was found at laparoscopy. Postoperatively, she developed septicaemic shock and was found to have a perforated sigmoid colon. She died despite intensive care. In this case insufficient information has been made available to the Assessors to permit comment on the standard of care.

In another case there was evidence of substandard care after appropriate initial treatment:

> A nulliparous woman with a history of pelvic inflammatory disease presented, shocked, with a ruptured ectopic pregnancy at eight weeks' gestation. She underwent laparotomy and salpingectomy without any apparent surgical or anaesthetic difficulties. She became unwell after 36 hours with evidence of sepsis and respiratory embarrassment. Despite vigorous intensive

care she died. Autopsy showed ARDS, sickle lung, endocarditis due to Candida, pulmonary embolism and myocardial infarction. There was nothing to suggest aspiration of stomach contents as the cause of respiratory disease.

Despite clinical evidence of serious decline postoperatively in this patient, there was no direct involvement of senior obstetric staff and requests to involve senior physicians were tardy.

In one further case, no information was available other than the death certificate which stated the cause of death as ectopic pregnancy.

It is again necessary to re-emphasise the conclusions in the previous Report. Ectopic pregnancy continues to be an important cause of maternal deaths and the need for early diagnosis is paramount. Awareness of the possibility of an ectopic pregnancy in any woman of reproductive age is essential. The emphasis is again placed on the importance of the history as well as suggestive signs on examination. Primary care doctors in particular must be constantly aware of the possibility of this diagnosis.

When a woman presents to her GP or to an A&E Department with unexplained abdominal pain, with or without vaginal bleeding, it is essential to exclude an ectopic pregnancy. The ready availability of sensitive β-hCG kits means that the diagnosis of early pregnancy can be made in GPs' surgeries or A&E Departments. The test itself is very reliable: the limiting factor is thinking of using it. If the diagnosis of ectopic pregnancy is likely then vaginal examination is best deferred until the patient is in hospital.

Abortion

This section discusses the three deaths related to spontaneous and legal abortion. This is the fifth successive Report in which no identified deaths from illegal abortion are reported. Table 6.2 shows data on abortion deaths from 1985, when the Report first covered the United Kingdom as a whole.

Spontaneous miscarriage

Although deaths from septic abortion have been rare in the UK in recent decades, this remains a very important cause of death globally[1]. When serious infection does occur, prompt action is necessary to minimise the risk to the mother. This includes appropriate antibiotic treatment, rapid removal of infected tissue, intensive care, and involvement of senior clinical and microbiological staff.

There is often uncertainty about the optimal timing of surgical evacuation of the uterus after initiating antibiotic treatment. The main initial aims of antibiotic treatment are to counter bacteraemia and to protect other tissues from becoming infected. Antibiotic penetration into necrotic, septic placental tissue is very limited and this is not the primary purpose of antibiotic treatment. It is therefore logical to perform evacuation when there are high levels of antibiotics in the bloodstream and increasing levels in normal tissues. With most antibiotics, blood levels are high around one hour after intravenous administration and then drop with increasing tissue uptake. The aim should be to perform surgical evacuation one hour after antibiotics are given. The timing of such procedures cannot, therefore, be left to the vagaries of the "emergency list" that

exists in many general hospitals. Nor should the operation be left to the most junior member of staff.
In the following cases, there seemed to be delay in appreciating fully the serious nature of the problem:

> A woman who had had several episodes of threatened miscarriage, re-presented to the hospital at 17 weeks' gestation with further bleeding. She miscarried nine hours later and a foul smelling discharge was noted, apparently for the first time. She was tachycardic, jaundiced, oliguric and anaemic. Disseminated intravascular coagulation was diagnosed, and appropriate therapy was initiated by a Consultant Haematologist. There was a delay of six hours before surgical evacuation of 'putrid' placental tissue by an obstetric registrar. Although intravenous antibiotic treatment had been started at the time of miscarriage, death occurred from *E. coli* septicaemia within hours.

> A parous woman was admitted with an incomplete miscarriage at 10 weeks' gestation. Although she was markedly tachycardic and hypotensive, her haemoglobin concentration was normal. Her vital signs improved after surgical evacuation of the uterus but she was readmitted three days later with further signs of shock, although apyrexial. Despite intravenous antibiotic treatment, intensive care and hysterectomy to remove the source of infection, she died. There is no record of the responsible organism but pathological findings were compatible with septicaemia with primary infection in the uterus.

Termination of pregnancy

The previous Report emphasised the need for laparoscopy or laparotomy if perforation of the uterus occurs during suction termination of pregnancy, because of the risk of bowel damage and life-threatening sequelae. In the following case this guideline was not followed, with fatal consequences:

> A young woman underwent a termination of pregnancy. The date of her last menstrual period was uncertain but, clinically, the uterus appeared to be 13-14 weeks' size. Ultrasound examination was not performed. Examination in theatre after Gemeprost pre-treatment showed the uterus to be 15 weeks' size. Dilatation and evacuation were performed followed by insertion of a suction catheter which was felt to pass through the fundus of the uterus. It was considered by the surgeon that no negative suction had been applied within the peritoneal cavity, and therefore no surgical inspection of intra-abdominal contents was performed. The patient was discharged home, apparently well, after overnight observation. She was admitted, moribund, to an A&E Department six days later and died despite attempts at resuscitation. Autopsy revealed two holes in the jejunum, and faecal peritonitis.

In addition to the need for laparoscopy after perforation, this case illustrates the value of ultrasound examination before termination if the gestational age is in doubt so that difficult and hazardous surgical terminations may be avoided. A policy of routine ultrasound would, in addition, allow the recognition of non-viable (or even non-existent) pregnancies thereby relieving some women of anxiety or a sense of guilt.

It was not clear if uterine perforation, in this case, occurred during dilatation and evacuation, or on insertion of the suction cannula. A similar death following dilatation and evacuation was reported in the 1988-90 triennium and raises questions as to whether this is an appropriate method of terminating second-trimester pregnancies when safe and effective medical alternatives exist. Research is required in this area.

Reference

1.   Royston, E. & Armstrong, S. *Preventing Maternal Deaths*. Geneva: World Health Organization, 1989.

REPORT ON CONFIDENTIAL ENQUIRIES INTO MATERNAL DEATHS IN THE UNITED KINGDOM

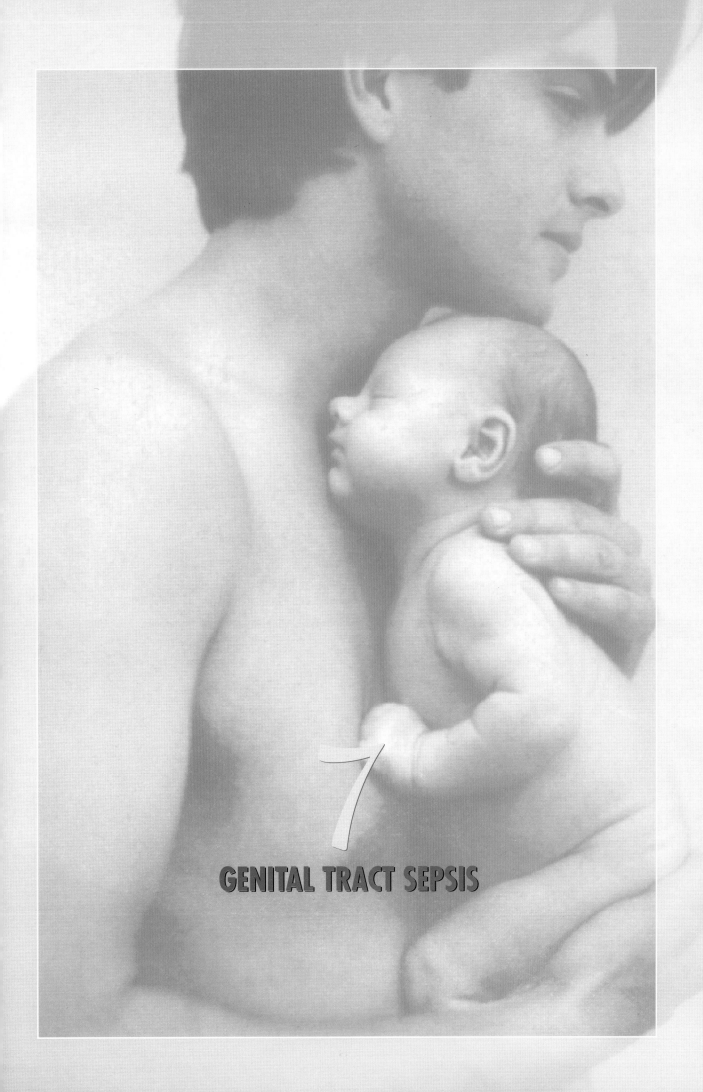

7

GENITAL TRACT SEPSIS

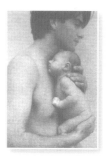

CHAPTER 7
GENITAL TRACT SEPSIS

Summary

There were 16 deaths due to genital tract sepsis, a similar number to those which occurred in the previous triennium. Fourteen of the deaths are counted in this Chapter. Two others followed spontaneous abortions and are counted in Chapter 6, which discusses deaths occurring before 24 weeks' gestation. There was also one *Late Direct* death, which is counted and discussed in Chapter 14. Substandard care occurred in five of the cases discussed in this Chapter.

Genital tract sepsis: key recommendations

Puerperal sepsis is not a disease of the past, and GPs and midwives must be aware of the signs and be prepared to institute immediate treatment and referral of any recently delivered woman with a fever and/or offensive vaginal discharge.

There is clear evidence from controlled trials showing the benefit of prophylactic antibiotics for caesarean section.

When infection develops and the patient is systemically ill, urgent and repeated bacteriological specimens, including blood cultures, must be obtained. The advice of a microbiologist must be sought at an early stage to assist with the use of appropriate antibiotic therapy. In serious cases doctors should be prepared to give parenteral antibiotics before the diagnosis can be confirmed.

The number of *Direct* deaths from sepsis compared with the previous two triennia is shown in Table 7.1

Table 7.1

	Maternal deaths from genital tract sepsis including abortion and ectopic pregnancy with rates per million maternities; United Kingdom 1985-96.						
Triennium	Sepsis after abortion	Sepsis after ectopic pregnancy	Puerperal sepsis*	Sepsis after surgical procedures	Sepsis before or during labour	Total	Rate per million maternities
1985-87	2	1	2	2	2	9	4.0
1988-90	7	1	4	5	0	17	7.2
1991-93	4	0	4	5	2	15	6.5
1994-96	2**	0	11	3	1	16	7.3

Note – this table includes only those deaths directly due to sepsis counted in Chapters 6 and 7.
* Puerperal sepsis includes deaths following spontaneous vaginal delivery. Deaths following caesarean section are included in "Sepsis after surgical proceedures"
** Two cases counted in Chapter 6

The 14 cases in this Chapter have been divided into sepsis before delivery, sepsis after vaginal delivery and sepsis after surgery. There were no cases of sepsis after ectopic pregnancy.

Sepsis before delivery

There was one case of sepsis before or during labour:

A grossly obese parous woman was admitted to hospital at 36 weeks' gestation with pyrexia and a 24-hour history of increasingly severe right-sided abdominal pain. On examination, the uterus was tender and there were no fetal heart sounds. A presumptive diagnosis of placental abruption or possibly a urinary tract infection was made. The initial coagulation screen was normal and the white cell count (WCC) was elevated. Intravenous antibiotics were administered and labour was induced with prostaglandin. During labour she developed peripheral cyanosis, hypotension, rapid respirations and coagulopathy. A stillborn infant was delivered vaginally. She then had a massive post-partum haemorrhage which responded to intensive treatment. Some hours later she had increasing respiratory difficulty and was transferred to an Intensive Care Unit (ICU) for elective ventilation. In spite of this she became bradycardic and hypotensive and had an asystolic arrest which failed to respond to resuscitation. It was later determined that blood cultures had grown Group A ß-haemolytic streptococcus. An autopsy was not performed.

Sepsis after vaginal delivery

Ten women died from sepsis of the genital tract after vaginal delivery:

A young woman who was 26 weeks pregnant developed severe shock and DIC some 12 hours after spontaneous labour and delivery of fresh stillborn twins. In spite of intensive treatment she died within six hours. A blood culture grew Group A ß-haemolytic streptococcus and autopsy findings supported the diagnosis of death from septic shock.

The pregnancy had been complicated by a twin-to-twin transfusion with polyhydramnios which was treated by intrauterine laser ablation of placental blood vessels. There had been no complications during or after this operation and it was considered to have been successful. It was most unlikely to have been associated with her death.

> A parous woman, who had intermittent episodes of vaginal bleeding from 14 weeks' gestation, was admitted to hospital at 26 weeks in spontaneous labour with an intrauterine death. She had a breech delivery and the placenta was said to be offensive. Twenty-four hours after delivery she developed jaundice, shock and DIC, was transferred to ICU and in spite of resuscitative measures had a cardiac arrest and died 13 hours later. At autopsy the appearances in the uterus were typical of clostridrial septicaemia and necrosis and this diagnosis was confirmed by microbiology.

The medical notes in this case provided no information about the observations which were made in the 24 hours after delivery. Furthermore, antibiotics were not prescribed prior to her transfer to ICU in spite of clinical evidence of intrauterine infection at the time of delivery. There was therefore substandard care in this case.

> A primigravida died from complications of necrotising fasciitis having had a normal pregnancy and delivery. She presented with a swollen left leg eight days after delivery and her GP arranged for immediate transfer to hospital. A provisional diagnosis of ileo-femoral thrombosis was made but her general condition rapidly deteriorated with extensive necrosis of the tissues extending from the vulva to the knee, confirming a diagnosis of necrotising fasciitis. Intensive antibiotic therapy and incision of the fascial planes of the leg were undertaken without maintained improvement. She subsequently had hyperbaric oxygen therapy, a hysterectomy to remove the focus of the infection and extensive debridement of the necrosed tissues. Her condition continued to deteriorate and she died 28 days post-partum. Histology of the excised uterus showed extensive haemorrhagic infarction and this was the presumed source of the infection. The organism identified from several tissues was Group A haemolytic streptococcus.

Necrotising fasciitis is extremely rare but similar cases in association with pregnancy have been reported in the last three triennial Reports.

> A parous woman had an uneventful pregnancy until 34 weeks' gestation when she was admitted 24 hours after spontaneous rupture of membranes. Labour was induced with prostaglandin pessaries a further 24 hours after admission and she had an uncomplicated assisted breech delivery of a live infant. She was discharged home a day later. On the third day post-partum she complained of some abdominal pain at home and was seen by her GP and midwife who were satisfied with her condition. The following morning she was found dead at home. An autopsy examination confirmed inflammation of the uterine cavity with Group B ß-haemolytic streptococcus. It was concluded that her death was due to septic shock.

A possible risk factor in this case was the delay between rupture of the membranes and delivery, but this was no longer than 48 hours. She developed lower abdominal pain without obvious evidence of infection, followed by sudden collapse and death. There was no element of substandard care in this case.

A young parous woman had a planned home confinement with an uncomplicated labour and delivery at 39 weeks' gestation supervised by a midwife. Postnatal observations were satisfactory for four days. She then had an isolated episode of severe diarrhoea for which she received treatment after a phone contact with a locum GP. She was seen by the midwife the next day and on examination her temperature was 40°C and the pulse rate was 140/min. The lochia were normal and not offensive and there was no abdominal tenderness. The midwife contacted the GP, who attended the patient and after an examination he considered her condition satisfactory. However, he failed to record her temperature. When the midwife revisited the patient later the same day her temperature and pulse remained elevated. The next morning the patient's husband called an ambulance as her condition had suddenly deteriorated. She died soon afterwards. An autopsy confirmed that she had died from Group A haemolytic streptococcal septicaemia.

This case emphasises the serious nature of post-partum infection, which can be insidious and can rapidly progress to fatal septicaemia. Although the midwife alerted the GP to the pyrexia it was not fully investigated nor was appropriate action taken with antibiotic treatment and transfer to hospital. This case represents substandard care.

A primigravida had an uneventful pregnancy with spontaneous onset of labour at 39 weeks' gestation and delivery by ventouse extraction. She was discharged well, four days post-partum. Two weeks later she was admitted to the Accident & Emergency Department with a 24-hour history of diarrhoea and vomiting. She was extremely shocked and had a cardiac arrest shortly after arrival at the hospital. She was successfully resuscitated and transferred to the ICU. She then developed marked abdominal distension with rigidity. A laparotomy was performed to exclude perforation of an abdominal viscus. At operation there were two litres of peritoneal fluid and an extremely bulky uterus. A sub-total hysterectomy was performed. Despite intensive therapy her condition did not improve and she died two weeks post-partum.

An autopsy showed evidence of terminal multi-organ failure. On histological examination there were no residual products of conception or intrauterine infection. It was assumed that the diagnosis was toxic shock syndrome but no organism was isolated from various cultures.

A parous woman with a history of premature labour and recurrent abortions was admitted to hospital at 23 weeks' gestation because of suspected spontaneous rupture of the membranes. She had a history of chorioamnionitis in a previous pregnancy. A cervical suture had been inserted in the first trimester of the present pregnancy and she had repeated vaginal infections treated by courses of antibiotics. The day after admission there was obvious evidence of ruptured membranes. Some six hours later she was pyrexial with clinical signs of systemic infection. The cervical suture was removed, with the release of pus from the uterine cavity. At this stage antibiotics were commenced. Her condition rapidly deteriorated and she was transferred to the ICU, where she died three hours later after a cardiac arrest. A vaginal swab taken on admission but not reported until three days after her death showed a heavy growth of *Escherichia coli*. An autopsy was not performed.

This patient had an overwhelming infection which progressed rapidly after the first clinical signs of the condition. In view of her past history antibiotic treatment should have been initiated at an earlier stage. There was no attempt to obtain an urgent report from the microbiology laboratory.

A primigravida had an uneventful pregnancy until 37 weeks' gestation when she was admitted to hospital with vomiting, pyrexia and a pulse rate of 136/min. There was no obvious source of infection and she was said to have a flu-like illness. Some six hours later she complained of lower abdominal pain and was transferred to the labour ward in established labour. Within two hours she developed peripheral cyanosis and shock, and fetal death *in utero* was confirmed by ultrasound scan. She was started on antibiotics and transferred to the ICU where she rapidly developed DIC. She had a forceps delivery without excessive haemorrhage, but her condition deteriorated and she died less than 18 hours after her initial admission.

A blood sample taken before delivery grew Group A ß-haemolytic streptococci. An autopsy examination provided no evidence of any other cause of death apart from septicaemia. The origin of the infection was not determined. There was no significant inflammation within the lungs or the uterine cavity.

A young multiparous woman was booked for confinement in a GP unit. She had an uneventful pregnancy, spontaneous onset of labour at 42 weeks' gestation and a normal delivery of a healthy infant following a short labour. She was discharged home 24 hours post-partum. Some seven days later she complained of feeling unwell and lost her appetite. She was again seen by her GP on the 18th day post-partum with a flu-like illness and had developed a rash. The next day her condition had deteriorated and she was admitted to an ICU with pulmonary oedema. In spite of artificial ventilation and antibiotics her condition deteriorated and she died several days later. Vaginal swabs grew Group A haemolytic streptococcus and the autopsy confirmed that death was due to septic shock.

One further case of overwhelming sepsis following a normal delivery was reported but no further details could be obtained. It is included in the figures.

Sepsis after surgery

Three women died after surgery:

A primigravida had an uneventful pregnancy and was admitted in spontaneous labour at 38 weeks' gestation. She was delivered by ventouse extraction because of fetal distress in the late second stage of labour. The immediate postnatal period was uneventful but on the second day after delivery she complained of abdominal pain. She was apyrexial but her pulse was 100/min. On the following day she remained apyrexial but complained of increasing abdominal pain. The episiotomy scar was reddened and lochia were offensive. A vaginal swab revealed a strong growth of ß-haemolytic streptococci. She rapidly developed septic shock and a total abdominal hysterectomy and vulval debridement were performed. In spite of intensive therapy including hyperbaric oxygen her condition slowly deteriorated with multiple organ failure. She died six weeks after delivery.

This case again illustrates the rapidity and seriousness of postnatal infection. The complaint of abdominal pain was assumed to be after-pains and the rapid pulse rate in the absence of pyrexia was not recognised as significant. There was therefore some delay in commencing appropriate antibiotic therapy.

> A primigravida was to have an elective caesarean section because of previous uterine surgery. She was admitted to hospital in spontaneous labour at 37 weeks' gestation and had an uncomplicated caesarean section without antibiotic cover. She was discharged on the fourth day post-partum but re-admitted three days later with a wound infection. This was treated with antibiotics and she was discharged after a few days. Four days later she was again re-admitted with abdominal pain and pyrexia and an ultrasound scan showed an intra-abdominal abscess. A laparotomy was performed and the abscess was drained. Her condition did not improve and she was found to have further abscess formation. Unsuccessful attempts were made to drain this by needle aspiration. A further laparotomy was performed, the abscess was drained and a sub-total hysterectomy was performed. She developed a post-operative haemorrhage and had a further laparotomy and splenectomy. In spite of intensive therapy her condition continued to deteriorate and she died several weeks later.

At autopsy there was massive liver necrosis. Both coliforms and streptococci were cultured from various sites. Prophylactic antibiotics would have been appropriate at the time of caesarean section. The attempt to drain the recurrent abscess by aspiration was inappropriate and as a result there was a delay in undertaking the repeat laparotomy.

> A young primigravida concealed her pregnancy until 37 weeks' gestation when she booked for hospital confinement. The progress of her pregnancy at that stage was satisfactory. She was admitted to hospital the following day in an agitated state complaining of backache and uterine contractions; her pulse rate was 140/min and an ultrasound scan confirmed fetal death. Some five hours later she had a mottled appearance and her temperature was 38.1° C. A blood test taken on admission was then reported as profound thrombocytopenia. Medical induction of labour was commenced but her condition deteriorated with a clinical diagnosis of severe DIC. She received intensive supportive therapy and a caesarean section was performed with delivery of a fresh stillbirth. Her condition continued to deteriorate and she died 15 hours after her admission to hospital. At autopsy there was no evidence of amniotic fluid embolism or placental abruption but group B streptococcus was cultured from an intrauterine swab. It was concluded that death was due to fulminating septicaemia.

The serious nature of this patient's condition was not recognised on admission. There was a delay in analysing the blood to confirm the diagnosis of severe thrombocytopaenia. In the face of her rapidly deteriorating condition induction of labour in this primigravid woman was unlikely to produce an improvement in the time scale necessary and an earlier caesarean section would have been more appropriate. It was a difficult diagnostic problem but on balance, there was a degree of substandard care.

Deaths counted in other Chapters

Two further cases of genital sepsis associated with early pregnancy are counted and discussed in Chapter 6. Neither was associated with substandard care:

> A young parous woman was seen by her GP at eight weeks' gestation with vaginal bleeding. On examination, the cervix was found to be 3 cm dilated and he assumed she had had a spontaneous abortion. A subsequent ultrasound scan, however, confirmed a normal intrauterine pregnancy. During the next 10 weeks she had intermittent episodes of vaginal bleeding but repeat ultrasound scans again confirmed normal progress of the pregnancy. At 19 weeks' gestation she was admitted to hospital with jaundice, further vaginal bleeding and uterine contractions. She delivered a macerated fetus and in view of a purulent vaginal discharge was started on intravenous antibiotics. Six hours later she underwent an evacuation of a retained placenta under general anaesthesia. Within 24 hours she developed DIC and severe shock and had a cardiac arrest which failed to respond to resuscitation. An autopsy confirmed that she had died from *E. coli* septicaemia of genital tract origin.

> A parous woman was admitted with an incomplete miscarriage at 10 weeks' gestation. She was tachycardic and hypotensive but her condition improved after evacuation of the uterus. She was readmitted a few days later with signs of septic shock. Despite all attempts at treatment, including antibiotics and hysterectomy to remove the source of infection, she died. The organism was not identified.

There was one *Direct Late* death counted in Chapter 14 but described here:

> A parous woman who had a completely normal pregnancy, delivery and puerperium was admitted to hospital six weeks post-partum with flu-like symptoms and a purpuric rash. Nothing abnormal was found on examination of the genital tract. Blood cultures grew Group A haemolytic streptococcus and appropriate antibiotic and supportive therapy was instituted. She fairly rapidly developed shock, DIC and multiple organ failure and died four days later despite intensive therapy. At autopsy a small amount of pus was expressed from the fallopian tubes and it was therefore assumed that the origin of the infection was the genital tract.

Comments

These cases demonstrate, once more, that infection must never be underestimated and that it continues to be an important cause of maternal mortality. The onset of infection, particularly after spontaneous rupture of the membranes, can be insidious and can rapidly progress to a fulminating septicaemia.

Puerperal sepsis is not a disease of the past, and GPs and midwives must be aware of the signs and be prepared to institute immediate treatment and referral of any recently delivered woman with a fever and/or offensive vaginal discharge.

As noted in the previous Report, **there is clear evidence from controlled trials showing the benefit of prophylactic antibiotics for caesarean section.** The Cochrane database [1] states:

> "Antibiotic prophylaxis markedly reduces the risk of serious postoperative infection, such as pelvic abscess, septic shock and septic pelvic vein thrombophlebitis. A protective effect of the same order of magnitude is seen for endometritis. The degree of reduction in risk of wound infection is somewhat less, but is still substantial. The evidence for these benefits is overwhelming."

When infection develops and the patient is systemically ill, urgent and repeated bacteriological specimens, including blood cultures, must be obtained. The advice of a microbiologist must be sought at an early stage to assist with the use of appropriate antibiotic therapy. In serious cases doctors should be prepared to give parenteral antibiotics before the diagnosis can be confirmed.

Clinicians must remain vigilant for early signs of invasive streptococcal disease. The signs of necrotising fasciitis are high fever plus swelling and marked tenderness localised to a muscle mass. Early treatment with antibiotics still seems to be the best way to prevent death.

There have been several recent reports [2] suggesting an increase in the number of cases of serious invasive streptococcal infections, with and without shock, suggesting spread of a more virulent clone. The course of these infections is dramatically rapid, as reflected in the cases reported here.

References

1.   Enkin, M., Keirse, M.J.N.C., Renfrew, M. & Neilson, J. *A Guide to Effective Care in Pregnancy and Childbirth* 2nd Edn. Oxford: OUP, 1995; 322-7.

2.   Holm, S.E. Invasive Group A streptococcal infections. *New England Journal of Medicine* 1996; **335**: 590-1.

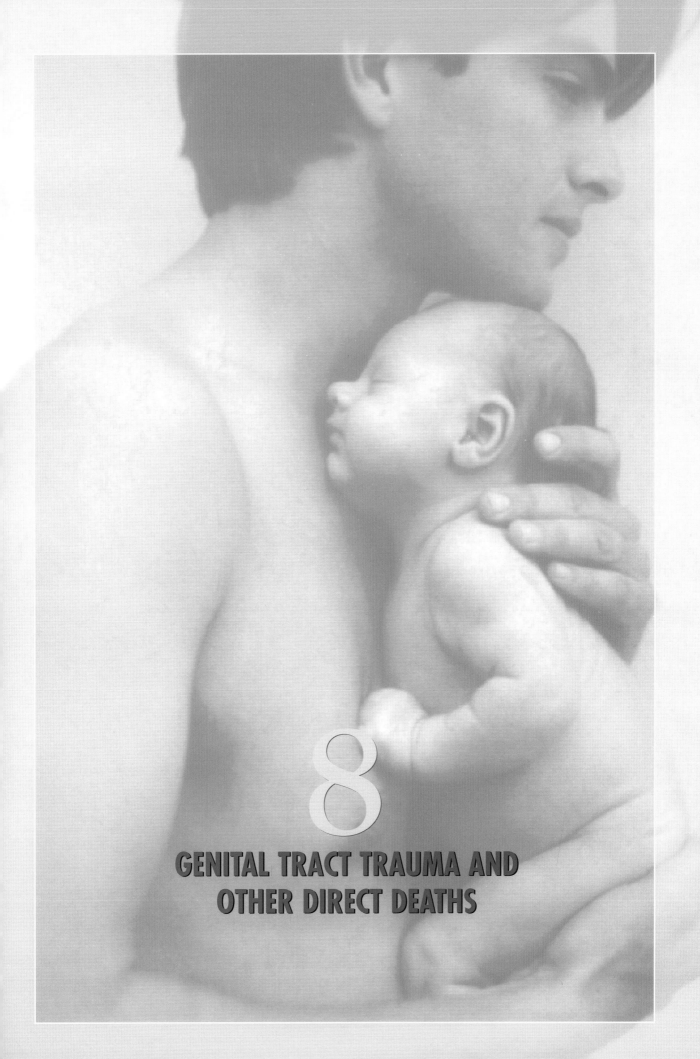

8
GENITAL TRACT TRAUMA AND OTHER DIRECT DEATHS

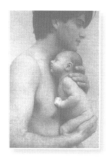

CHAPTER 8
GENITAL TRACT TRAUMA AND OTHER DIRECT DEATHS

Summary

There were seven deaths due to other *Direct* causes in this triennium compared with four in the previous Report. Five were due to uterine rupture, and two to fatty liver of pregnancy. A further case of uterine perforation occurred in association with termination of pregnancy and is discussed and counted in Chapter 6.

The overall maternal mortality rate was 3.2 per million maternities. The rate for uterine rupture was 2.3 per million maternities compared to 1.7 and 1.3 in the two previous Reports. It should be noted that due to the very small number of deaths from such trauma, it is not possible to draw any statistical inferences from these figures. The rates for "other *Direct* deaths" have fallen from 5.9 and 4.3 per million maternities in the two previous Reports, to 0.9 for the period of this Report.

Uterine rupture: key recommendations

Care is required in using prostaglandins for induction of labour because of the risk of hyperstimulation and uterine rupture. Recommendations from the CESDI 5th Annual Report[1] are endorsed and reproduced here:

Women with a previous uterine scar require:

- antenatal management including plans for delivery and induction involving a documented discussion with an experienced obstetrician,

- attentive intrapartum fetal and maternal surveillance in a setting where the baby can be delivered within 30 minutes,

- involvement of an experienced obstetrician in intrapartum management,

- no more than one dose of prostaglandin unless great vigilance is exercised, and

- information about relevant symptoms to be reported to those caring for them in labour.

Genital tract trauma

As in previous Reports, this section is concerned with maternal deaths directly due to genital tract trauma including vaginal, cervical and uterine lacerations, other than those following termination of pregnancy, which are discussed in Chapter 6 (early pregnancy deaths). One early pregnancy death, however, from spontaneous uterine rupture at 17 weeks' gestation, is counted and discussed in this Chapter. There was evidence of substandard care in two of these cases.

Spontaneous uterine rupture

There were four such cases:

> A multiparous women in her thirties was booked for confinement in a consultant unit. She had a previous elective caesarean section for a breech presentation because of her short stature. She had indicated her desire to have a vaginal delivery on this occasion. The pregnancy was uneventful until 37 weeks' gestation, when she developed mild pre-eclampsia and was admitted to hospital for bed rest. Three days later she felt unwell because of a headache and the obstetric registrar decided that she should be delivered. The fetal head was not engaged and the cervix was partially effaced. In the antenatal ward she had a 3-mg prostaglandin pessary inserted. As no uterine contractions occurred another 3-mg prostaglandin pessary was administered some seven hours later. Two hours after this she developed hypertonic uterine contractions and felt unwell with diarrhoea and vomiting. She was then transferred to the labour ward and reported tenderness over the caesarean section scar. The CTG showed baseline tachycardia and late decelerations. The contractions remained frequent and a vaginal examination showed no change in the cervix, with the presenting part unengaged. One hour later an epidural was sited but shortly after this she collapsed and had a cardiac arrest. Following resuscitation a caesarean section was performed and uterine rupture due to scar dehiscence was confirmed. No liquor was found and the fetus was dead. Postoperatively the patient was transferred to an Intensive Care Unit (ICU) when she developed severe haemorrhage from disseminated intravascular coagulation (DIC). Some six hours later, in spite of massive transfusion, she had a further, terminal, cardiac arrest. An autopsy examination confirmed that she had an amniotic fluid embolism.

The care of this case was considered substandard for several reasons. The decision to induce labour was probably unnecessary and should have been referred to the consultant. Induction of labour in this high-risk case should have taken place in the labour ward and not the antenatal ward. The dose of prostaglandin was high for a patient with a previous caesarean section and was probably responsible for the hypertonic contractions. In spite of evidence of fetal distress, uterine hypertonicity and no progress, the labour was allowed to continue. This decision may have been influenced by the patient's desire for a vaginal delivery. There was insufficient consultant supervision of this case, both regarding the decision to induce labour and its supervision.

> A parous woman, booked for confinement in a consultant unit, had an ultrasound scan at 16 weeks' gestation which suggested that there was an abnormality of the umbilical cord. It was considered insignificant and the pregnancy progressed normally until 36 weeks' gestation when

a repeat ultrasound scan showed nuchal oedema and duodenal atresia. A fetal blood sample was obtained and chromosome analysis confirmed the presence of Trisomy 13. When she re-attended the antenatal clinic two weeks later she complained that there were no fetal movements, and an ultrasound scan confirmed that intrauterine death had occurred. Labour was induced with prostaglandin pessaries but at 7cm dilatation the patient collapsed with vaginal bleeding. A laparotomy was performed which confirmed an anterior rupture of the uterus extending into the broad ligament. A hysterectomy was performed. There was massive haemorrhage due to DIC, and this was controlled by packs. She was transferred to an ICU but developed anuria and severe cerebral oedema. Her condition slowly deteriorated and she died from a cardiac arrest some days later.

A woman with a previous obstetric history of one normal delivery and several spontaneous miscarriages was seen for routine booking at 16 weeks' gestation. An ultrasound scan confirmed a single fetus and a normally sited placenta. One week later she developed severe abdominal pain and was attended by her GP, who diagnosed enteritis. Following a painful restless night with vomiting she was again seen by her doctor, who continued treatment for enteritis. Some four hours later her condition worsened rapidly. Her husband called the doctor, who arrived without delay, but by then she had died. At autopsy the abdominal cavity contained more than two litres of blood from a ruptured uterus. Histology confirmed a placenta percreta with total loss of full thickness myometrium over a large area around the site of uterine rupture.

Placenta percreta is a rare and dangerous complication of pregnancy. The GP did not establish the diagnosis but in the circumstances cannot be criticised, though an earlier transfer to hospital may have altered the outcome.

A primigravida was admitted to hospital at 38 weeks' gestation with a short history of epigastric pain. Her general condition was satisfactory and she had intermittent uterine contractions. It was assumed that she was in early labour and she was transferred to the labour ward for observation. Some seven hours later the epigastric pain became severe and she collapsed with hypovolaemic shock. Because of the severe peripheral vascular shutdown there was a delay of 50 minutes in achieving intravenous access even though senior medical staff were in attendance. There was a further delay in giving blood as the patient's religious beliefs did not permit blood transfusion and family consent to transfusion was being sought. A laparotomy was performed and she was found to have a massive haemoperitoneum from a large rupture in the left lateral wall of the uterus extending from the cervix to the fundus. The patient died during the operation. Histological examination of the uterine wall adjacent to the site of rupture showed that the myometrial thickness was only 1.5 mm and there was marked fibrous tissue mixed with the smooth muscle. The placenta was normally sited well clear of the rupture site and was not morbidly adherent. There was no past history of uterine surgery or evidence that this woman was in established labour at the time of uterine rupture.

Spontaneous rupture of an unscarred uterus in a woman who is not in established labour is an extremely rare complication. The patient was moribund from the time the medical team arrived and was unable to consent to treatment. In these circumstances, if she had not already made an advance directive stipulating she did not wish to receive blood products, then a doctor could lawfully carry out any treatment which he or she considered to be in the patient's best interests. It is also worrying that her care was delayed while "consent" was sought from her family, as no-one can lawfully give or withhold consent to treatment in respect of another adult, but earlier transfusion may not have made any difference.

REPORT ON CONFIDENTIAL ENQUIRIES INTO MATERNAL DEATHS IN THE UNITED KINGDOM

Traumatic uterine rupture

> A young primigravida had an uneventful pregnancy until 41 weeks' gestation, when she was admitted to a consultant unit for induction of labour. She had a failed forceps for fetal distress in the second stage of labour and proceeded to caesarean section with delivery of a live infant. This was performed by a registrar. There was significant vaginal bleeding in the immediate post-operative period and a laparotomy was performed to repair extensive lacerations of the bladder and vagina. During the operation she had a cardiac arrest. She was resuscitated but subsequently developed DIC and ARDS. She was transferred to an ICU but, in spite of intensive treatment, her condition deteriorated and she died two weeks later.

In this case there was limited information on which to make an assessment of the quality of care. The experience and skills of the registrar were not known, but it seems clear the attempted forceps delivery or subsequent operation were not performed to a satisfactory standard.

Comments

These cases emphasise the need for care in the use of prostaglandin for induction of labour because of the risk of hyperstimulation and uterine rupture. Although the British National Formulary identifies a previous caesarean section as a contraindication to the use of prostaglandins it is commonly used to induce labour in patients who have had this operation. Attention is drawn to the CESDI 5th Annual Report[1], which includes recommendations for practice with regard to induction of labour in women with a uterine scar. These are as follows:

Women with a uterine scar require:

- antenatal management including plans for delivery and induction involving a documented discussion with an experienced obstetrician (ideally a consultant but at least an SPR4 or higher),

- attentive intrapartum fetal and maternal surveillance in a setting where the baby can be delivered within 30 minutes,

- involvement of an obstetrician experienced in intrapartum management,

- no more than one dose of prostaglandin unless great vigilance is exercised, and

- information about relevant symptoms to be reported to those caring for them in labour.

These cases also reinforce the need for a team approach to the management of severe obstetric haemorrhage. All obstetric units should have a written protocol for this emergency and staff should be aware of contingency plans to cope with sudden unexpected haemorrhage. In two cases reported here junior staff assumed, or were given, too much responsibility in dealing with high-risk cases.

Other *Direct* causes of death: hepatic necrosis

There were two deaths in this triennium due to liver necrosis. In neither case was care considered to be substandard:

> A primigravida was admitted at 34 weeks' gestation complaining of epigastric pain. Investigation showed elevated liver enzymes but normal blood pressure and no proteinuria. Her symptoms worsened and the liver enzymes rapidly increased, necessitating delivery of the fetus by caesarean section one week after admission. She was transferred to a specialist liver unit but her condition deteriorated and she died a week later. Post-mortem confirmed acute fatty liver of pregnancy.

This condition, although rare, must rapidly be differentiated from the epigastric pain and mild, by comparison, alterations of liver enzymes seen in some patients with pre-eclampsia or in HELLP syndrome. Early delivery may sometimes reverse the progress although in some instances the only prospects of survival are following liver transplantation.

> The second woman had a history of alcohol abuse. She was admitted at 33 weeks' gestation with a poor appetite and weight loss. She rapidly became jaundiced, CTGs showed fetal distress and an emergency caesarean section was arranged. She collapsed during induction of anaesthesia and despite transfer to intensive care, never recovered consciousness and died a week later. Autopsy showed an almost complete necrosis of the liver.

This unusual case was one of liver failure rapidly progressing in a patient with known alcohol abuse but not the classical history of someone with cirrhosis. The contribution of added liver degeneration in pregnancy seems likely but the advanced stage of liver necrosis at post-mortem did not allow the specific diagnosis of acute fatty liver of pregnancy to be made.

Reference

1.   *Confidential Enquiry into Stillbirths and Deaths in Infancy*; 5th Annual Report. The Maternal and Child Health Research Consortium. London; July 1998. ISBN 0 9533536 0 5

9
DEATHS ASSOCIATED WITH ANAESTHESIA

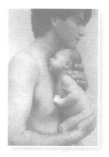

CHAPTER 9
DEATHS ASSOCIATED WITH ANAESTHESIA

Summary

Despite the increase in reported maternal deaths for this triennium, there is only one death directly attributable to anaesthesia, compared to eight in the previous Report. Figures for the previous three triennia are shown in Table 9.1. This is a considerable improvement on the last Report and a tribute to those responsible for provision of obstetric anaesthetic services.

The remainder of the deaths discussed in this Chapter are those in which the death was either associated with substandard anaesthetic care, or where the standard of anaesthetic care was satisfactory but the case may prove useful for trainee anaesthetists. As in the previous Report the cases are reported in some detail to allow evaluation of the problems encountered and assessment of how facilities could be improved.

In those cases associated with substandard care the key factors were:

- failure of communication and wise decision making,
- lack of consultant availability,
- failure of trainee doctors to recognise severity of illness,
- delay in providing adequate resuscitation,
- delay in obtaining blood products,
- delay or inadequate access to intensive and high dependency facilities when the obstetric unit is some distance from the main hospital, and
- split site working. This contributes to slow laboratory input, and slow access to medical staff and other emergency facilities.

Table 9.1

	Number of deaths directly associated with anaesthesia	Rate per million maternities	% of Direct maternal deaths
1985-87	6	2.6	4.3
1988-90	4	1.7	2.7
1991-93	8	3.5	6.5
1994-96	1	0.5	0.8

Deaths directly associated with anaesthesia (excluding *Indirect* and *Late* deaths), rate per million maternities and percentage of *Direct* maternal deaths; United Kingdom 1985-96

Death directly attributable to anaesthesia

Death associated with combined spinal/epidural anaesthesia

A woman of short stature was due to undergo an elective planned caesarean section as she was thought to have a big baby and had had a previous caesarean section for failure to progress in labour. The anaesthetist made several attempts to administer combined spinal and epidural anaesthesia. This consisted of spinal injection of 2.25 ml heavy bupivacaine, 125 μg alfentanil and 150 μg clonidine and 15 ml 0.375% bupivacaine into the epidural space. Shortly afterwards she complained of headache, shooting pains down her legs and difficulty with breathing. It was thought that the spinal injection might have been sited a little high so oxygen was given. Her blood pressure fell despite 2.5 L fluid and ephedrine, and oxygen saturation deteriorated despite her breathing 100% oxygen. She complained of tightness in her chest and increasing difficulty with breathing and a decision was taken to intubate and ventilate her. She then developed florid pulmonary oedema. It was decided that she should be transferred to a larger hospital for ventilation. Diuretics and glyceryl trinitrate were given, IV fluids were stopped, central and arterial lines were inserted and adrenaline was given with midazolam and ketamine for sedation. Whilst waiting for the ambulance she deteriorated and had a cardiac arrest. She was given adrenaline and isoprenaline and external cardiac pacing but could not be resuscitated.

The anaesthetic technique used was not common. Excessive doses of spinal anaesthetic were used and, coupled with a large volume of local anaesthetic injected into the epidural at the same time, led to hypotension due to extensive sympathetic block. The use of clonidine, which is still controversial, would worsen hypotension, especially at a high dose. Probably an epidural anaesthetic was not needed at all for the caesarean section. Her resuscitation was not conventional, particularly in relation to use of isoprenaline. The administration of 2.5 L of IV fluids probably did not have an adverse effect in this case. Care was clearly substandard.

Deaths associated with anaesthesia

In many cases in this Report the patient was anaesthetised without incident and these have not been included in this Chapter. However, there were 20 deaths in which anaesthesia was associated with the death, although only 12 involved substandard care.

Pulmonary hypertension and cardiac failure

There are five cases with pulmonary hypertension counted in Chapter 11. Anaesthetic care could be regarded as substandard in the first four of the following descriptions.

> The first woman had pulmonary hypertension, cor pulmonale and systemic lupus erythematosus. Caesarean section was performed by two consultant anaesthetists after which she was transferred to the intensive care unit (ICU) for monitoring, where her condition was stable. Oozing was noted from the wound and she returned to the delivery suite next day for exploration of a wound haematoma. She died on the operating table after collapsing during intubation and could not be resuscitated. Attempts were stopped after 50 minutes.

For her caesarean section she appears to have had routine general anaesthesia. Anticoagulation precluded a regional technique. She had full monitoring with a pulmonary artery (PA) catheter and received inhaled nitric oxide, which was without effect on her PA pressure. The consultant anaesthetist involved with the second operation had been present at the caesarean section and sought advice regarding the level of monitoring which would have been appropriate. As the patient was stable, a joint decision was made not to insert another PA catheter as nothing further could be done to modify PA pressures. However, this might have provided evidence of hypovolaemia if the PA occlusion pressure had been low.

There were small, but probably crucial, differences between the two anaesthetics. Quite a large dose of thiopentone was given for the second operation with a larger (2 mg instead of 1 mg) dose of alfentanil. No suxamethonium was given and a larger dose of atracurium (50 not 25 mg). On the first occasion the atracurium was given about the time of the skin incision so that the combination of surgery and a light anaesthetic might tend to counteract the peripheral vasodilatation and fall in systemic pressure, whereas on the second occasion there was a greater fall in blood pressure, reducing preload and cardiac output, with resultant hypoxia and worsening pulmonary hypertension.

The intravascular volume was probably depleted in view of the falling haemoglobin level and relatively low central venous pressure at the start of the second procedure, so a small change in technique might have resulted in a disastrous outcome in a patient with such severe underlying cardiac disease. Use of etomidate rather than thiopentone and vecuronium rather than atracurium might have been better, although the claimed advantage of etomidate is controversial.

> The second woman presented with cardiac failure at 14 weeks' gestation. A therapeutic termination of pregnancy was agreed, but there was inadequate cardiological assessment before surgery even though this was not an emergency procedure. During the course of the general anaesthetic her blood pressure fell despite intravenous fluids and adrenaline.

Her condition had not been optimal preoperatively and more aggressive treatment of her cardiac failure may have improved the outcome. Invasive monitoring may also have helped to optimise right ventricular filling pressure.

> The third woman was known to have pulmonary hypertension and requested a termination of pregnancy for medical reasons. She had a general anaesthetic but no anticoagulation was prescribed because the risk of bleeding was thought to exceed that of thromboembolic complications. She was readmitted as an emergency some days later when thromboembolism was diagnosed, and heparin was commenced. The next day she had a cardiac arrest and resuscitation was unsuccessful.

Part of the responsibility for ensuring long-term anticoagulation lies with the anaesthetist.

> In the fourth case of cardiac disease the patient had an emergency caesarean section under epidural anaesthesia for fetal distress. She was known to have cardiac disease but although she had been seen by a consultant anaesthetist in the antenatal period she was managed by trainees, despite requiring some high dependency care. She required readmission with progressive cardiac failure after delivery and died.

In this case communication between specialties was poor at a time when interventions might have helped.

> In one other case the woman had progressed rapidly to severe right ventricular failure. She was treated with nifedipine and warfarin and was awaiting heart-lung transplantation. When she became pregnant, termination by hysterotomy was advised. Her general anaesthesia was complicated by hypotension and hypoxia and these were treated by increased intravenous fluids, invasive monitoring and inotropic drugs, with little effect. She had a pulmonary artery catheter inserted in the ICU which showed the pulmonary pressures (90/50 mmHg) to be almost equal to systemic pressures (90/55 mmHg). Prostacyclin, glyceryl trinitrate and adrenaline produced no improvement and pulmonary vascular resistance increased until she had a cardiac arrest and could not be resuscitated.

Earlier PA catheterisation might have been valuable but in view of the lack of response to pulmonary vasodilators, the risk of endocarditis and the need for infection avoidance at that time, the decision was probably justifiable.

Amniotic fluid embolism

Five deaths from amniotic fluid embolism (AFE), counted in Chapter 5, will also be discussed here. Anaesthetic care was substandard in the first two:

> The first woman had a painful labour, and an epidural was requested after which fetal heart (FH) deceleration occurred. She was taken to the labour ward for a trial of forceps. She eventually had a caesarean section for which general anaesthesia was felt to be more appropriate to avoid further maternal distress. Anaesthesia was given by an Associate Specialist although a consultant was called when her blood pressure fell and DIC became apparent. Because of continued uncontrolled

bleeding the patient proceeded to hysterectomy when four units of blood, one litre of colloid and one litre of crystalloid were infused. A very severe contraction had occurred immediately before the insertion of the epidural and it seems likely that AFE occurred at that stage. A large dose (10 ml of 0.5%) of bupivacaine had been given for the epidural analgesia, which was likely to have produced hypotension. There is no record of attempts to control the pH of gastric contents or their volume. Only 500 ml of Hartmann's had been given by the time the consultant arrived and no attempts were made to give ergometrine or syntocinon. CVP access was not obtained until at least an hour later, there was no recorded blood pressure for 15 minutes and another 50 minutes passed before dopamine was started. There is no record of any urine output nor a record of blood loss. After delivery she was transferred, sedated, to the ICU where she died shortly after admission.

There was substandard care because of slow blood replacement, failure to reduce gastric acidity, failure to give oxytocic agents and a delay in starting inotropes. These factors are partly responsible, together with substandard obstetric care, for the fatal outcome. There was insufficient monitoring and lack of staff in the labour ward, and lack of consultant involvement so the severity of illness was not recognised.

The second woman had complex obstetric and medical problems and underwent caesarean section for fetal distress, during which she had a cardiac arrest and was initially resuscitated, dying an hour later in the ICU. The anaesthetic was administered by an SHO but was straightforward and incidental to the death, which was shown to be due to AFE by the presence of fetal squames in the pulmonary arteries.

There was lack of communication between departments and more senior anaesthetic help should have been provided.

In the third case the woman required anaesthesia for a caesarean section for fetal distress. She was well at induction but collapsed within minutes with asystole. The SHO anaesthetist had two and a half years' experience. There had been a small haemoptysis prior to induction and it was difficult to assess oxygenation, with the oximeter unable to detect SpO_2 because of movement artefact. Rapid sequence induction was used and she was attached to the capnograph but no trace was obtained. The ECG showed sinus tachycardia at 160/min and there was good air entry into both lungs. There was no bleeding at incision and no carotid pulse so ECM and 100% O_2 were started and emergency drugs were given with consultant anaesthetists now present. A diagnosis of pulmonary embolus (most likely with amniotic fluid) was made but despite resuscitation there was no response and the patient was declared dead one hour later.

Rather a large dose of thiopentone was given but this was immaterial to the outcome and there can be no criticism of the anaesthetic.

The fourth woman was an obese, asthmatic smoker who, after a previous caesarean section, had to be admitted to an ICU for aspiration pneumonia. She was noted to have polyhydramnios and elective delivery by a repeat caesarean was agreed. General anaesthesia was chosen because of her previous anaesthetic experiences and difficulty with lying flat. She suddenly collapsed after the delivery of the baby and failed to respond to resuscitation. DIC and EMD occurred and a clinical diagnosis of amniotic fluid embolus was made. She died on the labour ward two hours after delivery.

There is no evidence of substandard care. In fact thorough perioperative preparation and good anaesthetic techniques were used and recorded.

> The fifth woman had a general anaesthetic for emergency caesarean section for fetal distress. Three hours later she collapsed with a convulsion, severe DIC and hypotension. AFE was the most likely clinical diagnosis. She received blood products and was transferred to an ICU in another hospital where she spent several days with progressive multiple organ failure before she died.

There was no evidence of substandard care.

Eclampsia/pregnancy-induced hypertension

There were two deaths from eclampsia counted and discussed in Chapter 3. Substandard anaesthetic care was associated with the first:

> The first woman died two days after delivery with fulminant hepatic failure consequent on severe pregnancy-induced hypertension. She initially had an emergency caesarean section performed by the obstetric registrar for fulminating pre-eclampsia. General anaesthesia was given by an anaesthetic registrar and was unremarkable, but a rather large dose of thiopentone was used, presumably because her blood pressure was so high at induction (190/110 mmHg). Magnesium infusion was continued according to the protocol. She was transferred to a high dependency area in the labour ward but was only transferred to the ICU 16-20 hours later because of oliguria and a low platelet count diagnosed as HELLP syndrome. Her condition required transfer to a Liver Unit, where she died five days after delivery.

Care was substandard in so far as there was lack of expert consultant planning of her care when she was seriously ill and the severity of her condition was underestimated. There is no criticism of the anaesthetic registrar.

> The second woman was admitted unconscious to an Accident and Emergency (A&E) Department with sluggish pupillary reactions having been normotensive 11 days previously at an ante natal clinic visit. She had proteinuria and a blood pressure of 160/115 mmHg at admission, was assumed to have had an eclamptic fit and was delivered by caesarean section under general anaesthesia for fetal distress. The anaesthetist was a locum consultant who gave a routine general anaesthetic with the exception of neither giving antacids nor inserting a nasogastric tube, but there is no accompanying anaesthetic record. A subsequent CT scan showed a large inoperable intracerebral haematoma. She was managed on the ICU appropriately for two days but without improvement until brain stem death was diagnosed.

There is no record of her care on the ICU but it was unlikely to have affected the outcome.

Haemorrhage

Four deaths due to haemorrhage, counted in Chapter 4, are also discussed here. The first woman may have benefited from referral to a tertiary centre and in the other three cases there were delays in obtaining blood products:

> The first woman was a substance abuser and overweight. She developed hypertension and a low platelet count. Liver function tests were only minimally deranged but she was admitted to hospital with a diagnosis of HELLP syndrome. She was given steroids and delivered by elective caesarean section, with six litres of blood loss despite platelet transfusion. Both a consultant and a registrar anaesthetist were present, risk factors were identified and there were no administrative problems. The general anaesthetic was unremarkable. She did not recover from the anaesthetic and died two hours after induction. There is lack of documentation on the anaesthetic chart, in particular no evidence that blood was given or that additional intravascular lines were inserted. The case notes record platelet counts of 12 and later $10 \times 10^9 \, l^{-1}$ on the day of death. Apparently a 10-unit blood transfusion was given and hysterectomy was performed.

The patient was delivered in a small district general hospital whereas tertiary referral may have been more appropriate.

> In the second case there had been some bleeding during the woman's labour, which was assessed by the obstetric registrar. An IV line was set up and blood was cross-matched. An epidural was requested at which point her platelets were $118 \times 10^9 \, l^{-1}$. A forceps delivery took place for failure to progress in labour. For this, 10 ml 0.5% plain bupivacaine were given by the anaesthetic SHO. Twelve minutes later she became hypotensive and unresponsive and had a respiratory arrest. The placenta was undelivered and firmly attached. She was intubated and ventilated after transfer to theatre and underwent immediate laparotomy. The on-call consultant obstetrician records that he provided aortic compression whilst the anaesthetist was putting in lines, which took 20 minutes. No free blood was found at laparotomy but there was a very atonic abnormal uterus. The uterus was opened and placenta percreta was found. In view of profuse bleeding, hysterectomy was undertaken and this was straightforward.

> When she collapsed the anaesthetist gave oxygen and the head of the bed was lowered. Assisted ventilation with mask and Ambu bag was provided and colloid resuscitation was started whilst a second 14 g cannula was inserted by the obstetric SHO into the opposite arm. Ephedrine was given and the patient was intubated without any anaesthetic drugs. The patient was ventilated with 100% oxygen, the consultant was called, blood loss was reviewed and transfusion was commenced with four units of blood and then a further 10 units were requested. A CVP line was inserted when the consultant anaesthetist arrived. A clotting screen was requested. The CVP was +7 cm water. A dopamine infusion was set up and adrenaline was given. No peripheral pulses were palpable so no more attempts at arterial cannulation were tried. The SHO phoned the haematology technician to emphasise the urgency of blood requirement (it was on its way). The consultant anaesthetist phoned the consultant haematologist for platelets when FDPs were 4000, Hb 4.3 gdl^{-1} and platelets 33×10^9 l^{-1}. The ICU consultant arrived with femoral lines for arterial cannulation. Platelets arrived nearly two hours later and uncrossmatched blood, cryoprecipitate and further fresh frozen plasma (FFP) were also given but she still had a severe coagulopathy, became more hypotensive and had a cardiac arrest.

The cardiac arrest procedure was correctly carried out. Total measured blood loss was 15.5 litres and fluid administration was charted comprehensively. The anaesthetist comments that the delay in arrival of cross-matched blood, more than one and a half hours, was because the maternity hospital did not have cross-matching facilities so the blood sample was sent to the general hospital three miles away. The need for uncross-matched blood was not understood. Haemorrhagic shock, delayed arrival of blood due to the separate maternity hospital, and communications failure contributed to the fatal outcome. Care was substandard for organisational reasons.

> In the third case, caesarean section was planned for placenta praevia and twin pregnancy. The woman then presented with an ante-partum haemorrhage (APH). She was told she would have a GA and the risk of haemorrhage was explained. She had a straightforward anaesthetic with the consultant anaesthetist present throughout. The anaesthetists record that following delivery of the second twin there was uncontrolled bleeding and hypotension so a second IV line was sited to give blood, gelofusine and blood products to match measured losses.

> There were delays in obtaining blood and products and in obtaining results of clotting studies (two hours). Non-invasive blood pressure measurement became unreliable so an arterial line was inserted but her blood pressure was only 39/19 mmHg and the CVP was -5 cm water. Adrenaline was given. Arterial blood gases showed acidosis, with a poor response to bicarbonate. Adrenaline-soaked packs were used to try to control blood loss and the abdomen was closed but she died shortly afterwards. The total blood loss was 23 litres.

Death was due to profound hypovolaemia from haemorrhage. Cases of placenta praevia need two large bore cannulae in place before starting surgery. There was difficulty communicating between the haematology laboratory and operating theatre. It would have been wise for a consultant obstetrician to have performed the caesarean section with the combination of placenta percreta and DIC, which are very difficult to manage.

> The fourth patient developed eclampsia whilst awaiting ambulance transfer to a regional centre for further care and delivery. She was treated with diazepam and antihypertensive agents. During the journey intrauterine death occurred and on arrival she had severe coagulopathy precluding abdominal delivery. Vaginal delivery was followed by profuse bleeding and an emergency laparotomy was performed under general anaesthesia. Intraperitoneal bleeding could not be controlled so the patient was stabilised with intra-abdominal packing and transferred to ICU where she died. Autopsy showed a ruptured necrotic liver.

Lack of collaboration between hospitals and specialties also occurred in this case.

Sepsis

This case is counted and discussed in Chapter 7.

> After a spontaneous abortion at 17 weeks' gestation the patient complained of a foul smelling vaginal discharge. Appropriate IV antibiotics were started but she was noted to be jaundiced and was transferred to the ICU. She was oliguric with Hb 5.7 g dl^{-1}, and platelets 57 x 10^9 l^{-1}. Her case was discussed with a haematology consultant and she was given four units of FFP and six units of blood. Six hours after the fetus was passed she had suction evacuation of retained products under anaesthesia and was returned to the ICU, where she had a severe DIC and sustained a cardiac arrest. Despite full resuscitation, efforts were abandoned one hour later as she failed to respond.

There seemed to be very little input from any consultants in this patient's care, which was substandard. The anaesthetic chart has no physiological data entered at all. There was lack of awareness of the severity of her illness and great delay in dealing with the DIC.

Phaeochromocytoma

There are two cases which are counted in Chapter 11. Care was considered substandard in the first:

> The first woman complained of headache at 27 weeks' gestation, was found to be hypertensive, and was immediately admitted. Labour was induced for fulminating pre-eclampsia. About two hours later there was acute onset of visual disturbance, and her blood pressure was 210/140 mmHg, with fetal tachycardia. An immediate caesarean section was planned under GA. She was stable throughout and was extubated at the end of the procedure. She was returned, conscious, to the labour ward where she became hypotensive two hours later, had a cardiac arrest and died.

Investigations at the time of admission showed normal urate, liver function tests and platelet count. Hypertension was not controlled preoperatively. Surgery and anaesthesia were carried out by consultants, who considered the diagnosis of phaeochromocytoma and the advantages of transfer to ICU but the decision was that postoperative care would be managed by the obstetric anaesthetic team. She received labetalol for control of blood pressure but she became increasingly hypoxic and acidotic and required reintubation. Minutes later she had an asystolic cardiac arrest and despite conventional resuscitation she failed to respond. Death was confirmed after 30 minutes' resuscitation. In retrospect the patient should have gone immediately to ICU postoperatively for blood pressure control, haemodynamic monitoring and ventilation. To this extent care was substandard. Death was due to pulmonary oedema due to an extra-adrenal phaeochromocytoma found at autopsy.

> The second woman had a caesarean section for failure to progress in labour. The operation was carried out under general anaesthesia as the epidural block did not provide adequate pain relief. She was hypertensive at the time. An extended tear of the uterus was found but haemostasis was secured. During the repair arrhythmias were noted. She failed to wake up after surgery and was transferred to the ICU, where bleeding was still evident. She required further fluid resuscitation and inotropic therapy. She had fixed dilated pupils and died next day. Autopsy revealed no focal intracranial pathology, 2.5 L blood in the peritoneal cavity and a phaeochromocytoma.

Mitral valve disease

> A patient discussed in Chapter 11 had mitral valve disease with pulmonary hypertension and became pregnant although the risks to her health had been discussed with her by consultants in both cardiology and obstetrics. She was admitted with an antepartum haemorrhage, cough and tachycardia. She was anaesthetised by a staff grade doctor with a consultant anaesthetist and cardiologist present. The anaesthetists report a blood pressure of 96/75 mmHg, heart rate 133/min, APPT ratio 3.9, and K 5.8 mmol l[-1]. She was given sodium citrate and oral ranitidine and anaesthetised in theatre with etomidate, suxamethonium, atracurium and fentanyl, using CVP monitoring, She was then transferred, ventilated, to the ICU but was very unstable with a

low blood pressure. Adrenaline and dopamine were used. Echocardiography showed the mitral valve to be thrombosed or stenosed. By this time she was in cardiogenic shock so her transfer for cardiac surgery was arranged. She was accompanied by an anaesthetist, a nurse and an Operating Department Assistant. She died a few minutes after arrival at the receiving hospital.

Although this death was associated with anaesthesia no avoidable factors were identified, although it is not clear that she was fit to travel.

Deaths in which anaesthetists were involved in resuscitation

Amniotic fluid embolism

Three patients sustained cardiac arrest in the A&E Department and one in the labour ward. All had caesarean sections during the resuscitation. Problems identified by management of these cases include:

- the need for a non-kinkable cricothyrotomy cannula, and
- difficulty in communication between A&E, the resuscitation team and the obstetric team.

Haemorrhage

There were eight deaths in which resuscitation was required for massive haemorrhage in which the main factors are:

- delay in recognition of bleeding,
- inadequate fluid therapy,
- delay in institution of invasive monitoring, and
- failure of postoperative monitoring to detect ongoing bleeding.

Comments

There has been a great improvement since the last triennial Report, with only one *Direct* maternal death due to anaesthesia.

The anaesthetist plays a key role in the multidisciplinary team caring for patients who develop life-threatening complications of pregnancy.

Obstetric units which are isolated from main hospitals should always keep a large stock of group O Rhesus negative blood and ideally these units should be provided with their own blood transfusion laboratory to expedite delivery of blood and blood products.

Until patients can be transferred to an intensive care unit there should be good quality high dependency care on the delivery suite or in the labour ward theatre.

Monitoring of central venous, systemic and pulmonary artery pressure is not always well performed on an obstetric unit.

Failed forceps delivery often leads to an immediate caesarean section, for which the anaesthetist must be prepared either by good epidural top-up or by safe general anaesthesia, recognising the increased risk of hypotension.

In cases where the dose of thiopentone was thought to contribute to the outcome it is tempting to recommend an alternative shorter-acting drug but (especially in small doses) this alternative has the potential problem of awareness.

10
CARDIAC DISEASE

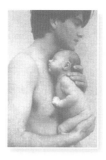

CHAPTER 10
CARDIAC DISEASE

Summary

There were a total of 39 *Indirect* deaths due to heart disease. In addition there are a further 10 cases where heart disease was a factor but which are counted in other Chapters. Substandard care was a factor in six of the cases counted in this Chapter.

Table 10.1 shows no consistent pattern of change since 1985. However, it is noteworthy that this is the first triennium in which there has been no death due to rheumatic heart disease, except in one or possibly two cases who had had valve replacements. By comparison, in the first three Reports of the CEMD series (1952-60) 86% of the 277 deaths ascribed to heart disease in pregnancy were thought to be due to rheumatic heart disease. In 1952-54, 96 of the 108 deaths from rheumatic heart disease were due to mitral valve disease. Not only have the absolute numbers of deaths from cardiac disease declined from an average of 35 per year to about 10 per year but the pattern of disease is completely changed.

Table 10.1

	Congenital	Acquired		Total
		Ischaemic	Other	Cases
1985-87	10(44%)	9(39%)	4(17%)	23
1988-90	9(50%)	5(25%)	4(25%)	18
1991-93	9(24%)	8(22%)	20(54%)	37
1994-96	10 (26%)	6 (21%)	23(53%)	39

Number of maternal deaths from congenital and acquired cardiac disease; United Kingdom 1985-96.

Congenital heart disease

There were 10 deaths from congenital heart disease. Care was substandard in two cases.

Aortic valve disease

Two of the deaths were from aortic valve disease with endocarditis:

> One multigravid woman was admitted urgently in a desperate condition at 29 weeks' gestation. She was known to have endocarditis on her aortic valve with possible additional mitral valve disease. She also had insulin-dependent diabetes mellitus. Emergency cardiac surgery was performed on arrival. This was followed by intrauterine death. The stillborn fetus was delivered following ARM and Syntocinon. The mother died soon afterwards and within 24 hours of surgery.

> The second patient was diagnosed as having endocarditis when she became disorientated two days after delivery. The attending SHO in neurology noted a heart murmur, and echocardiography showed a large vegetation on the aortic valve. She became comatose and died soon after transfer to a tertiary centre. Cerebral haemorrhage was demonstrated on a CT scan. No autopsy was performed. She had had multiple admissions for headache and other pains before delivery and the significance of a blood culture showing Gram positive cocci about two weeks before delivery was not appreciated. Presumably because examination of the heart was normal, endocarditis was discounted if it was ever considered.

This case represents substandard care. In any patient with vague undiagnosed illness, positive blood cultures always raise the possibility of endocarditis.

Pulmonary hypertension

There were seven deaths from pulmonary hypertension in pregnancy, three due to Eisenmenger's syndrome, three due to primary pulmonary hypertension and one due to secondary pulmonary hypertension.

> A woman with known Eisenmenger's syndrome due to ventricular septal defect (VSD) became pregnant and declined termination despite being informed of the 30-40% risk of maternal mortality. At 26 weeks' gestation she developed fulminating pre-eclampsia and was delivered by caesarean section under general anaesthesia. Fourteen days after delivery, while still an inpatient at a tertiary referral centre, she became increasingly hypoxic and died, a common pattern of death in Eisenmenger's syndrome in relation to pregnancy. Autopsy showed that the terminal event was pulmonary haemorrhage related to plexogenic arteriopathy of the pulmonary arterioles.

This woman received exemplary care at world class cardiac and obstetric centres as did the other woman with Eisenmenger's syndrome:

> This woman had residual pulmonary hypertension despite having had a VSD repaired. This may have related to the persistence of a small residual defect. She had been on the waiting list for heart-lung transplantation but was removed from the list because of her lack of symptoms. The risks of pregnancy were discussed with her but she chose to become pregnant. She was referred to a tertiary referral centre at 21 weeks' gestation and was followed up very closely. At 35 weeks' gestation she developed systemic desaturation on exercise and was delivered by elective caesarean section. Two days later she became desaturated at rest and Swan-Ganz pulmonary artery monitoring showed a progressive rise in pulmonary vascular resistance. She died three days later despite treatment with inhaled nitrous oxide and prostacyclin given both intravenously and by nebuliser. Autopsy confirmed the clinical diagnosis.

These two cases illustrate the continuing danger of Eisenmenger's syndrome in pregnancy, particularly in association with pre-eclampsia. However, there were also three deaths in association with termination for pulmonary hypertension in pregnancy, one in relation to Eisenmenger's syndrome and two related to primary pulmonary hypertension (see page 107).

> A patient with Eisenmenger's syndrome had a patent ductus arteriosus ligated in childhood but was known to have residual pulmonary hypertension. Previously she had had one successful pregnancy delivered at 33 weeks' gestation because of pulmonary hypertension, one earlier termination on medical grounds and then became pregnant again. She was referred for termination of pregnancy at eight weeks' gestation by her cardiologist. She had a vacuum aspiration of pregnancy and laparoscopic sterilization. Eight days later she suddenly became breathless and died. Pulmonary embolism was queried, particularly since no short-or long-term anticoagulant cover was given. However, no autopsy was performed.

Primary pulmonary hypertension

A multigravid woman was admitted to the medical ward of a local hospital at 12 weeks' gestation because of breathlessness which she had had for four months. Pulmonary embolism was excluded and she was discharged only to be readmitted at 13 weeks' gestation with vaginal bleeding and increasing breathlessness with ankle oedema. She was discharged again when the bleeding stopped but was again readmitted a week later with spontaneous rupture of membranes. Because of gross ankle oedema an echocardiogram was performed which showed pulmonary hypertension. Termination of pregnancy was agreed and a hysterotomy was performed on the day of admission. She died during the procedure. Autopsy confirmed pulmonary hypertension with plexogenic pulmonary arteriopathy.

This case represents substandard care. The breathlessness present before pregnancy was not adequately investigated on the first admission. Furthermore only a medical registrar assessed the patient from a cardiological point of view once the diagnosis of pulmonary hypertension had been made. These cases are so difficult to manage that a consultant, preferably cardiological, opinion and in a tertiary centre should be sought wherever possible.

Another woman with known primary pulmonary hypertension became pregnant inadvertently while on the waiting list for heart lung transplant. She had only been using sheaths for contraception because her menstrual periods had been infrequent since menarche and she had needed fertility treatment to conceive her previous pregnancy. Because of the gross pulmonary hypertension with a huge right ventricle, termination of pregnancy was advised and accepted. At 15 weeks' gestation a hysterotomy was performed. The postoperative period was complicated by mild disseminated intravascular coagulopathy. Four days later she became markedly hypoxic with pulmonary artery pressure equal to systemic (90/55 mmHg). She died despite prostaglandin and trinitrin infusion.

Termination of pregnancy is not without risk in patients with pulmonary hypertension and again the typical mode of death appears to be increasing pulmonary resistance occurring either at delivery or a few days after the uterus has been emptied.

Another woman died from primary pulmonary hypertension. Details available are sparse but she was known to have primary pulmonary hypertension since adolescence and had refused a heart lung transplant. Caesarean section was performed at 34 weeks but the indication is not known. Again, as typically occurs in pulmonary hypertension in pregnancy (see before) she became more hypoxic five days after delivery and died four days later.

These cases of primary pulmonary hypertension have been counted among congenital heart disease for consistency with previous Reports but the precise aetiology remains obscure.

Hypertrophic Obstructive Cardiomyopathy

There was one death from this condition in which, five days after an uneventful pregnancy and delivery, the woman was found dead at home. Autopsy showed that the patient died from hypertrophic obstructive cardiomyopathy. Sudden death is a recognized feature of this condition.

Anomalous coronary arteries

A primipara in her thirties was admitted with severe breathlessness and chest pain. The fetus was already dead and the woman died within 24 hours despite all resuscitative measures. Autopsy showed the origin of the coronary arteries to be normal but thereafter their courses were extremely anomalous. They were tiny and no specific artery could be identified, rather a leash of very small arteries. The myocardium was normal. There was no atheroma. A family history of possible Duchenne muscular dystrophy may be relevant.

Table 10.2

Maternal deaths due to cardiac diseases; United Kingdom 1994-96.	
Congenital	
Aortic valve disease	2
Ventricular septal defect, Eisenmenger's syndrome	3
Primary pulmonary hypertension	3
Hypertrophic obstructive cardiomyopathy	1
Anomalous coronary arteries	1
Total	10
Acquired	
Aneurysm of thoracic aorta and its branches	7
Puerperal cardiomyopathy	4
Cardiomyopathy and myocarditis	4
Myocardial infarct	6
Pericarditis	1
Thrombosed mitral valve replacement	1
Secondary pulmonary hypertension	1
Left ventricular hypertrophy,	1
Total	25
Inadequate details	4
Overall total deaths	39

Acquired heart disease

There were 29 deaths from acquired heart disease (see Table 10.2). Substandard care was present in four cases.

Puerperal Cardiomyopathy

There were four deaths from puerperal cardiomyopathy recorded in this Chapter and five *Late* deaths are recorded in Chapter 14. One *Late* death, also mentioned in Chapter 12, was considered *Direct* because of death from widespread thromboembolism secondary to dilated cardiomyopathy. In addition one patient recorded in Chapter 2 died from pulmonary embolism but autopsy showed evidence of cardiomyopathy which may have been ischaemic or puerperal.

> A woman weighing 110 kilograms, presented at 30 weeks' gestation with gross pulmonary oedema. Echocardiography showed poorly contracting ventricles with no evidence of pericardial disease. After transfer to a regional cardiac centre she initially responded well to delivery but subsequently deteriorated and died three days later. Autopsy was declined.

> Another woman weighing 147 kg presented with a twin pregnancy and hypertension at 32 weeks' gestation. Four weeks later she was delivered by elective caesarean section. On the third postoperative day she became breathless and her condition rapidly deteriorated. Despite very intensive measures she died on the next day. At autopsy she had a grossly enlarged heart with histology typical of puerperal cardiomyopathy.

In two other cases no details are available other than the cause of death. One woman died after delivery. The timing of the other woman's death and all other details are unknown to the Enquiry.

> One of the *Late* deaths occurred in a woman who developed puerperal cardiomyopathy in her previous pregnancy. She had subsequent problems with dysrhythmias and was advised against further pregnancy. She became pregnant again and declined termination of pregnancy. She had an uneventful pregnancy with no evidence of further deterioration of cardiac function. Ten weeks after delivery she collapsed, presumably because of another episode of dysrhythmia. She was admitted to hospital and died soon afterwards. No autopsy was performed.

> Another woman, though technically a *Late* death, developed breathlessness and cardiac failure a few days after delivery. She was treated medically at her local hospital for about six weeks. When her condition continued to deteriorate she was transferred to a cardiac transplant centre. She arrived in a parlous state with impalpable peripheral pulses. Despite implantation of two different ventricular assist devices she died three days later. In retrospect she should have been transferred earlier for consideration of cardiac transplantation.

Other forms of cardiomyopathy and myocarditis

There were four deaths in this group:

One woman was found dead at home by her husband at 16 weeks' gestation. After an autopsy showing pulmonary congestion, death was certified as due to cardiomyopathy. Histology showed a very focal myocarditis with acute and chronic components. Because of the latter it is unlikely that this was puerperal cardiomyopathy.

Another primigravid woman was found dead at home in the third trimester. At autopsy the heart was macroscopically normal but histology showed myocardial fibrosis involving the conducting system. In such cases death has been described due to ventricular arrhythmia. There may be a family history, as was the case in this instance.

A further primigravid woman suddenly became unwell six days after caesarean section for failure to progress in labour. She suffered a cardiac arrest in the ambulance and could not be resuscitated. The autopsy showed an enlarged heart with an infiltrate characteristic of acute myocarditis. Blood counts taken after delivery and at the time of resuscitation showed marked anaemia and thrombocytopaenia. It is likely that the myocarditis was infectious in origin.

In addition there were two *Late* deaths from myocardial fibrosis counted in Chapter 14. In one of these the woman died seven weeks after delivery. The condition may have been related to varicella virus infection earlier in pregnancy.

One further patient, also counted in Chapter 14, died suddenly 11 months after delivery. At autopsy she was found to have cardiomyopathy, though from the description given, the diagnosis could have been viral myocarditis. Nevertheless it is difficult to believe that either of these conditions was connected with pregnancy.

Myocardial infarction

There were six cases in this group. All except one were multigravid women in their thirties and all except one were known to have smoked, three heavily. One also abused various substances including alcohol. One death occurred before delivery at 34 weeks, one occurred after termination of pregnancy and one occurred 10 days after treatment of ectopic pregnancy. The other deaths occurred after delivery at six, 29 and 39 days respectively. All the deaths were sudden and unexpected.

One woman, however, had a sudden episode of central chest pain and left arm numbness while she was an inpatient after delivery, and again six days before death. The autopsy was in keeping with myocardial infarction occurring at this time. This represents substandard care. This obese cigarette smoking patient was at high risk for myocardial infarction. The condition could have been diagnosed at presentation. Chest pain must always be taken seriously in pregnant women.

Dissection of the thoracic aorta and its branches

There were seven cases in this group:

> A multigravid woman in her late thirties was admitted at term with epigastric pain. There was a strong family history of death from dissecting aneurysm at this same age. Differential diagnoses considered were peptic ulcer, pancreatitis, cholecystitis, or abruption. It was decided to deliver her and then sort out the pain later. Forty-eight hours after delivery she collapsed and could not be resuscitated. Autopsy revealed dissection from the aortic root into the pericardium and beyond the renal arteries. Histology showed cystic medial necrosis characteristic of an arteriopathy such as Marfan's syndrome. However, there were no other phenotypic features of Marfan's.

In an obscure emergency at term it is often sensible to deliver the woman first and sort out the underlying condition afterwards, but not in aortic dissection. It is likely that dissection started when she presented with epigastric pain. Had dissection been considered at that time, her life might have been saved. In the last Report there were nine deaths from dissection. In three of these cases care was judged to be substandard, partly because this diagnosis was never considered.

> Another multigravid woman was delivered by caesarean section for abruption. Three days later she developed chest pain and was thought to have had a pulmonary embolus. She was given heparin but her condition deteriorated. The heparin was stopped and the ventilation perfusion scan was negative for pulmonary embolus. Shortly after this she collapsed and died. Autopsy showed dissection of the aorta distal to an undiagnosed coarctation of the aorta.

It is difficult to know what was the contribution of the coarctation proximal to the dissection. However, there is no comment about any chest X-ray which should have been taken at the time of the suspected pulmonary embolism and might have shown mediastinal widening. **Chest X-ray should always be performed in sick pregnant women with chest pain.**

There were two deaths from dissection of the coronary arteries. Both occurred within two weeks after delivery:

> A woman in her twenties who had no past medical history had an uncomplicated delivery at term. Nine days later she complained of chest pain and her breathing became erratic. An ambulance was called and the crew considered she was hyperventilating. Shortly afterwards she collapsed. The ambulance returned and took her to hospital where she was found dead on arrival. Autopsy showed that death was due to coronary artery dissection. There were no other abnormalities in the blood vessels or myocardium.

Although in retrospect the patient should have been admitted to hospital when the ambulance first called, it is unlikely that admission one hour later would have made much difference to the outcome.

Substandard care was present in one further death from aortic rupture:

> A woman who had a renal transplant was treated with antihypertensive and immunosuppressive drug therapy throughout her pregnancy. At 32 weeks' gestation the membranes ruptured spontaneously and she was delivered by caesarean section because of failure to progress in labour. Blood pressure control was a problem for four days after delivery and she remained on the Delivery Suite. On the fifth day she developed such severe back pain that she was given parenteral opiates and then was treated by local anaesthetic injection. No investigations appear to have been performed. Ten hours later she collapsed and could not be resuscitated. Autopsy showed a rupture in the ascending aorta which had dissected back into the pericardium. Death was due to cardiac tamponade.

Pain as severe as this should have been investigated more thoroughly. The past history of hypertension should have suggested a vascular cause.

In two cases of ruptured aorta no details are known except that one had Marfan's syndrome.

Pericarditis

> An older multigravid woman booked for private care with a consultant who practised 30 miles from her home. At 32 weeks' gestation she became unwell and refused to see any doctor other than the GP and the obstetrician, who visited her at home. She died undelivered at home at 36 weeks' gestation. Autopsy showed that death was due to cardiac tamponade subsequent to haemorrhagic pericarditis, possibly of viral origin.

This is a very unusual set of circumstances. It is uncommon for patients to die from viral pericarditis but possibly that is because they are usually admitted to hospital. The patient's refusal to leave home was a major factor in the outcome of this case.

Thrombosed mitral valve replacement

> A woman in her twenties became pregnant against medical advice. She had had a mitral valve replacement (type unknown) inserted in childhood and also had aortic valve disease. Following a termination of pregnancy some years previously she had had several spontaneous pregnancy losses, perhaps associated with her long-term warfarin therapy. She had also attended a specialist miscarriage clinic. At six weeks' gestation warfarin therapy was changed to subcutaneous heparin (dose unknown). She declined to attend her cardiac centre and was managed at the local hospital. She was well until 28 weeks' gestation when she had to be delivered by caesarean section because of bleeding from placenta praevia. She collapsed during general anaesthesia and eventually echocardiography demonstrated that the mitral valve was thrombosed. She died on transfer to another cardiac centre for valve replacement.

This case represents substandard care primarily because the patient was not receiving tertiary care for one of the most difficult medical problems to manage in pregnancy. But it may be that she did not want to attend her specialist centre because she had been advised against pregnancy. The manner in which this was done should be reviewed in view of the fact that she had shown determination to have children by getting pregnant five times and by seeking advice from a specialist miscarriage clinic. Thrombosis of valve prostheses is a recognised complication of subcutaneous heparin therapy in pregnancy. The dose given in this case is not known but it is unlikely to have been adequate to prevent this fatal complication. In retrospect the valve thrombosis may well have occurred before the patient started bleeding from placenta praevia and would have contributed to the haemodynamic instability that forced the obstetricians to operate. It is unusual for this to be necessary in patients bleeding from otherwise uncomplicated placenta praevia at 28 weeks' gestation.

Secondary Pulmonary Hypertension

Another patient had pulmonary hypertension due to systemic lupus erythematosus (SLE). Caesarean section was performed with two consultant anaesthetists after which she was transferred for monitoring to the intensive care unit (ICU) where her condition was stable. Oozing was noted from the wound and she returned to the delivery suite next day for exploration of a wound haematoma. She died on the operating table after collapsing during intubation and could not be resuscitated; attempts were stopped after 50 minutes.

A number of questions arise, in particular whether she should have had a further operation for the wound haematoma. General anaesthesia is very dangerous in patients with pulmonary hypertension.

Miscellaneous

One patient died from pulmonary oedema due to left ventricular hypertrophy of unknown cause. Pre-eclampsia may have contributed.

Inadequate details for classification

In four cases, details available to the Assessors were inadequate to allow further classification.

One patient died 4 weeks after delivery by caesarean section because of presumed sepsis, fetal tachycardia and failure to progress. Ten years earlier she had had a tricuspid valve replacement in another country. She spoke no English but appeared well, both before and immediately after her delivery. The circumstances of her death are unknown and the coroner's autopsy does not give an adequate explanation of her death. There was pulmonary oedema but there were no abnormalities on the left side of the heart, only right ventricular hypertrophy. The leaflets of the prosthetic (xeno?) graft were calcified. Death was classified as due to acute heart failure due to tricuspid incompetence but this would not give left-sided heart failure.

Another woman, a known diabetic, who had had a myocardial infarct in the past was found by her GP to be in left ventricular failure at home about two weeks after delivery. She was treated medically and there were no abnormalities when she was examined three days later. Two days after this she was found collapsed and could not be resuscitated. No autopsy was performed.

Two days after a spontaneous miscarriage and evacuation of retained products a woman in her thirties collapsed and died at work. Autopsy showed pulmonary oedema, non-atherosclerotic coronary artery stenosis and fatty infiltration of the right ventricle. The mechanism of death remains unclear.

In one case death was simply ascribed to hypertension.

Another patient counted in Chapter 11 with known systemic lupus became very ill in a non-specific way and died while aborting a non-viable pregnancy. The cause of death was not clear despite a very comprehensive autopsy, but it did show Libman-Sacks endocarditis and the patient had very poor left ventricular function at the time she died. However there was no autopsy evidence of myocarditis.

Comment

Endocarditis remains a fatal complication of heart disease in pregnancy. Over the last 12 years 11 (10%) of the 115 cardiac deaths reported to the CEMD have been due to endocarditis. Endocarditis is not necessarily contracted at delivery and the high incidence is not an argument for routine antibiotic prophylaxis for delivery in all patients with heart disease. Rather, attendants should be aware of the risk of endocarditis in pregnancy, particularly in patients with non-specific illness.

Pulmonary hypertension is also a common cause of maternal mortality in heart disease. In previous Reports, clinicians have been criticized for not appreciating its significance. In this Report at least three patients who died from pulmonary hypertension chose to become pregnant or to continue with their pregnancy when the considerable risks to their health had been explained and discussed with them.

The manner in which such advice is given is very important. The patient with the obstructed mitral valve prosthesis discussed above may have been alienated from the highly specialised care she needed by advice not to get pregnant. Whenever such advice is given, it should be done so in a supportive manner, with counselling offered as necessary. It must be made clear to the woman and her partner that whatever decision she makes will be respected and this should be coupled with encouragement to return for specialist care as soon as possible should she become pregnant either as a positive choice or inadvertently.

Dissection of the aorta and its branches, above the diaphragm (discussed here) or below the diaphragm (discussed in Chapter 11), was responsible for seven and three deaths respectively. In none of the cases described in this Chapter was the diagnosis considered before death. In at least two cases a chest X-ray could have given a clue to the diagnosis, though for dissections occurring around the heart echocardiography is more specific. The radiation risk from chest radiography with modern equipment is trivial by comparison to the benefit to the patient, not only in dissection but in other conditions such as pulmonary embolism.

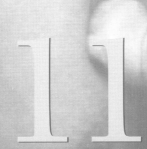

11
OTHER INDIRECT DEATHS

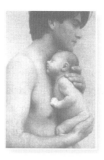

CHAPTER 11
OTHER *INDIRECT* DEATHS

Summary

In this triennium there were a total of 86 other *Indirect* deaths compared to 63 in 1991-93. Although there have been minor decreases in some causes of death, the major change was an increase in death from epilepsy from six cases in 1991-93 to 19 in the period of this Report. Table 11.1 gives a breakdown of cases counted in this Chapter. There were 17 cases of substandard care.

Indirect deaths due to suicide consequent on postnatal depression or other psychiatric causes are now counted and discussed in Chapter 12. In addition there were 32 *Late Indirect* deaths counted in Chapter 14.

Indirect deaths: key recommendations

Epilepsy is a potentially fatal disease whether the patient is pregnant or not. GPs and midwives should check with relatives that they know what to do in the case of a fit and should provide instruction, particularly on the need to place the patient in the recovery position once the fit is over. Pregnant women who are at risk of fits should be advised not to bathe alone, or should use a shower instead.

Sepsis arising outside the genital tract continues to kill women in pregnancy. In serious cases doctors should be prepared to give parenteral antibiotics before the diagnosis can be confirmed.

Patients with life threatening diseases such as cystic fibrosis (or pulmonary hypertension, see Chapter 10) should be aware that it is not possible to predict the maternal outcome of pregnancy with accuracy.

Obstetricians and midwives should liaise early with other health care professionals when patients have non-obstetric illness.

Maternity health care professionals should ensure that their services are as approachable as possible for all ethnic groups.

Table 11.1

Causes of *Indirect* deaths; United Kingdom 1994-96.		
Disease	**Number**	**Total**
Infectious diseases		
Streptococcus pneumoniae	3	
Streptococcus other	1	
Meningococcus	1	
Toxoplasmosis	2	
Varicella pneumonia	1	
Organism unknown	1	9
Neoplastic diseases		
Colon	1	
Brain (not specified)	1	2
Endocrine, metabolic and immunity disorders		
Diabetes mellitus	2	
Phaeochromocytoma	5	
Systemic lupus erythematosus	4	
Primary antiphospholipid syndrome	1	12
Diseases of the blood		
Acute myeloid leukaemia	1	
Neutropaenia	1	2
Diseases of the central nervous system		
Subarachnoid haemorrhage	15	
Intracerebral haemorrhage	9	
Cerebral thrombosis	2	
Epilepsy	19	
Guillain-Barré syndrome	1	
Hypoxic brain damage	1	47
Diseases of the circulatory system		
Splenic/renal artery aneurysm	2	
Air embolism	1	
Renal artery aneurysm	1	
Ruptured epigastric artery	1	
Ruptured iliac vein	1	6
Diseases of the respiratory system		
Asthma	3	
Cystic fibrosis	2	
Pneumonia	2	7
Disease of the gastrointestinal system		
Angiodysplasia	1	1
Total		**86**

Infectious diseases

Nine deaths relating to infectious disease are counted in this Chapter. Two were thought to be due to pneumococcal sepsis:

> An older woman who had previously had a splenectomy was admitted moribund at 30 weeks' gestation after a two day history of diarrhoea, vomiting and abdominal pain and died two hours later. At autopsy both adrenal glands were haemorrhagic and Gram-positive cocci were seen in post-mortem blood cultures. Although these did not grow, probably due to antibiotic therapy, they tested positive for pneumococcal antigen. The causative organism could have been pneumococcus or streptococcus but in view of the previous splenectomy, the former seems more likely.

This case represents substandard care. Perhaps because the patient had been given pneumococcal vaccine she was not offered penicillin prophylaxis. All patients who have had splenectomy or who have sickle cell disease (autosplenectomy) should be offered both regular phenoxymethyl penicillin 500 mg twice daily and pneumococcal vaccine, but pneumococcal vaccine should not be administered in pregnancy.

> A multigravid woman had previously been diagnosed as having vasculitis and chronic active hepatitis. Early in pregnancy she was referred to physicians because of heavy proteinuria: systemic lupus erythematosus (SLE) was probably the unifying diagnosis. She had ceased steroid therapy six months before her sudden terminal illness, which occurred at 29 weeks' gestation when she complained of an upset stomach with vomiting. The next morning she appeared disorientated: an ambulance was called but before it arrived she sat down, stopped breathing and died.

At autopsy the only macroscopic abnormality was a small spleen. Histology showed that the spleen was atrophic with marked loss of lymphoid tissue. The kidneys showed glomerular loop basement membrane thickening. Culture of amniotic fluid grew *Streptococcus pneumoniae*. Blood cultures were not taken. This patient almost certainly did have SLE with hyposplenism either due to the disease or to steroid treatment. This, plus the possible immune-compromised state of pregnancy, led to the overwhelming pneumococcal infection.

> An obese grandmultipara with non-insulin-dependent diabetes was admitted in the mid trimester with severe headaches and earache. She suffered a cardiac arrest on admission and was resuscitated. However, her deteriorating condition led the obstetricians to perform an emergency caesarean section at 26 weeks' gestation, to improve her oxygenation. The baby suffered an early neonatal death and the woman herself succumbed to overwhelming pneumococcal septicaemia shortly afterwards.

> A young woman became ill in the latter half of pregnancy. She initially called her GP who diagnosed a flu-like illness and when her condition deteriorated she was admitted to the labour ward of a consultant unit. There she was found to be short of breath with headache, vomiting, blurred vision and fever. She had a purpuric rash all over her body. Intrauterine death was diagnosed by ultrasound. She was seen by obstetric and medical Registrars who noted cyanosis

and the worsening rash. She was initially thought to have pulmonary embolism or overwhelming sepsis with disseminating intravascular coagulopathy (DIC). The Intensive Care Unit (ICU) Registrar thought that the very high levels of fibrin degradation products were due to DIC secondary to intrauterine death. She was transferred to an ICU and died very soon afterwards. Blood cultures later confirmed meningococcal septicaemia.

This represents substandard care. A purpuric rash, in particular in a patient who is ill, represents meningococcal septicaemia until proven otherwise and should be treated with high-dose antibiotic therapy before the results of blood cultures are available. The delay in therapy might not have made any difference in this case but in addition, intrauterine death of recent onset could not have been the cause of her disseminated intravascular coagulopathy, which generally does not occur until about two weeks after an intrauterine death. Disseminated intravascular coagulopathy is a well-known complication of meningococcal septicaemia.

> One death was due to streptococcal sepsis. The patient was apparently well until she developed severe diarrhoea at 35 weeks' gestation. She died undelivered 12 hours later. Autopsy showed ß haemolytic streptococci at all sites sampled. The portal of entry was not defined.

There were five similar deaths in the last Report. It is not clear whether pregnancy increases the risk of these overwhelming infections. If treatment is to be effective, high-dose antibiotics must be given parenterally on clinical suspicion and before the results of any investigations are available.

There were two deaths from cerebral toxoplasmosis. Both were in women who had recently moved to the United Kingdom from parts of the world with a higher prevalence of Human Immunodeficiency Virus (HIV).

> The first case was a multiparous woman whose haemoglobin (Hb) at booking was 7.9g%. She was seen a week later for further investigations, and shortly afterwards admitted as she was complaining of severe headaches. A CT scan that day showed a cerebral abscess, diagnosed as toxoplasmosis by Magnetic Resonance Imaging (MRI) guided biopsy. She was found to be HIV positive. Despite intensive efforts she became comatose and died, undelivered at 24 weeks' gestation, of pneumonia.

In the opinion of the Assessors the care she received at all times was exemplary.

> The second woman, also multiparous, was admitted towards the end of her pregnancy with a very severe headache. An MRI scan showed a space occupying intracerebral lesion. Her condition deteriorated and she was delivered by caesarean section. After transfer to a neurosurgical unit a brain biopsy was not helpful in obtaining a firm diagnosis and her increased intracerebral pressure could not be controlled. She died eight days after delivery. Autopsy demonstrated a cerebral abscess due to toxoplasmosis.

In this case it is possible that HIV infection may also have been the underlying cause but there was no record of antenatal HIV testing. Her care was also not substandard.

A young woman contracted chicken-pox from a child. She presented to her GP with varicella rash at 28 weeks' gestation and was treated symptomatically. Two days later she was admitted to hospital because of breathlessness, vomiting and dehydration. Pneumonitis was diagnosed and acyclovir was given. She rapidly deteriorated despite intensive care. The fetus died. Five days after admission it was decided to deliver her in the hope that this would improve matters, but she died during the caesarean section. Autopsy confirmed varicella pneumonia.

It is recognised that varicella pneumonia is a potentially fatal complication of chicken-pox and is more common in pregnancy. Acyclovir treatment is advised for all who develop chicken-pox in pregnancy or the puerperium. The patient should have been given acyclovir when she first presented to her GP and the failure to do so represents substandard care.

In one woman the autopsy diagnosis was "shock lung" presumed due to sepsis though there was no specific evidence of infection. The patient had been discharged home following delivery. The only abnormality had been anaemia (haemoglobin 8.5 g%) discovered in the puerperium and for which she had been transfused. On day 26 she complained of pyrexia and vomiting and following the GP's second visit that day, hospital admission was refused by the patient. By the next day her condition had deteriorated. An ambulance was called and fatal cardiac arrest occurred on the way to hospital. Autopsy showed "hyaline membrane" in the lungs which were grossly oedematous. No other specific abnormalities were seen. No samples were taken for culture. Substance abuse was queried and traces of amphetamine and benzodiazapines were found in the blood, not enough to be a cause of death unless by an idiosyncratic reaction.

Neoplastic diseases

Two cases of neoplastic disease are counted in this Chapter as *Indirect* deaths. There were five *Late Indirect* deaths discussed in Chapter 14. *Fortuitous* deaths from malignant disease are counted in Chapter 13: these are deaths where pregnancy did not affect the outcome of the disease.

A patient with abdominal pain was admitted and transferred to the care of gynaecologists when she was found to be 13 weeks pregnant with bilateral ovarian masses. At laparotomy she was thought to have stage 1 ovarian cancer but she made a slow recovery and two weeks later there was bowel obstruction. This was treated conservatively until she collapsed and was found to have faecal peritonitis due to carcinoma of the ascending colon with perforation. She then aborted and died the next day. The colectomy specimen was mislaid. No autopsy was performed.

This represents substandard care. Primary cancer in the colon was missed at the original laparotomy for removal of the ovarian masses which presumably were secondary, not primary cancer. There is no comment with regard to peritoneal washings which should have been performed at the time of the first laparotomy for presumed primary ovarian cancer. There was delay in performing the second laparotomy. Mislaying the colectomy specimen meant that histology was not performed. This could have been an example of the colloid carcinoma of the right colon which occurs predominantly in young females and has a genetic basis. This diagnosis would have had implications for screening the rest of the family.

A young primiparous woman from an ethnic minority group received regular antenatal care. All seemed well until she was admitted at 29 weeks' gestation after a sudden collapse. She had not told anyone about headaches which she had suffered for the preceding three weeks. She suffered a cardiac arrest but was resuscitated and transferred to the ICU where a CT scan showed a large haemorrhagic brain tumour in the left fronto-parietal region, causing brain stem distortion. Brain stem death was diagnosed because of the lack of brain stem reflexes. She had a classical caesarean section with delivery of a live baby and ventilator support was then withdrawn from the woman. Autopsy was refused.

This case has been included amongst *Indirect* deaths because of the tendency of some tumours such as meningioma and arterio-venous malformation to increase in size in pregnancy. It is disturbing that this patient did not report the headaches which had been present for three weeks before death and which are likely to have been severe. Maternity health care professionals should ensure that their services are as approachable as possible for woman from all ethnic groups.

The five *Late Indirect* deaths counted in Chapter 14 are mentioned here because in each case diagnosis was delayed by pregnancy. There was one small cell carcinoma of the bladder, one carcinoma of the caecum, one metastatic carcinoma, one carcinoma of the ovary (possibly squamous carcinoma arising in an endometrioma) and one carcinoma of the cervix .

Endocrine, metabolic and immunity disorders

Diabetes

Two women died because of diabetes:

> In one, a known diabetic, a missed abortion was diagnosed at 12 weeks' gestation. She refused an evacuation of the uterus. One week later she was found dead at home. No abnormalities were found at autopsy apart from a blood glucose of 2.3 mmol/L.

This is in keeping with hypoglycaemia although post-mortem samples from the anterior chamber of the eye or the cerebrospinal fluid would have made the diagnosis more reliable.

> The other woman spent most of her pregnancy in hospital. She was known to have retinopathy, nephropathy, neuropathy and asthma which was thought to be due to pulmonary vasculitis (Churg Strauss Syndrome). Her membranes ruptured spontaneously at 34 weeks' gestation and she had a ventouse delivery of an appropriately grown infant. Eight days later while still in hospital she collapsed and was found to be severely hypoglycaemic. She was resuscitated and transferred to an ICU where she was ventilated. She developed renal failure and remained de-cerebrate, dying three weeks after the collapse. Autopsy revealed myocardial necrosis and review of the medical record suggests that she had a myocardial infarct two days before the collapse.

The combination of hypoglycaemia and myocardial infarction is particularly dangerous, as is complicated diabetes in pregnancy. For example, another patient with diabetic nephropathy deteriorated and received haemodialysis during pregnancy, before being delivered of a stillborn fetus at 25 weeks' gestation. She developed infection at the shunt and died of endocarditis seven months after delivery. This case is counted in Chapter 14 amongst other *Late* deaths.

One further insulin-dependent diabetic died from subacute bacterial endocarditis and is therefore counted in Chapter 10. Her insulin-dependent diabetes mellitus is likely to have increased the risk of endocarditis. Another diabetic patient is recorded later in this Chapter as dying from epilepsy, and a further non-insulin-dependent diabetic has already been mentioned as dying from pneumococcal septicaemia.

Phaeochromocytoma

There were five deaths from phaeochromocytoma:

> A multigravid woman had an uneventful pregnancy until she was admitted at 37 weeks' gestation with a blood pressure 170/100 mmHg and headache. She also had proteinuria and was hyper-reflexic so labour was induced two hours later. Two hours after induction, when the blood pressure rose to 210/140 mmHg and she developed visual symptoms, she was delivered by caesarean section. Liver function tests, uric acid level and platelet count were normal. Because of intense tachycardia and vasoconstriction, phaeochromocytoma was considered at the time of surgery but nevertheless she returned to the labour ward rather than an ICU for the recovery period. About two hours later her blood pressure fell to 70/40 mmHg and she had a terminal cardiac arrest. Autopsy showed that death was due to pulmonary oedema. There was a para-aortic mass below the left kidney which histology showed to be a paraganglionoma, i.e. an extra-adrenal phaeochromocytoma.

Phaeochromocytoma can mimic all features of pre-eclampsia but the diagnosis had been considered in this patient. Patients with undiagnosed, and therefore untreated, phaeochromocytoma have a very high mortality. In retrospect, the absence of any abnormality in her blood tests given the severity of her hypertension is striking. There was also evidence of hypoxaemia before her final cardiac arrest. Therefore this management plan represents substandard care. The patient should have been transferred to an ICU for more intensive monitoring after delivery.

There were really no clinical features to suggest phaeochromocytoma in the following patients:

> A multigravid woman also had an illness suggesting pregnancy-induced hypertension. She developed a blood pressure of 160/90 mmHg at 30 weeks' gestation which settled. She was admitted at 37 weeks with headache and a blood pressure of 180/110 mmHg, which again settled. When the blood pressure again rose to 180/100, labour was induced. After the membranes ruptured she was found to have a prolapsed cord. At extubation following caesarean section she collapsed. Autopsy demonstrated phaeochromocytoma.

Another multigravid woman was admitted because of hypertension which only developed at the end of pregnancy. She was soon delivered by caesarean section because of fetal distress. Epidural block failed and she had a general anaesthetic. During the anaesthetic she became markedly hypertensive and after the procedure she had fixed dilated pupils and did not wake up. She was transferred to an ICU and died six hours later. Autopsy showed that one adrenal gland had been replaced by a 4-5 cm phaeochromocytoma.

Eight days after an uneventful pregnancy and delivery a young woman was readmitted because of severe headache of sudden onset. Lumbar puncture was equivocal for subarachnoid haemorrhage (92 cells). Following a negative CT scan, a cerebral angiogram showed widespread abnormalities, possibly due to "vasculitis". On day 12 her headache returned and she was thought to have a cerebral haemorrhage, following which she deteriorated and died four days later. There was no hypertension in pregnancy and she only became hypertensive on the day of her death. At autopsy there was a haemorrhagic phaeochromocytoma in the left adrenal gland. There was no gross brain lesion but histology showed very acute hypoxic and ischaemic changes throughout the cerebral cortex. This was thought to be due to intracranial arterial spasm.

This last case is a very unusual presentation and mechanism of death for phaeochromocytoma. Presumably the cerebral blood vessels were particularly affected by catecholamines released from the phaeochromocytoma.

One further woman is known to have died from phaeochromocytoma in association with pregnancy but no other details are known to the Enquiry.

Systemic Lupus Erythematosus (SLE)

There were four deaths from SLE counted in this section. The first case is also mentioned in Chapter 10 because of the cardiac involvement:

A multigravid woman with known SLE became very ill in a rather non-specific way and died while aborting a non-viable pregnancy. The cause of death was not clear despite a very comprehensive autopsy. The clinical immunologist caring for her suggested sepsis, Addisonian crisis or a primary cardiac problem. Sepsis was excluded at autopsy. Addisonian crisis is clearly a possibility in view of the manner of her death (severe hypotension), previous prednisolone treatment and the thin adrenal cortex found at autopsy. With regard to a primary cardiovascular event, previous pulmonary embolus was excluded at autopsy despite thrombi in the pelvic veins. Pulmonary hypertension was a further possibility excluded at autopsy. The autopsy did show Libman-Sacks endocarditis and the patient had very poor left ventricular function at the time she died. However there was no autopsy evidence of myocarditis.

Clearly acute SLE was the cause of her death and Addisonian crisis may have been an additional factor. Perhaps the acute exacerbation of SLE caused her death by affecting left ventricular function, possibly before there was time for histological evidence of myocarditis.

Another woman with known SLE eventually had a successful pregnancy following six miscarriages. The pregnancy had been supported with aspirin and subcutaneous heparin injections and she was delivered at 34 weeks' gestation by elective caesarean section because of fetal growth restriction. She was discharged home on the fourth day apparently well but with a haemoglobin concentration of 8 g%. The puerperium was initially complicated by backache and constipation from which she recovered. Eleven days after delivery she became delirious and was eventually readmitted to the specialist unit where her pregnancy had been managed. She died four days later from acute cerebral lupus with two large cerebral infarcts with brain haemorrhage, cerebral oedema and coagulopathy.

Flare up after delivery is a well recognised complication of lupus in pregnancy. The community midwife was not told of this woman's anaemia at discharge and this represents substandard care. It is possible that the flare up of lupus would have been detected earlier by routine blood tests if the hospital team had been monitoring the patient either as an inpatient or as an outpatient.

Another patient with known SLE with renal involvement received substandard care because of failure to involve a tertiary centre. The degree of renal impairment at the beginning of pregnancy is not known but at that time the local general physician discontinued hydroxychloroquine and azathioprine, limited prednisolone therapy to 5 mg daily and withheld low-dose aspirin or heparin presumably in the (unfounded) interests of the fetus. As early as 19 weeks' gestation intrauterine growth restriction was demonstrated at the local tertiary referral centre but care was not transferred. At 25 weeks' gestation she was admitted to the local tertiary centre with uncontrolled hypertension and nephrotic syndrome. She then developed pulmonary oedema and was delivered by caesarean section, the infant dying on the same day. Her condition deteriorated relentlessly after delivery and she died about four weeks later.

In effect this patient had all her treatment withdrawn in early pregnancy and did not receive the treatment (aspirin and heparin) that might have helped the fetus. All of this substandard care appears to have been given because of lack of knowledge of the effect of maternal medication on the developing fetus. Whether this would ultimately have made any difference to the maternal or fetal outcome is uncertain but women with such serious medical and fetal complications must be offered specialist care in tertiary centres.

One other patient with SLE is known to the Enquiry, having died from cytomegalovirus pneumonia in association with steroid and azathioprine treatment. Caesarean section at 26 weeks at the time of her death allowed her child to survive. No other details are known. In addition, one case, described earlier, of probable SLE, died from pneumococcal septicaemia.

Primary antiphospholipid syndrome

One patient was considered to have primary antiphospholipid syndrome because of her history of eight previous miscarriages, a very high titre of lupus anticoagulant and no other clinical or laboratory features of SLE. She initially elected to be treated by aspirin alone but later in pregnancy accepted steroid treatment and plasmapheresis. Nevertheless the fetus died at 25 weeks' gestation. Following induced labour and delivery she had an epileptic fit and developed very severe disseminated intravascular coagulation. This proved very difficult to control and she died a few days later of cerebral haemorrhage.

Diseases of the blood

There were two maternal deaths counted in this category:

> A young primigravid woman was known to have acute myeloid leukaemia and is included as an *Indirect* death because of the possibility that pregnancy delayed her treatment. Myeloid leukaemia had been diagnosed and treated one year previously but she then relapsed. While preparations were being made for a bone marrow transplant she was discovered to be 24 weeks pregnant, having conceived while taking the progesterone-only pill. After this, plans for bone marrow transplantation were abandoned. She miscarried nine days after the pregnancy was diagnosed and then developed a fever. In spite of antibiotic treatment she deteriorated and died of sepsis.

It was considered that her care was substandard because pregnancy was not diagnosed between the time that she relapsed and the time of her miscarriage three months later; but it is doubtful if earlier diagnosis would have affected the outcome.

> A multigravid woman had been found to be neutropaenic in her fourth pregnancy and bone marrow examination showed dysplasia with myeloid arrest. She remained well in the (index) pregnancy except for mild infections at various sites including the urinary tract. The neutrophil count varied between 2.3 and 3.2 x10^9/L during pregnancy. She was discharged 12 hours after normal delivery. On day 14 she developed bronchitis and was given antibiotics by her GP. Two days later she was very unwell, was admitted with presumed septicaemia and died the next day despite intensive care therapy. Autopsy confirmed death from septicaemia although no organisms were ever isolated. There were some retained fragments of placenta which may have contributed.

This case is included amongst *Indirect* deaths because of the possibility that pregnancy may have further compromised her existing immunodeficiency.

Diseases of the blood were also involved in two other cases mentioned elsewhere. A case of probable pneumococcal sepsis following splenectomy has already been cited under Infectious Diseases in this Chapter. In addition, one patient with a congenital abnormality of platelet function died from postpartum haemorrhage following caesarean section and is therefore counted in Chapter 4.

Diseases of the central nervous system

Intracranial haemorrhage

There were 24 deaths from intracranial haemorrhage. In addition there were three deaths from cerebral haemorrhage and one from a subarachnoid haemorrhage in association with eclampsia or severe pre-eclampsia counted in Chapter 3. One *Late* death from subarachnoid haemorrhage due to ruptured berry aneurysm is counted in Chapter 14.

Subarachnoid haemorrhage

Fourteen of the deaths were from primary subarachnoid haemorrhage. Eight cases presented before delivery at 15, 16, 22, 27 (two cases), 29, 32 and 34 weeks. One of these had her berry aneurysm clipped at 23 weeks, made a good recovery and then died from a separate brain stem haemorrhage at 29 weeks. Another had a berry aneurysm clipped on the day of her bleed but she suffered a perioperative brain infarct and died 19 days later. In another, mild pre-eclampsia may have been a factor. The remaining cases presented after delivery at between 5 and 23 days. Berry aneurysm was identified in four cases at autopsy or surgery but in the remaining cases no autopsy was performed. This is regrettable and, in at least one case, represents poor care:

> A multigravid patient with known essential hypertension booked in early pregnancy with a blood pressure of 190/140 mmHg. However, this rapidly came under control with antihypertensive drugs and when last checked by her physician at 29 weeks the blood pressure was 130/85 mmHg. Three days later she collapsed and was admitted following a cardiac arrest at home. She was thought to have had a cerebrovascular accident and was certified brain dead on the following day. Death was certified as due to subarachnoid haemorrhage and hypertensive disease of pregnancy. No autopsy was performed.

This is very unsatisfactory since the cause of death is quite unclear. Although the severe essential hypertension was probably a causal factor in the presumed subarachnoid haemorrhage, it was treated appropriately in pregnancy and there was no evidence of hypertensive disease of pregnancy separate from her underlying essential hypertension.

In another patient hypertension was likely to be a causative factor:

> Some years before her pregnancy a woman had received a renal transplant because of end-stage renal disease. During pregnancy her condition deteriorated with hypertension, proteinuria and worsening renal function, and she was delivered by caesarean section at 37 weeks' gestation following a failed induction. She was treated with six different antihypertensive drugs in the puerperium, some in combination. She was discharged 18 days after delivery with her blood pressure "controlled". No details are available of her blood pressure at that time. Five days later she collapsed at home. CT scan on admission showed a subarachnoid haemorrhage with secondary hydrocephaly. She died 12 days later.

The records indicate that the patient often did not take the treatment that had been prescribed for her. One factor may have been the lack of a combined obstetric and medical or renal clinic. The patient was therefore given many hospital appointments, several of which she did not attend.

> In one further case, where the woman presented two days after delivery, death was certified as due to ruptured berry aneurysm caused by hypertension due to unilateral renal agenesis. There is no doubt about the ruptured berry aneurysm or the absent kidney but the maximum blood pressures recorded during antenatal care were 130 mmHg systolic and 90 diastolic and the Assessors have criticised the quality of the autopsy, so renal agenesis may have been an incidental finding.

REPORT ON CONFIDENTIAL ENQUIRIES INTO MATERNAL DEATHS IN THE UNITED KINGDOM

The other patients were not hypertensive or had probably recovered from pregnancy-related hypertension by the time of their subarachnoid haemorrhage. For example:

> One patient was admitted at 36 weeks' gestation because of blood pressure 140/85 mmHg. There was no proteinuria. The serum uric acid rose from 0.40 to 0.44 mmol/L and induction was planned but she went into spontaneous labour. During labour her diastolic blood pressure rose to 105 mmHg and she developed heavy proteinuria. She was delivered by forceps of a healthy child. She was discharged home five days later with blood pressure 110/80 to 135/90 mmHg. She was admitted 10 days after delivery with headache and drowsiness. CT scan showed a large subarachnoid haemorrhage. She rapidly deteriorated and died on the day after admission.

Although this woman had pre-eclampsia it had settled by the time of her discharge and the subsequent subarachnoid haemorrhage was probably not connected.

Substandard care was present in one case, if only because of the lack of information available:

> Following an uncomplicated pregnancy and delivery, a woman went to her GP complaining of headache. Her symptoms were dismissed as minor. Two days later she collapsed and was sent home from the Accident and Emergency department. The next day she was admitted with subarachnoid haemorrhage. A few days later she re-bled and quickly became brain-stem dead.

It may be that she was carefully assessed on the two occasions that she was seen prior to her admission but that seems unlikely. Had subarachnoid haemorrhage been suspected earlier, she could have been admitted sooner and may possibly have had life-saving surgery.

> One patient had a previous postpartum haemorrhage, 18 units of blood transfused and a hysterectomy. Five days later she collapsed and died from a ruptured berry aneurysm. Autopsy also showed that 50% of the pituitary gland was infarcted, presumably consequent on the postpartum haemorrhage. However it is difficult to connect the death from subarachnoid haemorrhage with the traumatic events at the time of delivery.

There was inadequate information to assess one further patient who died 21 days after an uncomplicated delivery and one patient who died at 15 weeks' gestation. The only information given was that they died from subarachnoid haemorrhage.

Cerebral haemorrhage

There were nine deaths thought to be due to primary intracerebral haemorrhage. Six of the haemorrhages occurred before delivery at between 18 and 31 weeks. Two occurred peripartum and one occurred three weeks after delivery. No autopsies were performed on seven of these cases so the diagnoses are insecure and each death could have been caused by subarachnoid haemorrhage. The lack of autopsy information is particularly pertinent in the first two patients:

A young multigravid woman had a normal pregnancy and spontaneous delivery at term. One hour after delivery she developed chest pain and was found to have a blood pressure of 170/120 mmHg. An opiate was given and her symptoms initially settled. Six hours later she collapsed and CT scans showed extensive intracerebral haemorrhage. She died soon after. Her hypertension at presentation could have been due to pre-eclampsia, and without autopsy data pre-eclampsia cannot be excluded.

A multigravid woman with a longstanding psychiatric disorder spent most of her pregnancy in a psychiatric hospital. She was delivered at term and then returned to inpatient psychiatric care. Twenty days later she collapsed and was admitted to a general hospital. She died soon afterwards and death was certified as due to ruptured cerebral aneurysm; but with no autopsy the cause of death is not known with any degree of certainty.

A young woman died from a ruptured cerebellar arterio-venous malformation:

A young primipara collapsed at work at 18 weeks' gestation from a large cerebral haemorrhage secondary to a cerebellar arterio-venous malformation. She was resuscitated but on arrival in A&E it was clear she was profoundly comatose. She was transferred to the care of the neurosurgeons, who drained the haematoma but she did not regain consciousness. She remained unconscious for several months, receiving parenteral support until 34 weeks' gestation, when her condition suddenly deteriorated. An emergency caesarean section was performed with the delivery of a live infant. However, her condition worsened and she died shortly afterwards.

There was no substandard care in this case.

Another woman was noted to have telangiectasia on her lips, so abnormal cerebral blood vessels may have been a factor. However, there was no autopsy.

A woman with known Moya Moya disease had a stroke in labour caused by massive intracerebral haemorrhage. She never recovered and died six weeks later.

In one case where an autopsy was performed it was of poor standard and was not helpful:

The woman had had bronchiectasis and a psychotic illness in the past but her pregnancy seems to have been uneventful. Thirteen hours after a rapid labour and delivery she complained of chest pain and headaches, vomited, developed left-sided weakness and collapsed, dying soon after. Autopsy showed a large intracerebral haemorrhage but there was also extensive intraperitoneal haemorrhage, brain-stem bleeding and "streaky haemorrhage" in the endocardium and first part of the duodenum. There was no comment in the autopsy as to the cause of this widespread haemorrhage. Perhaps the patient had an amniotic fluid embolus.

A Late death counted in Chapter 14 followed pontine haemorrhage from an arterio-venous malformation at 18 weeks' gestation, persistent vegetative state, delivery at 30 weeks and death six months after delivery.

Cerebral thrombosis

There were two deaths from cerebral thrombosis, occurring 6 and 10 days after delivery. No autopsy information is available for either case. It is possible that one case had a post-mortem examination; the other certainly did not. Indeed, it is striking that in the 25 deaths from cerebrovascular disease, there were only five autopsies performed.

Both deaths from cerebral thrombosis were unexpected and there were no risk factors apart from obesity and mild hypertension in one case:

> This occurred suddenly 10 days after a caesarean section for breech presentation in a patient with sickle cell trait. The caesarean section is unlikely to have been related since surgery in general predisposes to venous, not arterial, thrombosis and there was no suggestion that there were abnormal communications between the right and left sides of the heart, such as patent foramen ovale. Sickle cell trait causes thrombosis in association with hypoxia such as may occur with general anaesthesia, but the operation occurred too long before the incident and in any case a spinal anaesthetic was given.

Epilepsy

There were 19 deaths from epilepsy compared to nine in the last Report. There is no obvious reason for this sudden increase. The majority of deaths (14) occurred antenatally, three in the first trimester, one in the second trimester and 10 in the third trimester. The high proportion in the third trimester is likely to be due to multiple factors, such as increased physical stress and the metabolic effects of pregnancy, which in general decrease effective blood levels of anticonvulsant drugs.

Eight of the patients were obese, weighing 80-110 Kg. Although 10 of the patients died from aspiration, including one drowned in the bath, there was no evidence of asphyxiation in the remaining nine. It is poorly appreciated by medical and lay personnel that epileptic fits can be fatal in themselves.

Four patients took no treatment. Carbamazepine monotherapy was used in three patients, and valproate in six patients. The remaining six patients took mixtures of carbamazepine, valproate, vigabatrin, phenytoin and phenobarbitone.

A consultant neurologist or physician was involved in the care of 11 patients during their pregnancy, and drug levels were estimated in at least 10 patients. Four of the patients had major social problems. Although five of the patients had poor control of their epilepsy, this was a minority. For example, two patients died not having had a fit for the previous two years. One patient died having only ever had two minor seizures and these started in the index pregnancy.

Diabetes was an additional factor in one case:

> A known poorly controlled insulin-dependent diabetic who also had epilepsy was found dead in bed at 12 weeks' gestation. Autopsy indicated death from epilepsy without asphyxia but the vitreous humor blood glucose was < 1 mml/L. Since the normal blood glucose in plasma is 3-8 mmol/L, this suggests that hypoglycaemia may have been an additional factor.

One patient may have stopped medication electively:

> The patient was being treated with sodium valproate and had had a previous pregnancy terminated because of a neural tube defect, a known teratogenic effect of the drug. She had been counselled by a consultant neurologist that one option was to taper valproate therapy and then become pregnant once valproate treatment had been discontinued. The patient may have just decided to stop all treatment once she knew that she was pregnant. It should be appreciated that sudden cessation of anticonvulsant drugs can precipitate seizures or even status epilepticus.

Substandard care was present in five cases:

> The hospital was responsible for substandard care in a woman who was living with her extended family and who had had very badly controlled generalised epilepsy since a young age. Her epilepsy was being managed by the GP alone. She became pregnant and continued to take carbamazepine and vigabatrin but the fits remained poorly controlled. At 33 weeks' gestation she was found dead on the floor of her bedroom, having aspirated vomit. Earlier that day the GP had contacted the hospital because the patient had already had eight fits, but her admission was refused.

Earlier CEMD Reports have drawn attention to the dangers of epilepsy in pregnancy. Much less severe epilepsy than this would be an indication for admission.

The emergency services were deficient in the case of a multigravid woman who also had poorly controlled epilepsy and was having fits every day:

> The woman was delivered at term and discharged herself the next day. Fourteen days later she had a series of fits and developed status epilepticus. Her partner called the ambulance service. The ambulance crew arrived 13 minutes later but they estimated her weight to be >100 Kg and did not think they could safely carry her down a narrow staircase whilst she was still fitting. They were not authorised to use Diazemuls (diazepam) in adults, but only in children. An emergency doctor arrived two hours after the 999 call and gave Diazemuls intravenously. On the stretcher she suffered a respiratory arrest and when she was admitted to the A&E Department she was in cardiopulmonary arrest from which she died, having had four further seizures in the next 24 hours.

The emergency service should have been (and is now) authorised to give intravenous Diazemuls in an emergency. It is unfortunate that she did not receive midwifery care in the puerperium and that she had not had specialized medical care for epilepsy in pregnancy but these factors are unlikely to have affected the outcome.

The patient's actions may have contributed to another death from epilepsy:

> She developed epilepsy and was found to have an arterio-venous malformation in the right frontal lobe. She then became pregnant and refused medical and surgical treatment throughout the pregnancy. She was found dead in bed at 37 weeks' gestation. Autopsy showed that there had been no gross acute intracerebral bleeding and there was no brain swelling. Therefore death was considered to be due to an epileptic seizure.

The refusal of anticonvulsant medication and surgery may have led to her death. Her refusal may have been due to the way in which the risks were explained to her.

In two cases it was considered possible that the patients' relatives may have been able to help the woman further if they had had the knowledge and the skill to apply basic first aid principles. It is not clear whether they knew what to do in these circumstances:

> The GP of a known epileptic was called by a relative who said that his patient was having one of her fits and was "slow coming out of it". When he arrived within five minutes, the patient who was 36 weeks pregnant, was lying flat on her back, her airway choked with vomit, and with fixed dilated pupils.

> In another case relatives called the ambulance service because the patient, a known epileptic, was having a seizure. When the ambulance men arrived 10 minutes later, they also found the patient lying face up, "full up with vomit". She too could not be resuscitated.

With knowledge and application of elementary first aid, the relatives might have been able to place the women in the recovery position.

> A known epileptic had her carbamazepine increased from 600 to 800 mg per day when she had two seizures at 27 weeks' gestation. After delivery she was told to decrease her medication by 100 mg/day each week to 400 mg/day. At 17 days she was found dead at home and could not be resuscitated. The post-mortem blood level of carbamazepine was 1.5 mg/Litre, well below the accepted therapeutic range of 4 - 12 mg/Litre.

This is less than optimal care though not substandard. Changes in anticonvulsant therapy should be monitored by blood levels and the reduction in dose after delivery was too rapid. Pre-pregnancy dose requirements are not achieved until 6-8 weeks after delivery.

Guillain-Barré syndrome

> In the second half of her pregnancy a young multigravid woman developed Guillain-Barré syndrome, which was later shown to be due to cytomegalovirus. She was transferred to a neurological unit, where she received immunoglobulin and naso-gastric feeding to protect the airway. Although respiration was impaired, she just avoided elective ventilation and improved sufficiently to allow a vaginal delivery, assisted by ventouse after a three-hour second stage. This occurred in her original obstetric hospital. Later that evening she became very weak and was transferred back to the neurological unit, where she was unable to talk. She was no better the next day and a consultant neurologist sought admission to an ICU without success. On the next day

another neurologist was concerned about her breathing and the possibility of aspiration. An anaesthetist did not think that she required transfer to intensive care. On the next day the patient was very breathless and distressed. Even though she was exhausted and barely able to whisper, she was still not transferred to the local ICU although the staff there did start trying to clear a bed. A few hours later she required emergency intubation on the ward and was transferred to the ICU in a third hospital. She died about two weeks later from adult respiratory distress syndrome (ARDS).

ARDS is not a complication of Guillain-Barré Syndrome *per se*. It arises as a consequence of some insult to the lungs, in this case most likely aspiration. This case represents substandard care. In Guillain-Barré Syndrome, as well as in other conditions, patients should not have to stop breathing before they are intubated and ventilated. It should be possible to anticipate the need but in this case the pressure on ICU beds was too great.

Hypoxic brain damage

A *Late* death occurred in a multigravid woman found unconscious at home and admitted to hospital. There she had several epileptic fits which had not been recorded before. A CT brain scan showed diffuse brain swelling. She died one week later having never regained consciousness. Autopsy showed that she was approximately 18 weeks pregnant, which had not been noted before.

There were no features of eclampsia, either clinically in retrospect, or histologically at autopsy. Brain histology showed features in keeping with severe ongoing hypoxic brain damage, in particular within the cerebellar hemispheres where there was selective loss of Purkinje cells. The cause of hypoxic brain damage was unknown. An extensive toxicological screen was negative. Carbon monoxide poisoning was discounted on clinical grounds.

Diseases of the circulatory system

Aneurysms

Deaths from four aneurysms of the aorta and its branches below the diaphragm are described here. Aneurysms of the aorta and its branches above the diaphragm are described in Chapter 10. There were two deaths from ruptured splenic artery aneurysm:

Substandard care was present in the case of a multigravid woman who collapsed two minutes after spontaneous vaginal delivery at term. Blood loss at delivery was recorded as only 50 ml. The Senior Registrar in anaesthesia was called and resuscitated the patient. Ten minutes later she had recovered and was able to tell of central chest pain at the time of delivery. Blood was taken which showed normal blood gas estimation and no evidence of coagulopathy, but the haemoglobin concentration was 6.2 g%. There was no overt bleeding and the abdomen was soft. The electrocardiogram was normal. A diagnosis was made of amniotic fluid embolism. The consultant in obstetrics visited 40 minutes after the collapse and concurred. Two attempts at central venous pressure line insertion failed. An hour and a half after the initial recovery, she had a cardiac arrest from which she could not be resuscitated. Autopsy showed that death was due to massive intra-abdominal bleeding which was mainly retroperitoneal. The bleeding came from a ruptured aneurysm of the splenic artery. No cause was found for the splenic artery aneurysm. The coronary arteries showed minimal atheroma though the opening of the left coronary artery was small and narrowed. There was no evidence of acute myocardial infarction.

Amniotic fluid embolism is almost invariably accompanied by disseminated intravascular coagulopathy caused by thromboplastins released from the amniotic fluid. The very low haemoglobin concentration was a clue to blood loss that should not have been ignored. Had the clinicians been successful with central venous pressure line insertion, it would have read very low giving a further clue to hypovolaemia, but they should have been prepared to proceed to laparotomy without this information. The chest pain was probably due to cardiac ischaemia secondary to the acute anaemia and low cardiac output.

> An older multigravid woman who stopped smoking in pregnancy booked at 14 weeks' gestation. Her blood pressure was 160/110 mmHg and she started taking methyl dopa with good effect. Subsequent blood pressures were no higher than 150 mmHg systolic and 100 mmHg diastolic. At 32 weeks' gestation her husband telephoned the midwife saying she was in agony with back pain. The midwife could hear her crying in the background so she advised the husband to take the patient into hospital. She arrived in the evening and remained in pain. A "full admission procedure" was undertaken by the midwifery staff. A medical review was requested 90 minutes after admission. She was examined by the doctor ten minutes later, during which examination the patient fainted. At this time the working diagnosis was urinary tract infection. A catheter specimen of urine showed 4+ proteinuria and the obstetric Registrar, reviewing her three hours after admission, added pre-eclampsia to the differential diagnosis, though she was not hypertensive. One hour later pethidine was given for pain relief and she then became pale and clammy, rolling around the bed in pain. Half an hour later the systolic blood pressure was 50 mmHg, the fetus was dead and abruption and amniotic fluid embolism were added to the differential diagnoses. The consultant on call was finally summoned and arrived 5½ hours after she was admitted. He decided to evacuate the uterus by caesarean section. At laparotomy one hour later a large retroperitoneal haematoma was noted. The vascular surgeon was called but cardiac arrest occurred during exploration of the bleeding point. Autopsy showed that she had ruptured an aneurysm of the renal artery.

This represents substandard care. A patient who was clearly so ill should not have waited nearly two hours to see a doctor, a further one hour to see the Registrar and a further 2½ hours to see the consultant. However, the diagnosis was clearly difficult and speedier referral to a more senior doctor might not have made any difference to the eventual outcome.

> An obese multigravid woman who was a heavy smoker was admitted to hospital in the third trimester because of hypertension. While in hospital she woke up with right-sided chest and abdominal pains. She was treated for pulmonary embolism with heparin. Later the same day she collapsed and could not be resuscitated. Autopsy showed that death was due to retroperitoneal haemorrhage from a ruptured aneurysm of the inferior epigastric artery.

Heparin treatment must have contributed to the bleeding that eventually killed the patient but without further knowledge of the clinical circumstances the presumptive diagnosis of pulmonary embolism seems highly plausible.

Ruptured iliac vein

A patient being treated with heparin for proven iliac vein thrombosis collapsed with signs of intra-abdominal bleeding. She died following laparotomy, during which her abdomen was found to be full of blood coming from a spontaneous rupture in an iliac vein. This is a very unusual case.

Air embolism

A couple resumed sexual intercourse five days after the woman had a spontaneous vaginal delivery. During the act of intercourse in the "missionary" position the woman collapsed, had some vaginal bleeding and died. Autopsy showed that death was due to air embolism: on opening the right atrium under water air bubbles were released and there were also air bubbles mixed with blood in the interstices of the right ventricular wall. Numerous tiny air bubbles were found in abdominal and pelvic veins and froth was present in the inferior vena cava.

The blood vessels in the placental bed lining the uterus do not undergo complete involution immediately after childbirth, and sexual intercourse can force air into these vessels in the raw placental bed allowing air bubbles to enter the general circulation. An almost identical case was noted in the last Report. In that case however, the couple were having intercourse in the rear entry position 10 days after delivery and it was postulated that the uterus being above the heart, air may be sucked into the venous circulation. From the current account this is not a necessary factor. Death from air embolism during sexual intercourse is exceptionally rare but these two cases raise the possibility that the early puerperium, when the uterus is not involuted and the cervix is open, may be a particularly risky time for sexual intercourse.

Diseases of the respiratory system

Asthma

There were three deaths from asthma:

A woman with very severe asthma had pregnancy diagnosed during one of her admissions to hospital. Her asthma was being treated with all standard therapies in high dosage, including prednisolone. She had several admissions to hospital during pregnancy, including one precipitated by respiratory arrest. Nevertheless she had a vaginal delivery of an appropriately grown infant at term. She was readmitted with asthma 21 days after delivery, had a cardio-respiratory arrest seven days later and died from hypoxic brain damage 33 days after delivery. Pregnancy probably did not influence her very severe disease.

The second death occurred in a woman who had suffered from asthma as a child but then had no problems until after delivery in the index pregnancy. She became wheezy on day eight and was treated by her GP with antibiotics and inhaled bronchodilators and glucocorticoids with apparently good effect. Six days later she collapsed and died very suddenly. Autopsy showed the typical features of acute severe asthma. The bronchi were plugged with mucus containing eosinophils and Charcot-Leyden crystals. This case illustrates the well-known unpredictable nature of bronchial asthma.

Information is inadequate about the third case. She is known to have died from asthma at 23 weeks' gestation. She also had diabetes and was an infrequent attender; but no further details are available concerning the manner of her death.

Cystic fibrosis

There were two cases counted in this Chapter and one *Late* death is counted in Chapter 14.

A young woman with cystic fibrosis had been under the care of a national centre where she had many admissions for chest infections before and during pregnancy. She was ambivalent about continuing her pregnancy. In the second trimester her chest condition deteriorated during a further episode of infection and she died immediately after a spontaneous abortion, while preparations were being made for termination of pregnancy.

Another patient with cystic fibrosis had been advised of the risks of pregnancy. Her weight at booking was only 44 Kg and forced expiratory volume in one second (FEV_1) was 65% of the predicted value. There were recurrent problems with chest infection. At 24 weeks' gestation she became markedly hypoxaemic despite aggressive antibiotic treatment. She was therefore electively delivered but nevertheless she died about 10 days later from bronchopneumonia.

The *Late* death occurred in a woman who did not always choose to accept her doctor's advice. She had reasonable lung function before pregnancy (FEV_1 1.94 L and vital capacity 3.1 L). She was not unduly thin (54 kg). Nevertheless in pregnancy she dictated her medication, her attendances and nutrition and it was particularly difficult for the physicians to give what they considered to be optimal care. She refused naso-gastric feeding when her weight loss became quite acute. Total parenteral nutrition was considered but she refused this also. From 22 weeks' gestation her respiratory function deteriorated and by 34 weeks' gestation she was transferred from the cystic fibrosis unit to the obstetric ward for an elective caesarean section in an attempt to improve oxygenation and to secure a live child. She received ventilator support for six weeks after delivery and eventually died of septicaemia and acute renal failure.

Because of intensive care in specialist centres, patients with cystic fibrosis are now surviving longer and many women with the condition will wish to have children. It is difficult to predict the maternal outcome in patients who have more than mild disease. In a recent British study[1] of 22 pregnancies in 20 women with cystic fibrosis, four died, up to 3.2 years after delivery. The best predictor of bad maternal outcome was considered to be $FEV_1 < 60\%$. Probable adverse effects of pregnancy are the nutritional demands of pregnancy and the fetus in cystic fibrosis patients who have malabsorption, and the 50 ml/minute extra oxygen consumption of pregnancy, which can be critical in patients with severely limited ventilation. Patients and their attendants need to be aware of the adverse effects of pregnancy on the survival of women with cystic fibrosis.

Pneumonia

A woman was delivered in the private sector and had a postpartum haemorrhage due to atony of the uterus. She was transfused one unit of blood. Three days later she developed a cough and was diagnosed as having lobar pneumonia. She was said to be sensitive to most commonly used antibiotics and so was treated with cotrimoxazole. Two days later a consultant physician saw her and additional bronchodilator drugs were added. She was transferred from the obstetric ward to a medical ward. Although she was thought to be improving, she had a cardiopulmonary arrest two days after transfer. At autopsy she was found to have bilateral lobar pneumonia.

This represents substandard care. Patients should not die in hospital from lobar pneumonia at least without full monitoring in an intensive care environment. Much more aggressive antibiotic therapy should have been given notwithstanding her previous purported antibiotic sensitivity. It is likely that the management of this patient in the private sector contributed to her death: no intensive care facilities were available in the hospital at which she was delivered. Patients who become severely ill in any hospital, including those in the private sector, should be transferred to a hospital where such facilities are available, even if this entails transfer from private to National Health Service facilities.

A woman in a methadone maintenance programme developed, and was treated for, acute bronchitis during the second trimester of her pregnancy. She then developed pneumonia and died shortly after admission to an ICU.

General issues relating to substance abuse and pregnancy are discussed further in Chapter 12.

Diseases of the gastrointestinal system

A woman was readmitted 10 days after delivery because of vaginal bleeding due to retained products of conception. Before she was discharged home she suffered from melaena. She continued to bleed despite multiple surgical procedures and transfusion of about 50 units of blood and died 10 days later. An autopsy demonstrated angio-dysplasia of the ileum and colon. This case is included as an *Indirect* rather than a *Fortuitous* death because of the tendency of blood vessels to rupture and bleed more easily in pregnancy.

Comments

Vascular disease remains an important cause of mortality in pregnancy. In the previous Report there was a total of 20 deaths due to rupture of blood vessels at all sites. In this triennium there were seven aneurysms of the aorta and its branches above the diaphragm and four aneurysms below the diaphragm. At least six of the subarachnoid haemorrhages were due to ruptured berry aneurysm, giving a total of at least 17 cases. The health care team must be aware of this risk and be prepared to act appropriately.

The increasing mortality from epilepsy is worrying. Health care workers should be aware that epilepsy is a potentially fatal illness that can kill even if the patients do not aspirate. The public, and in particular relatives of those suffering from epilepsy, need better instruction in basic first aid. GPs and midwives could check with relatives that they know what to do in the event of a fit and provide instruction. In addition, one case mentioned in this Report was found dead in her bath, as was one patient in the 1991-93 Report. Patients are at increased risk of syncope during and after pregnancy and hot baths can precipitate syncope which, in itself, can cause epileptic seizures. Epileptic seizures while bathing carry the obvious risk of drowning. If possible, women with epilepsy should shower rather than take baths during pregnancy.

Overwhelming sepsis from pneumococcal, streptococcal and meningococcal infection continues to kill pregnant women. The four cases reported in this triennium died very quickly. Only high-dose antibiotic therapy with penicillin, or erythromycin for those sensitive to penicillin, given before the results of microbial investigation are available could have saved them, though one patient who had a splenectomy probably would not have got the infection if she had been given prophylactic penicillin.

Lack of intensive care beds remains a factor in these *Indirect* deaths but so too does lack of communication between obstetricians and intensive care unit staff. Early communication in patients who are sick will optimise the use of such scarce resources. This is particularly important for young pregnant women, such as the one dying from Guillain-Barré Syndrome, who have the capacity to make a complete recovery.

As in other cases of maternal mortality, substandard care was evident when experienced personnel were not called in quickly enough to see women who were obviously ill. To obtain experienced consultant advice from disciplines other than obstetrics, such as medicine and anaesthesia, better links will have to be established between obstetric and other departments. This will involve appointing more consultant anaesthetists and physicians with special interests in pregnancy.

Reference

1.   Edenborough, F.P Stableforth, D.E. Webb, A.K. Mackenzie, W.E. & Smith, D.L. Outcome of pregnancy in women with cystic fibrosis. *Thorax* 1995; **50**:170-4.

12

DEATHS FROM PSYCHIATRIC CAUSES:
SUICIDE AND SUBSTANCE ABUSE

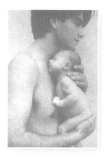

CHAPTER 12
DEATHS FROM PSYCHIATRIC CAUSES: SUICIDE AND SUBSTANCE ABUSE

Summary

This new Chapter discusses all maternal deaths notified to the Enquiry due to psychiatric causes. It probably does not cover all such deaths which occurred during this triennium, as some may not have been coded, or considered, as primarily having a psychiatric cause, and others may not have been notified as maternal deaths and may thus remain unknown to the Assessors. However, valuable lessons may be drawn from the cases discussed in this Chapter. It is hoped that all similar deaths will be reported to future Enquiries and better information will be provided about the non-obstetric care in each case. This Chapter aims to identify possible common factors underlying the reported deaths and to suggest ways in which improvements in care may be implemented.

Twenty-eight deaths are reviewed in this Chapter and the likely cause in almost all cases was an intentional act, although in cases of overdose in the context of substance abuse it is not always possible to exclude an accident.

Psychiatric causes of death: key recommendations

A relatively simple procedure should be instituted in every antenatal clinic to identify women at risk of postnatal depression and/or self harm.

Commissioners and providers of primary care, maternity and psychiatric services should consider the identification in each district of a clinician who would be responsible on a sessional basis for managing a perinatal mental health service.

In future, the collection of pertinent psychiatric and other relevant information about cases of completed maternal suicide may be greatly improved by the adoption of the classic method of psychological autopsy .

Details were available for eight cases of suicide considered to be *Indirect* maternal deaths, and there was only a death certificate for a ninth, and hence unevaluated, case. Five of the *Indirect* deaths occurred during pregnancy. Fourteen deaths are counted in Chapter 14 as *Late Indirect* because they occurred after 42 days post-partum, but little or no information was available for three of these. Furthermore there were five cases of substance abuse which are also discussed here and counted by convention either in Chapters 13 or 14 as *Fortuitous* or *Late Fortuitous* deaths. Overall, there seems to have been a slight increase since 1991-93 when 19 of 228 maternal deaths were linked to psychiatric illness and substance abuse. This change is probably due to improved ascertainment.

In relative numerical terms, therefore, *Indirect* and *Late Indirect* deaths due to psychological causes including substance abuse (classed as *Fortuitous*) are at least as important as those directly due to hypertensive disorders of pregnancy, of which there are 20 in this triennium. In the opinion of this Enquiry, classification of such deaths as *Indirect*, *Late* and *Fortuitous* can result in misleading first impressions of apparently low maternal mortality rates from psychiatric causes (see Table 1.1) and it can also be argued that such conventions do not meaningfully apply to such deaths. An important objective of future Enquiries should be to improve the identification of risk factors for maternal suicide during pregnancy and the entire first postnatal year. In some instances the mental illnesses may have their origins in the childbearing process, in others, pregnancy and childbirth may provoke a recurrence of illness or they may exacerbate problems associated with chronic mental illness, disability, or substance abuse. The presence of mental illness is a significant risk factor but, as with the assessment of suicide risk generally, there are additional factors which must also be taken into account.

Psychiatric illness is implicated in about 10% of maternal deaths and, given that pregnancy and the puerperium are times of repeated contact with health professionals, it should be possible to identify vulnerable women most at risk and to prevent at least some maternal deaths in this category. Childbearing, and particularly the post-partum period, are associated with a steep rise in the incidence and prevalence of both psychotic[1] and non-psychotic affective illness[2]. About 2 in every 1,000 mothers experience a psychotic breakdown, with an onset mainly in the first two weeks after delivery, almost always necessitating psychiatric intervention and usually admission to hospital[3]. Non-psychotic depressive disorder begins most commonly in the first month after delivery[4], but the onset is more insidious and spread out in time in comparison with psychotic breakdowns, and the contributory causal factors are predominantly psychosocial, i.e. early childhood traumas, disturbed family relationships, marital problems, lack of support, social adversity, or stressful life events. Post-partum psychosis, on the other hand, appears primarily to arise out of a physiological vulnerability[5,6] and the most powerful predictor is a previous history of affective psychosis, which elevates the risk of post-partum breakdown from 0.2% to between 25 and 50%[7,8]. The third group of childbearing women 'at risk' comprises those who suffer from chronic mental and behavioural illnesses and in whom the difficulties of being the primary carer for the newborn baby may cause concern, especially if the mother is single and unsupported. Commonest among such cases are women with disorders such as chronic schizophrenia, substance abuse, severe learning disability and personality disorders[9].

The most striking fact is that despite the clearly elevated rates of mental illness in childbearing women, the risks of completed suicide and of self harm are markedly reduced[10,11]. The presence of a young and dependent child is therefore probably protective. In spite of this, suicide continues to account for a significant proportion of maternal deaths. Childbearing women who do complete suicide tend to do so by violent means and, as with most cases of suicide, there are warning signals beforehand, such as severe depression with suicidal ideation, a recent attempt at self-harm and evidence of planning, as well as a clutch of associated risk factors, e.g., recent adverse life events, social isolation and lack of support. Furthermore, the suicide rate amongst intravenous drug users is raised thirtyfold and substance misuse in patients with histories of self-harm is a powerful predictor of eventual suicide[12]. Some, at least, of these deaths may be preventable.

During pregnancy and after childbirth a mother regularly has contact with obstetricians, midwives, GPs, health visitors, paediatricians, occasionally social workers and, rarely, psychiatrists. For a variety of reasons, e.g. failure to recognize psychiatric disorder, lack of communication, or lack of resources in the context of other priorities, there is a risk that many mental health problems in childbearing women will remain undetected, or if they are picked up, there is no obvious mechanism or line of responsibility for dealing with them. Vigorous efforts are being made to develop obstetric services that are more sensitive and responsive to women's needs and there is, therefore, an opportunity to improve the detection of risk not only to prevent some of the tragic loss of life but also to improve the welfare of mentally ill mothers and their babies generally. Suicide prevention cannot work in isolation from efforts to improve prevention and treatment of maternal psychiatric disorders and their sequelae.

Deaths from suicide

Deaths during pregnancy

There were five *Indirect* deaths recorded during pregnancy:

> The first was that of a woman who was admitted in a coma in the first trimester of pregnancy, having taken an overdose of paracetamol. She aborted while unconscious and died of acute cardio-respiratory and liver failure. She had been seen only once prior to the overdose, in the previous week, for booking by a community midwife. From the little information available it appeared that she had previous pregnancies that had not gone to term, but her records provided no further information. There was a mention in the various post-mortem reports that she was in a relationship and that there was a history of domestic violence.

In the absence of information about her previous gynaecological, medical, social and psychiatric history it is impossible to know what were the underlying causes of death, or whether her care was in any way substandard through lack of identification of, or inadequate liaison about, a possible suicide risk.

> The second woman was experiencing domestic difficulties and had a young child. She had a history of substance abuse and was maintained on methadone but, in addition, was HIV positive. She had been admitted to a medical ward in the early weeks of this pregnancy and a termination was being arranged. Despite her problems she was receiving good support from her family and the community AIDS team and during her brief stay in the medical ward she gave no indications of depression or of suicidal ideas. A week after admission she was found hanged.

In the third case, an older single primiparous woman had a long history of depression, alcohol dependence and substance misuse. She had taken several overdoses in the previous few years and several days before her death, early in her pregnancy, had been admitted to hospital unconscious, having taken another overdose. She had been followed up regularly by her GP and daily by the community drug and alcohol team and she was ambivalent about accepting admission for detoxification. She was unemployed and in debt and although it was recorded that she had an earlier long-term relationship, there was no information about the circumstances of this conception and pregnancy. She had not yet started antenatal care. She was found dead at home by a friend and there appears to have been no post-mortem examination. Therefore the most likely cause of death was probably an overdose of drugs and or alcohol.

She appeared to have received intensive support from her GP and community team in the time leading up to her death, but there is very little information about what might have precipitated the two overdoses nine days apart, the last being fatal.

Similarly, little information is available concerning the fourth case. This was a young primipara with a recent history of depression, who was taking antidepressant medication at the time of conception. She had discontinued this by the time of booking. She was not perceived as being depressed at this stage in her pregnancy, either by her GP or community midwife, who, presumably, were responsible for much of her antenatal care. Apparently she did not seek specific help. She hanged herself in the second trimester of pregnancy.

The report form for this case provides no information about her previous history or mental health, or her social circumstances, and it is not possible to rule out substandard care in this case.

The fifth case was that of another single primigravida who was known to suffer from schizophrenia. She was receiving depot antipsychotic medication from her GP and was being monitored by the community psychiatric team. She appeared happy to be pregnant but in the midtrimester she was admitted to a psychiatric hospital having taken an overdose following an argument with her boyfriend. Five days later she left hospital against advice and was followed up by a community psychiatric nurse. Her dose of antipsychotic medication had meanwhile been slightly reduced, but it is doubtful whether this would have had any significant detrimental effect on her mental state or whether the drug was rendered any less potentially harmful to the fetus. This patient was known to have taken overdoses in the past and she had previously threatened to kill herself by jumping from a height. She was found dead from head injuries, some weeks later, having fallen from the building in which she lived.

It seems likely that in this last case there was inadequate liaison between the various professionals engaged in her care, for example, the GP, community psychiatric social worker, community psychiatric nurse (CPN), community midwife and hospital-based obstetric and midwifery services. The risks of suicide do not seem to have been fully recognised and managed in someone with a history of self harm and at least one threat of death by violent means. She was also someone who was suffering from a chronic and severe mental illness, living alone and coping with pregnancy and possible single parenthood.

Comments on deaths occurring during pregnancy

The information that is available to Assessors is often sketchy and is at times entirely lacking. Such a paucity of information is entirely understandable if the mother has not yet made contact with antenatal services or has only just booked. In other cases there is evidence of a lack of liaison between various professionals and thus, although there may have been awareness of problems in one part of the health care system, e.g. the GP, the health visitor, the community psychiatrist, the CPN, or the community drug team, there is often a failure to articulate the various components of the service. Similarly, obstetricians and midwives may not recognise possible added pressures on a mentally ill mother during a pregnancy which often occurs in the context of marital problems. In this small series, substance abuse was prominent in the histories of two of the five women who died in pregnancy but the lack of an autopsy makes the precise cause of death uncertain. Two of the women also had recent histories of parasuicide or serious threats, and three deaths were by violent means, hanging or falling from a height.

Deaths after delivery

There were four *Indirect* deaths within six weeks of delivery and 14 *Late Indirect* deaths. No details, other than the death certificate, were available for one *Indirect* and two *Late Indirect* cases. A depressive illness was noted in 11 cases as a significant background factor and in five instances there may have been associated psychotic symptoms. In many cases there were warnings which seemed to have been unheeded.

Indirect deaths

> In the first, a woman became very depressed and suicidal in the second week after a forceps delivery. She had been anxious about the baby's feeding but had been reassured by the midwife. Some days later her husband called the community midwife for help; because she was depressed and suicidal and during the night she had tried to hang herself. The onset had been ominously sudden. The next day the GP found her mood to be inappropriate and blank . A psychiatrist assessed her and she refused the offer of admission to a general psychiatric ward. A bed was found in a nearby mother and baby unit and she again refused this. She was not felt to be psychotic. Her family offered to be with her at all times and visits by a CPN were arranged. The next day, she slipped out of home alone and jumped to her death from a tall building.

It is difficult to evaluate the standard of care given in this case. With hindsight one might say that she should have been admitted compulsorily under a section of the Mental Health Act. She had already tried to hang herself at home the day before her death, had become suddenly and severely depressed and her mood had been noted at one time to be odd and blank. There was also a family history of suicide. On the other hand, she was thoroughly assessed by her GP and by a psychiatrist, her family were willing to be with her at all times and plans were made to monitor her with daily visits by the CPN and midwives. It is considered that, overall, a balanced decision was made and a thorough assessment and care plan were undertaken.

The second case was that of an older primipara who delivered her first baby at term. There was a reference in her notes that she had been depressed, but no relevant information was available. It is not known whether she had a history of previous suicide attempts. She drowned herself six weeks after the delivery, having left a suicide note.

Like other cases, there was a lack of information about the nature and severity of depression or about the personal, social and domestic context in which the mother became depressed and then suicidal. It is not possible, therefore, to comment on the standard of non-obstetric care in this case.

A young married woman who had a history of depression was found dead some days after the birth of her first child, having fallen from a multi-storey car park. There were no comments about her mental condition following the birth and it is not meaningful to assess the standard of her care.

The only information regarding the fourth case was that given on the death certificate.

Late Indirect deaths

A woman with a history of infertility and a previous miscarriage after assisted conception, had a pregnancy following a normal conception which resulted in the birth of a healthy child. It appears she was not living with the father of the child. The notes make reference to social isolation, previous work stress and a lack of pleasure in motherhood. At two months postpartum she was prescribed an antidepressant of the serotonin selective reuptake inhibitor type (SSRI). There appeared to have been no warning of any suicidal act but four months after the birth she hanged herself.

It is likely that the standard of care was adequate, but in the absence of a detailed history this is not certain.

A young single woman died by hanging a few months after the birth of her first baby. There was very little information about this case. She had had two antenatal admissions, one for abdominal pain following an altercation with the police and one following postcoital vaginal bleeding. She rapidly discharged herself against advice after the latter admission. There was a history of several previous overdoses of paracetamol and one of wrist cutting.

The lack of details relating to this case makes it impossible to draw any conclusions as to why she committed suicide. Little seems to be known of her current circumstances, her mental state and her psychiatric history. Nor is there a record of any post-natal care. She is grouped with cases of 'postnatal depression', but this is based on inference. The lack of information may possibly reflect sub-standard care by professionals involved in this woman's care.

A multiparous mother had a long history of episodic psychotic depression which had recurred after previous births. She became severely depressed again following the birth of her next child and was admitted to a mother and baby unit. She tried to electrocute herself and admitted to staff that she felt like throwing herself under a car. Pharmacological and psychological treatment and rehabilitation were started. Following discharge home she received intensive community support, but she remained depressed and coped poorly, expressing intermittent suicidal ideas. About five months after the birth of the baby neither she nor another of her children could be found at home and they were both later discovered drowned.

REPORT ON CONFIDENTIAL ENQUIRIES INTO MATERNAL DEATHS IN THE UNITED KINGDOM

There may have been a delay in engaging the help of social services and her care package in the community may have been unfocused. Only a more detailed enquiry might show whether her psychiatric care had, in general terms, been of an adequate standard and whether sufficient heed had been paid to her impulse to kill herself by violent means.

A woman had an uncomplicated pregnancy until the eighth month, when she was briefly admitted under the care of a psychiatrist with an acute depressive illness. This was treated by a tricyclic antidepressant, and she received follow-up and support. She delivered the baby normally, but some months later she again became severely depressed. There may have been some associated psychotic symptoms as she was treated with haloperidol in addition to the antidepressant which she was taking when discharged home. Seven months postnatally she died of an overdose of her antidepressant and of procyclidine which she usually took to counter extrapyramidal symptoms due to haloperidol.

Again the records do not give full details of her social and family history, her current circumstances, or whether she had shown psychotic features before. One does not know if she had expressed suicidal ideas or impulses, or had a previous history of self-harm. It is not clear how this *Late* death was related to pregnancy and childbirth, or whether her psychiatric care was of an adequate standard.

A woman who had children by a previous relationship had an unplanned but eventually wanted pregnancy. She had a history of an overdose. She became depressed three months after the delivery and was prescribed an antidepressant which was changed following partial improvement and then maintained, possibly by repeat prescription, as it was recorded that she was not seen again. Several months later she was found dead of carbon monoxide poisoning.

A married woman had suffered from postnatal depression after earlier pregnancies and had been depressed at the beginning of the next pregnancy. She had been taking an antidepressant which she stopped on discovering the pregnancy. She was noted to be anxious during the pregnancy, but not pathologically so. She declined genetic investigations which had been offered on account of her age. A week after delivery there was a mention of altered affect and a "hint of elation", but no signs of depression were noted within the next month. There were no further records but her autopsy report mentioned that she had been admitted to hospital four months postnatally for treatment of depression and two weeks later, while still in hospital, was found dead, hanged.

A multiparous woman who had a history of anaemia, depression, overdoses and alcohol dependence gave birth to a baby who required admission to the neonatal unit for some days. The pregnancy had been monitored, having been considered to be "at risk". In the two weeks following delivery there were notes of several rows with the baby's father, and an attendance at the Casualty Department where a psychiatric referral was requested, possibly because she had resumed heavy drinking. She left before seeing anyone. Two days later, because she had not been seen, her partner contacted social services and on breaking into her flat they found her alone, dead for some time of an overdose of chlormethiazole.

It is not clear what arrangements had been made for the care of her other children, or the extent of the involvement of social services. It would be helpful to know what follow-up had been arranged of this volatile, and probably difficult, alcohol-dependent patient with a low birth weight baby. It is difficult to believe that the care of this case, and probably the two preceding ones, had been of an acceptably high standard.

> A multipara died of multiple injuries including skull fractures following a fall from the roof of her home. There was no information about her obstetric or postnatal care, the delivery or the age of her baby at the time of her death. This case is categorised as a *Late Indirect* death. A psychiatric report to the Coroner recorded that the patient had been known to psychiatric services for about five years, having developed postnatal depression following the birth of her first child. She responded well to treatment which included antidepressants. She had a recurrence of depression after her second child was born and she received counselling and antidepressants for much of the next two years. She then had a miscarriage, became severely depressed and was admitted to a psychiatric hospital following an overdose of antidepressants and paracetamol. Following a consultation with a private practitioner she received a course of progesterone with apparent initial benefit during her third pregnancy. She was readmitted postnatally to hospital as a suicide risk and progesterone was restarted. Her mood seemed to be improving and she appeared to be coping well with her baby. It is not clear whether she was still an inpatient when she killed herself.

The information supplied in the report gave no indication that suicidal risk had been fully assessed. Furthermore, the use of progesterone as an antidepressant gives serious cause for concern as, in this context, the hormone is of unproven efficacy. Its use during pregnancy can also be questioned. The non-obstetric care of this patient was probably substandard.

> A very young woman, who was seriously overweight and had a history of epilepsy and associated auditory and visual hallucinations, was seen repeatedly by midwives in her second pregnancy. Her partner was much older than she was. She presented at 30 weeks' gestation claiming to be in labour and delivered a placenta but denied having delivered a baby. She was treated pharmacologically for depression. One week later she complained of double vision and, following investigation, a diagnosis of benign intracranial hypertension was made. One month later she was found lost and confused. She had further investigations but a week later, three months after the delivery of the placenta, she doused herself with petrol, set fire to herself and died.

This was not a case of concealed pregnancy but the baby was not found. The causes for many of her actions are not clear. There are no notes describing her premorbid personality nor her level of comprehension. Neither is much information available about her relationship with her partner. It is not clear if the subsequent police investigation placed her under severe stress and one can only speculate about the part that her previous and current organic brain syndrome might have played in her suicide. There is insufficient information to comment with certainty about the adequacy of care. However, there did not seem to be any urgency to try to tie together the unusual circumstances of the delivery of the placenta, her personal and psychiatric history and the organic brain syndrome. Thus it is likely that investigation and management of this case were sub-standard.

Only the death certificate was available for the other cases of *Late Indirect* deaths due to suicide.

REPORT ON CONFIDENTIAL ENQUIRIES INTO MATERNAL DEATHS IN THE UNITED KINGDOM

Death following termination of pregnancy

In this case a woman killed herself by inhaling car exhaust fumes some months after a termination of pregnancy for severe chromosomal abnormality at 19 weeks' gestation. There was a clear background history of family and marital problems, of adjustment problems, of previous terminations for psychological reasons, of depression and of suicidal threats for which she had seen a psychiatrist about two months after the most recent termination. She had been counselled about the chromosomal abnormality and had been offered support after the termination but did not take this up. The suicide was premeditated but in the days leading up to it the family were unaware of any depression or of suicidal intent. She had been discharged back to the care of her GP by the psychiatrist some three months previously.

Chronic mental illness

Two cases differ from the others reported here in that both had histories of chronic mental illness:

The first was a multiparous woman with several children, whose partner suffered from schizophrenia. There was a suggestion that she was also a schizophrenic but her summary notes suggest otherwise. She seemed to have suffered from recurrent depression for many years with numerous hospital admissions. She had, however, occasionally been treated with antipsychotic drugs. On this occasion she was admitted some days after delivery because she had become depressed and suicidal when her partner left her. She was discharged after a month of intensive rehabilitation and treatment with antidepressant and antipsychotic medication. However, three months later she was readmitted following a family dispute. She was depressed but her consultant psychiatrist did not judge her to be suicidal or psychotic. She was prescribed antidepressants, went home on leave and brought back a bottle of antipsychotic tablets (chlorpromazine) which she took as an overdose while in hospital. She was transferred to the local general hospital but went into a coma and subsequently died of cardiac arrest. She was receiving appropriate care and although she had previously presented risk factors for suicide she had not apparently been considered to be actively at risk at the time she was allowed home and following her return to the psychiatric ward.

Clinical staff are required regularly to balance risk against efforts to rehabilitate patients and from the available information it does not seem that her care was substandard.

The second case was a woman who had a longstanding history of manic depressive illness and of several overdoses. She became depressed about six months after delivery and when she was seen by her GP she was felt not to be suicidal. She was referred to a CPN but died of an overdose of tricyclic antidepressant medication the day before the appointment. She had come off her maintenance lithium three months before she conceived this pregnancy, and given the risks of postnatal relapse of manic depression it is unclear why this was not restarted.

Given her history of chronic mental illness it is surprising she was not being monitored routinely by her community psychiatric team. There are sufficient causes for concern to suggest that from a psychiatric point of view the care of this woman was substandard.

Comments on deaths after delivery

These cases exemplify the importance of taking seriously suicidal ideation and histories of self-harm, substance abuse, depression, chronic mental illness, severe environmental stress, disturbed close interpersonal relationships, isolation and lack of support. Plans to kill oneself, especially by violent means, are also a grave warning sign. Seven of the cases reviewed died by violent means.

Substance abuse

Recreational or regular substance misuse was implicated in five deaths.

Butane poisoning

Two teenage mothers died of butane poisoning:

> In the first, both she and her partner were unemployed and lived in a friend's flat. She had been delivered by elective caesarean section. She was found dead in bed following a fall when her baby was three months old. The baby had been in hospital for some time due to congenital malformations and it is unclear whether the baby was back with the mother when she died. The precise cause of death was uncertain; there were no external signs of head injury and the presence of butane in the blood was thought to have been responsible. There was no information recorded about previous substance abuse or about her psychiatric or medical history, family and social circumstances.

> The second teenager was of school age and had booked late at the antenatal clinic. She had attended an educational unit for teenage mothers in the last trimester of pregnancy and returned to the parental home one day after a normal delivery. There was no record of any special postnatal follow-up, e.g. from social services, which might have been expected given the antenatal referral for special schooling. About five months after delivery she and a friend obtained a butane gas lighter cylinder and they both sniffed it. She rapidly became ill and could not be resuscitated. As with the other case of butane poisoning there was no known history of substance abuse and no outstanding warning signs indicative of suicide risk. It is not clear if this was an isolated incident of solvent abuse that went tragically wrong or part of a pattern of regular use.

Overdose of heroin/methadone

The other three deaths occurred in women who were known heroin users being maintained on methadone. One death occurred during pregnancy. In the two cases occurring after delivery there is a suspicion that the overdose may have been intentional.

> The woman who died during pregnancy was a multipara who had been deserted some years earlier, her partner having taken the child. Several years later she had a second child but the available records do not record paternity, or the child's whereabouts. She had a history of IV drug abuse but was now maintained on methadone. The father of the expected baby was also

a drug user and was living with her. She received shared GP and hospital antenatal care and had been seen several times antenatally. The consultant obstetrician judged the pregnancy to be high risk, warranting monitoring by the hospital. At about 20 weeks' gestation she was admitted semi-conscious, with pneumonia, and she died a week later. There was no autopsy. It was considered that she may have been using IV drugs again and may have taken an overdose.

The cause of the pneumonia is not clear, nor is it known whether there was any liaison between staff at the drug clinic, who must have been regulating her methadone, and the obstetric and medical team. Her GP recalled her as being a helpless and fatalistic individual, but it is unclear whether she was receiving any form of psychological support or whether she had expressed any suicidal ideas prior to her death. Once again, the lack of relevant information militates against attempts to judge whether her non-obstetric care was of an adequate standard.

> The first of the two opiate-dependent women who died after delivery was in her mid-twenties She had had a previous miscarriage and had booked early and attended the antenatal clinic regularly. She was maintained on methadone but continued intermittently to use IV heroin. Despite intensive supervision from her consultant obstetrician the baby died *in utero* at 39 weeks and was delivered stillborn following induction of labour. The mother expressed guilt about her part in the baby's death but her partner blamed the staff. Her partner was then arrested in connection with drugs and she was victimised by neighbours. She continued to receive maintenance methadone but there was no evidence of any bereavement counselling following the stillbirth, or of liaison between the drug services, GP, health visitor and obstetrician. She was still using heroin and six months after the stillbirth she died of heroin overdose, confirmed on post-mortem examination. It is not clear if this was intentional or an accident.

Her obstetrician, who had provided exemplary personal care throughout, had thought she was not suicidal when he saw her some weeks after the delivery, but she was exposed to severe stress and was apparently not receiving support and counselling. She had lost a baby, her partner was in prison, she was under pressure from neighbours and she was maintained on methadone and was injecting heroin as well. As with all such cases a fuller enquiry would almost certainly be helpful but it seems reasonable to regard this as a *Late* death, indirectly related to the stillbirth. It is not possible meaningfully to comment on the standard of non-obstetric care other than to suspect that there had not been effective liaison between the various agencies and professionals involved in her care.

> The final woman was single and a known heroin addict, maintained on methadone. She booked very late and next turned up in labour. She was later found dead at home of a methadone overdose four months after the birth of the baby. The information on her family and social background was limited. She had declined an offer of paediatric follow-up, but it is not clear whether there had been any concerns on the part of social services about the safety and welfare of the baby. It is quite possible the overdose was intentional and the very large plasma concentration at autopsy supports this supposition.

Comments

Psychiatric illness leading to suicide is a significant factor in at least 10% of maternal deaths.

Suicide was four times more likely to occur in the nine months after childbirth than during pregnancy.

In this triennium, as in more robust epidemiological studies[10,12], there was no clear preponderance of early deaths, i.e in the first month after birth, but the numbers are small. The majority of postnatal suicides were *Late,* by which time these women had left the obstetric and midwifery services. Nevertheless, given that most of them had been in repeated contact with maternity services there may have been opportunities for prevention that were missed.

Violent suicides appear more common in childbearing women who commit suicide than in the population generally.

In many cases suicides were successful despite awareness of recognised risk factors (e.g. severe depression, substance abuse, chronic mental illness, recent attempts at self-harm). This profile is similar to that found generally among mentally ill patients who kill themselves [13,14]. Suicidal ideation, threats and recent acts appeared often in the current small sample of childbearing women who went on to complete suicide.

In many cases there appeared to have been inadequate liaison between the various agencies involved in a woman's care, and very often the evidence was not available to judge whether care provided by relevant non-obstetric services was substandard. Given the lack of information it would be unsafe to assume that there was an adequate standard of care in all cases and it is likely that there were failures to recognise and respond to suicide risk.

Recommendations

A relatively simple procedure should be instituted in every antenatal clinic to identify women at risk of self harm. At booking, brief details should be taken by the midwife about the presence or history of maternal psychiatric disorder, alcohol and substance abuse, severe social problems and previous self harm. Such techniques are currently being piloted in selected hospitals, and evidence of their efficacy or otherwise should be available in the relatively near future. There is, however, little point in screening for mental health problems in childbearing women if specialist support services are not in place.

Commissioners and providers of primary care, maternity and psychiatric services should consider the identification in each district of a clinician - probably, but not necessarily, a psychiatrist - who would be responsible on a sessional basis for managing a perinatal mental health service. With limited infrastructure support, such a person would have the responsibility for putting in place procedures for screening and subsequent evaluation of cases, followed, where appropriate, by effective liaison, i.e., with existing primary care, community mental health and social services, linking these up with maternity care. The size and nature of such a liaison service for childbearing women will depend to some extent on local demographic factors but it is not difficult to estimate the need, based on current knowledge of prevalence of mental illness in childbearing women.

REPORT ON CONFIDENTIAL ENQUIRIES INTO MATERNAL DEATHS IN THE UNITED KINGDOM

A liaison service of this nature cannot be expected to carry a large case-load but rather it should serve as a resource to which difficult cases may be referred for assessment and also as a focus for co-ordinating the efforts of relevant clinical and other services in the community, for example in relation to women with chronic psychiatric illnesses, histories of substance abuse etc. The presence of such a service will also heighten awareness of postnatal depression amongst professionals in the primary care sector. One of the main objectives must be to avoid and overcome discontinuities of care as a mentally ill woman and her baby pass through maternity and paediatric services and back into the community.

In future, the collection of pertinent psychiatric and other relevant information about cases of maternal suicide may be greatly improved by the adoption of the classic method of psychological autopsy [15,16].

References

1. Kendell, R. E. Chalmers, J. C. & Platz, C. Epidemiology of puerperal psychosis. *British Journal of Psychiatry* 1987: **150**: 662-73.

2. O'Hara, M. W. & Swain, A. M. Rates and risk of postpartum depression - a meta-analysis. *International Review of Psychiatry* 1996: **8**: 37-54.

3. Oates, M. Psychiatric services for women following childbirth. *International Review of Psychiatry* 1996: **8**: 87-98.

4. Cox, J. L., Murray, D. & Chapman, G. A controlled study of the onset, duration and prevalence of postnatal depression. *British Journal of Psychiatry* 1993: **163**: 27-31.

5. Kumar, R. Postnatal mental illness: a transcultural perspective. *Social Psychiatry and Psychiatric Epidemiology* 1994: **29**: 250-64.

6. Wieck, A., Kumar, R., Hirst, A. D., Marks, M. N., Campbell, I. C. & Checkley, S. A. Increased sensitivity of dopamine receptors and recurrence of affective psychosis after childbirth. *British Medical Journal* 1991: **303**: 613-16.

7. Brockington, I. *Maternal Mental Health*. Oxford: Oxford University Press; 1996.

8. Marks, M.N., Wieck, A., Checkley, S.A., Kumar, R. Contribution of psychological and social factors to psychiatric and non-psychiatric relapse after childbirth in women with previous histories of affective disorder. *Journal of Affective Disorders* 1992: **29**: 253-64.

9. Kumar, R. & Hipwell. Implications for the Infant of Maternal Puerperal Psychiatric Disorders. In Rutter, M., Taylor, E. & Hersov, L. (eds) *Child & Adolescent Psychiatry 3rd Edition*. Oxford: Blackwell. 1994: 759-75.

10. Appleby, L. Suicide during pregnancy and in the first postnatal year. *British Medical Journal* 1991: **302**: 137-40.

11. Appleby, L. & Turnbull, G. Parasuicide in the first postnatal year. *Psychological Medicine* 1995: **25**: 1087-90.

12. Hogberg, U., Innala, E. & Sandstrom, A. Maternal mortality in Sweden. *Obstetrics and Gynecology* 1994: **84**: 241-44.

13. Hawton, K., Fag, J., Plait, S. et al. Factors associated with suicide after parasuicide in young people. *British Medical Journal* 1993: **306**: 1641-44.

14. Appleby, L. *National Confidential Inquiry into Suicide and Homicide by people with Mental Illness*. Progress Report 1997. London: Department of Health.

15. Barraclough, B., Bunch, J., Nelson, B. et al. A hundred cases of suicide: Clinical aspects. *British Journal of Psychiatry* 1974: **125**: 355-73.

16. Medical Research Council. *Suicide and Parasuicide*. MRC Topic Review. London: MRC: 1995.

13
FORTUITOUS DEATHS

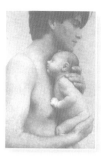

CHAPTER 13
FORTUITOUS DEATHS

Summary

In this triennium 36 *Fortuitous* deaths occurring during pregnancy or within 42 days of delivery or termination were notified to the Enquiry. These are shown in Table 13.1. In addition, there were 36 *Late Fortuitous* deaths discussed in Chapter 14. The figures for the previous triennium were 46 *Fortuitous* and 15 *Late Fortuitous* deaths.

Fortuitous deaths are coincidental deaths unconnected with pregnancy or the puerperium which occur before delivery or up to 42 days postpartum. By international definition they are not considered maternal deaths and do not contribute to maternal mortality statistics. However, *Fortuitous* deaths still have important implications for the management of certain non-pregnancy related conditions, such as co-incidental carcinomatosis, or for more general public health issues such as guidance for the use of seat belts in pregnancy. They also highlight the fatal outcome of some episodes of domestic violence. For these reasons, this Chapter, for the first time, includes sections on road traffic accidents and domestic violence. Issues for the training of midwives, such as in caring for women with terminal cancer, are discussed in Chapter 16.

Annexes to this Chapter contain recommendations on the identification and management of women who suffer domestic violence and on the need for all pregnant women to be given appropriate information on the correct use of seat belts.

Fortuitous deaths: key recommendations

All health professionals should make themselves aware of the importance of domestic violence in their practice.

Enquiry about violence should be routinely included when taking a social history.

Local trusts and community teams should develop guidelines for the identification and provision of further support for these women, including developing multi-agency working to enable appropriate referrals or provision of information on sources of further help.

Women should be educated that it is important to wear a seat belt during pregnancy and in the correct method of doing so.

This Chapter traditionally also contains descriptions of the small number of deaths for which, despite intensive investigations and assessments, no obvious cause of death could be found.

Table 13.1

Fortuitous deaths; United Kingdom 1994-96.	
Cause of Death	**Number**
Cause of death undetermined	7
Unnatural Deaths	
Road Traffic Accident	13
Murder	3
Overdose of dothepin	1
Burns	1
Neoplastic Disease	
Carcinoma of the ovary	1
Carcinomatosis (unknown primary)	2
Carcinoma of the stomach	1
Lymphoma	2
Carcinoma of the pancreas	1
Malignant melanoma	1
Infectious Disease	
Creutzfeldt-Jacob Disease	1
Other	
Alcohol	2
TOTAL	**36**

Cause of death undetermined

There were seven cases in which the cause of death could not be accurately ascertained:

A multiparous woman in her twenties was admitted to hospital in the second trimester with basal pneumonia. This was treated and she was discharged home a few days later. After approximately two weeks she collapsed at home and was in cardiac arrest when the ambulance arrived. Efforts at resuscitation were not successful and she was certified dead on arrival in A&E. At autopsy she was found to have aspirated gastric contents and have minor signs of pneumonia. Despite intensive investigations the cause of death could not be established although it was mooted that she may have suffered spontaneous fatal aspiration.

In another case the Coroner recorded the cause of death of a young woman in early pregnancy as unascertainable. The woman was known to have depression, was alcohol dependent and was in the care of her GP and the community alcohol and drug service. Several days prior to her death she had been admitted to hospital with a drug overdose and refused the offer of admission to a detoxification unit. She remained under the close supervision of the community alcohol and drug nurses and had just agreed to be admitted when she was found dead at home. The full post-mortem report was not released. This case is discussed in Chapter 12.

In one unusual case a primigravida, in the later stages of a twin pregnancy, collapsed at home, some minutes after complaining of pain in her thighs. She apparently arched her body and twitched her arms during her fatal collapse. Cardiopulmonary resuscitation (CPR) was sustained for 45 minutes without effect, by which time she had arrived at the A&E Department. Whilst she was in asystole an emergency caesarean section was performed to no avail. During her pregnancy she had shown no signs of pre-eclampsia, and although eclampsia was the stated cause of death on the death certificate, in the opinion of every Assessor who reviewed the case, this cause of death must be in doubt. There was no evidence at autopsy of eclampsia, although minimal pre-eclamptic signs were reported. The gross description of the brain and lungs gave the impression of an acute anoxic death so a fatal dysrhythmia was clearly possible, and this is considered the most likely cause of death. The "twitching" reported at the time of collapse was most likely agonal.

In another case, where the absence of key documentation has not enabled a full assessment, an older multipara was found collapsed on the toilet at about six weeks' gestation. The ambulance crew found her asystolic and CPR was commenced. She never regained consciousness. On admission to hospital a CT scan showed cerebral oedema but no underlying cause for this was found. She continued to deteriorate and died six days after her collapse. Despite the uncertainty of her death no autopsy results were available to the Enquiry although the case appears to have been referred to the Coroner. No inquest was held. The death certificate states the cause of death to be "brain death" due to anoxia and vaso-vagal attack. In the opinion of the Central Pathology Assessor, this is not an acceptable description without further supporting evidence.

Poor pathological investigations meant that the cause of death of a woman who died in early pregnancy and who had a history of cardiac disease could not be accurately classified. There was no attempt to examine the cardiac conducting system.

A young woman collapsed at home in very early pregnancy. She sustained cerebral anoxia, failed to recover consciousness and died shortly afterwards. As an autopsy was not performed it was not possible to establish the cause of death.

The last woman died at home late in the first trimester. She had had a DVT nine years previously. No further details are known to the Enquiry.

Domestic Violence/Murder

Murders by a partner or ex-partner are the extreme end of the spectrum of domestic violence. This is a very important, but often overlooked, cause of maternal and child morbidity and mortality, which is said to affect one in 10 women at any one time. It is associated with severe morbidity, fetal death, miscarriage, depression, suicide and alcohol and drug abuse as well as having important effects on other family members, especially children. Annex 1 to this Chapter discusses the impact of domestic violence during pregnancy and suggests steps to help identify women who are, or are at risk of, being abused.

From this Report it has not been possible to ascertain how many women were murdered by their husband or partner since these cases, to date, have not been considered by the Enquiry, although the association between pregnancy and increasing domestic violence is well known. From the few cases that were reported, the all too obvious warning signs were present in all cases. Because some cases are still *sub judice* it is not possible to give details of the exact circumstances, but they identify valuable pointers to include in the educational initiatives suggested in Annex 1 and they underline the need for vigilance, especially when there may be a high index of suspicion.

Of the six women who died (three are counted in Chapter 14 as *Late* deaths occurring some months after delivery), all were apparently murdered by husbands or male partners:

A woman who spoke no English had been admitted earlier during her pregnancy "having fallen down stairs". She was strangled by her husband shortly before delivery. She had been seen regularly throughout her pregnancy by a midwifery team but her husband acted as her interpreter.

Two other women, also undelivered but in the later stages of pregnancy, were murdered. In one her ex-partner was convicted but the other case was closed following the suicide of the possible suspect and it was not proved that any identifiable or named person was responsible.

In a fourth case a woman was repeatedly physically abused by her husband during her pregnancy and prevented from attending antenatal appointments. She was murdered some months later.

In the other two *Late* cases the women were killed by their partners some months after delivery, and a strong history of violence then emerged.

Road Traffic Accidents

Thirteen women died as a result of road traffic accidents.

Two women died prior to 24 weeks' gestation. One was travelling unrestrained in the back of a van which collided with a concrete central reservation and she died at the roadside of multiple injuries, having been forcibly ejected from the van. The other was a front seat passenger who died of head injuries some days after the accident, having suffered a spontaneous miscarriage of a dead fetus shortly before her death. The use of a seat belt in this case was not recorded.

Two women died at around six months of pregnancy. In neither case was the use of a seat belt mentioned or reported in the autopsy. Both were in cardiac arrest on arrival in the Accident and Emergency (A&E) Department and emergency explorative surgery was performed. In one case an attempt was made to undertake an emergency caesarean section but this was discontinued when both the mother and baby died during the procedure.

Seven women died in the last trimester of their pregnancy:

> In four cases the uterus was ruptured and all these women were front seat passengers. Of these, three women died at the scene of the accident and the use of seat belts was not recorded, although there is post-mortem evidence to suggest their use. The fourth woman who ruptured her uterus was wearing a seat belt, but arrived at A&E in cardiac arrest and a post-mortem caesarean section was performed with the delivery of a dead infant. In none of these cases was the ruptured uterus the main cause of death.

> In the fifth case a post-mortem caesarean section was carried out by a surgical registrar on a woman admitted to A&E in asystole having sustained multiple injuries. She was a front seat passenger and wearing a seat belt. The baby was dead.

> In the sixth case the woman was driving the car and wearing a seat belt. She too was in cardiac arrest on arrival at A&E and a post-mortem caesarean section was performed with the delivery of a dead fetus.

> In another incident a woman was a front seat passenger trapped in a burning car. The use of seat belts was not recorded. She was certified dead at the scene of the accident and the baby, who was undelivered, died of anoxia.

Four women died after delivery. All were front seat passengers wearing seat belts and died instantaneously from multiple injuries.

These cases highlight the poor success rate for fetal survival in post-mortem caesarean sections, which, unless performed immediately after the maternal death, are almost invariably associated with severe fetal anoxia and consequent stillbirth.

Annex 2 to this Chapter contains further discussion about the use of seat belts during pregnancy and contains important recommendations for education and their correct use.

REPORT ON CONFIDENTIAL ENQUIRIES INTO MATERNAL DEATHS IN THE UNITED KINGDOM

Neoplastic disease

Eight deaths due to neoplastic disease were considered to be *Fortuitous* in that the pregnancy had no effect on the underlying pathology. In six cases the malignancy was identified in the first trimester and in two of these termination of pregnancy was performed to enable chemotherapy to be instituted. One woman died before delivery and in the fourth case an emergency caesarean section was performed due to deterioration of the mother's condition. Two women delivered spontaneously around 28-30 weeks' gestation. The aggressive nature of these tumours, which obviously predated the pregnancy but may have been hastened by the physiological effects of pregnancy, meant that these women died shortly after chemotherapy had commenced. Some of these cases are described more fully:

> In one case a woman in very early pregnancy was admitted with a deep vein thrombosis (DVT) which was successfully treated. She was then readmitted complaining of abdominal pain. An ultrasound scan revealed a large ovarian mass which, on laparotomy, was found to be malignant. After the termination of pregnancy the rapidly growing tumour failed to respond to treatment and she died a month later.

> A second woman was admitted at three months' gestation with epigastric pain and jaundice. An adenocarcinoma was diagnosed, although the primary site was not ascertained, and she died shortly after termination of pregnancy.

> In a third case a metastatic adenocarcinoma in the liver with an unknown primary site was diagnosed in the first trimester. The woman wished the pregnancy to continue, but despite a laparotomy to establish whether the tumour could be resected her condition continued to deteriorate. She had an emergency caesarean section at about 28 weeks' gestation and she and the baby died a few days later.

> A fourth, multiparous, woman, who had previously been treated for gastric carcinoma, suffered a recurrence in her third trimester. She rapidly developed jaundice and an emergency caesarean section was performed at 30 weeks' gestation. Her condition continued to deteriorate and she died a few days later. The baby survived.

Infectious disease

There was one death due to infectious disease:

Creutzfeldt-Jacob Disease (CJD)

> A multiparous woman in her twenties was thought to be depressed during the early part of her pregnancy and was referred for psychiatric care. She was cared for jointly by an obstetric consultant, the team midwives, her GP and the psychiatric department of her local hospital. She was subsequently admitted to the neurology ward with progressive encephalopathy and recurrent convulsions and CJD was suspected. She was transferred to the ICU for stabilisation prior to a caesarean section, performed at 30 weeks' gestation, and a live infant was delivered. She was subsequently managed on ICU and the neurology ward, where she died three weeks after delivery. In view of the possible diagnosis a limited autopsy was performed and the Medical Research Council (MRC) CJD unit in Edinburgh subsequently confirmed she had died of new variant CJD.

Overdose of dothepin

A woman in her thirties and with a long standing history of manic depression and alcohol dependency took a fatal overdose of dothepin in the mid-trimester of her pregnancy. She had been referred back to the psychiatric services for care (by telephone and fax from the GP) but died before the Community Psychiatric Nurse could visit to assess her. It is not clear whether this was an intentional act. This case is discussed in Chapter 12.

Possible substance/alcohol misuse

Two women died of possible alcohol misuse. One woman died of cirrhosis of the liver. In the other case a woman in the last trimester of pregnancy was found dead at a social function. She had aspirated vomit. No initial cause of death was given and the pathologist reported it as "undetermined pending further laboratory investigations".

In the latter case, despite the circumstances, toxicology, which should have been mandatory, was not performed and the autopsy itself was considered by the Assessors of this Enquiry to be totally inadequate. In the absence of any other findings, in the opinion of the Assessors this death is consistent with substance or alcohol misuse.

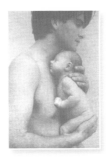

ANNEX 1 TO CHAPTER 13
GUIDELINES FOR DOMESTIC VIOLENCE

Violence against women encompasses physical, sexual, emotional and psychological abuse. It is rarely an isolated event and usually escalates in severity and frequency. It is a serious and common offence. In the context of obstetric care it can cause recurrent miscarriage, stillbirths and maternal deaths.

It is difficult to ascertain the prevalence of domestic violence as it remains largely unrecognised, but various reports, listed in the reference section, estimate that:

- one in three women experiences domestic violence at some point in their lives (perhaps one in 10 in the last year);

- over one million incidents of domestic violence are recorded by the police each year (one in four of all assaults);

- about 30% of domestic violence starts during pregnancy;

- it can often escalate during pregnancy or after birth; and

- two in five women who are murdered are killed by a current or ex-partner.

The impact of violence upon the health of women and their families, and the burden placed on the National Health Service as a whole, is becoming increasingly recognised, by Government and by the medical and nursing professions. Attention was drawn to this in the Chief Medical Officer for England's Annual Report 1996[1] in which he said health and social services staff can play a role in:

- helping women to disclose domestic violence,

- providing support and practical advice about the options available, and

- demonstrating continuing understanding and a source of help whatever initial decision is made.

To be able to do this, staff need:

- a better understanding of the nature of domestic violence,

- the professional skills and compassion to help women address the implications and options, and

- the capability to provide support over what may be a long period of time.

The Royal College of Obstetricians and Gynaecologists[2] (RCOG), the Royal College of Midwives[3] (RCM) and the British Association of Accident and Emergency Medicine[4] have issued, or are in the process of issuing, guidelines for the detection and management of women who may have been abused. The Royal College of General Practitioners published guidelines in their Members' handbook in 1992[5] which are shortly to be revised. Apart from management strategies, all recommend the use of simple screening questions, for example at routine antenatal clinics and whenever there may be an index of suspicion. Further information can be obtained from the references cited at the end of this Chapter.

Domestic violence in pregnancy and the postnatal period

Studies have shown a variable incidence of abuse amongst pregnant women. One survey in the US showed 37% of obstetric patients were at risk of abuse[6] and another survey that 48% of abused women were assaulted during pregnancy[7]. Apart from showing that violence worsens during pregnancy, a further study showed the risk of miscarriage may double[8] and a recent study in Yale found abused women were 15 times more likely to suffer a miscarriage than non-abused women[9].

The Yale trauma study also showed that victims of domestic violence are:

- fifteen times more likely to abuse alcohol,

- nine times more likely to abuse drugs,

- three times more likely to be diagnosed as depressed or psychotic, and

- five times more likely to attempt suicide.

Characteristics, particularly in the context of obstetric practice

These include:

- repeated attendance at antenatal clinics, the GP's surgery or A&E for minor injuries or trivial or non-existent complaints,

- constant presence of partner at examinations, who may answer all the questions for the woman and be unwilling to leave the room (this may have particular relevance in situations where the woman cannot speak English and her partner acts as her interpreter),

- non-attendance through lack of money for travel expenses, not being allowed out of the home, or not being given access to a telephone,

- non-compliance with treatment,

- the woman may be evasive or reluctant to speak or disagree in front of her partner, and

- minimalisation of signs of violence on the body.

Physical manifestations during pregnancy and postnatally:

These include[3]:

- Gynaecological problems, such as frequent vaginal and urinary tract infections, dyspareunia and pelvic pain,

- frequent visits with vague complaints or symptoms without apparent physiological cause and recurring admissions for abdominal pain/reduced fetal movements or "? urinary tract infection",

- injuries that are untended and of several different ages, especially to the neck, head, breasts, abdomen and genitals,

- repeated or chronic injuries, and

- postnatally, removal of perineal sutures.

There may also be a history of :

- repeated miscarriage or terminations of pregnancy,

- stillbirth,

- preterm labour/prematurity,

- intrauterine growth retardation/ low birth weight,

- preterm labours,

- drug or alcohol abuse,

- depression or suicide attempts, and

- unwanted or unplanned pregnancy.

Recommendations

These are based on the main recommendations from the RCOG[2] and RCM[3] reports. All health professionals who care for pregnant women are strongly urged to read these reports more fully.

All health professionals should make themselves aware of the importance of domestic violence in their practice. They should adopt a non-judgemental and supportive response to women who have experienced physical, psychological or sexual abuse and be able to give basic information to women about where to get help. They should provide continuing support, whatever decision the woman makes concerning her future.

Local trusts and community teams should develop guidelines for the identification and provision of further support for these women, including developing multi-agency working to enable appropriate referrals or provision of information on sources of further help.

Information about sources of help and local telephone help lines should be displayed in clinics, including the Ladies' toilets.

Enquiry about violence should be routinely included when taking a social history. Obstetricians and gynaecologists should consider introducing questions about violence during the course of all consultations. In General Practice and midwifery, this could be at the booking visit. There are a number of useful documents explaining how this can be achieved through the use of sensitive questions.

If routine questioning is introduced, this must be accompanied by the development of local strategies for referral, which should be accompanied by an educational programme for professionals, in consultation with local groups, and preferably delivered by those already working in this area.

Where the woman is unable to speak English an interpreter should be provided, and not a partner, friend, or family member.

The RCOG recommends that all women are seen on their own at least once during the antenatal period to enable the disclosure of such information.

Useful Contacts

Women's Aid

Women's Aid Federation of England
(refuge, legal advice and emotional support)
PO Box 391, Bristol BS99 7WS
0117 944 4411 (office)
0345 023468 (24-hour national helpline)

London Women's Aid
0171 392 2092 (24 hours)

Northern Ireland Women's Aid Federation
129 University Street, Belfast BT7 1HP
01232 249 041 or 01232 249 358

Scottish Women's Aid
13/9 North Bank Street, Edinburgh EH1 2LP
0131 221 0401

Welsh Women's Aid
01222 390 874 (Cardiff)
01970 612748 (Aberystwyth)
01745 334767 (Rhyl)

Victim Support

National Association of Victim Support Schemes
National Office
Cranmer House, 39 Brixton Road, London SW9 6DZ
0171 587 1162 (referrals)
0171 735 9166 (enquiries)

Victim Support Northern Ireland
Annsgate House, 70/74 Ann Street, Belfast BT1 4EH
01232 244039

Victim Support Republic of Ireland
29/30 Dame Street, Dublin 2
(00 343) 1 6798673

Victim Support Scotland
14 Frederick Street, Edinburgh EH2 2HB
0131 225 7779

Other Groups

Rape Crisis (support/counselling)
PO Box 69, London WC1X 9NJ
0171 837 1600 (24-hour helpline)

Refuge

2-8 Maltravers Street, London WC2R 3EE

0171 395 7700 (office)

0990 995443 (24-hour crisis line)

Rights of Women (ROW) (advice and referral)

52-54 Featherstone Street, London EC1Y 8RT

0171 251 6575 (office)

0171 251 6577 (advice)

Samaritans

0345 909090

References

1. The Annual Report of The Chief Medical Officer of the Department of Health for 1996. *On The State of the Public Health.* London: The Stationery Office; 1997.

2. Bewley, S., Friend, J. & Mezey, G. (eds). *Violence against Women.* London: The Royal College of Obstetricians and Gynaecologists; 1997.

3. The Royal College of Midwives. *Domestic Abuse in Pregnancy.* Position paper No 19. London Royal College of Midwives. Nov 1997.

4. British Association of Accident and Emergency Medicine. *Domestic Violence; Recognition and Management in Accident and Emergency.* 1994.

5. Heath, I. Domestic violence: the general practitioner's role. In: *The Royal College of General Practitioners Members' Reference Book,* 283-5. London: Sabrecrown; 1992.

6. Helton, A.S, Anderson, E. & McFarlane, J. Battered and pregnant: a prevalence study with intervention measures. *Am J Public Health* 1987; **77**: 1337-9.

7. Bowker, L.H. & Maurer, L. The medical treatment of battered wives. *Women and Health* 1987; **12**: 25-45.

8. Andrews, B. & Brown, G.W. Marital violence in the community. *Br J Psychiatry* 1988; **153**: 305-12.

9. Stark, E. & Flitcraft, A. *Women at Risk.* London: Sage; 1996.

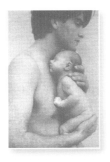

ANNEX II TO CHAPTER 13
SEAT BELTS IN PREGNANCY

Although it is not possible to be sure how many women who died as a result of road traffic accidents were wearing seat belts, autopsies show that some of those who did not rupture their uterus had transected their aorta, indicating a sudden deceleration injury whilst most likely restrained by a seat belt.

Nevertheless, studies have shown that maternal mortality associated with road traffic accidents was 33% for pregnant women thrown from the car compared to 5% who were not ejected. Fetal mortality was 47% and 11% respectively[1,2,3]. A recent survey in the Republic of Ireland[4] showed that either many women did not routinely wear seat belts or they were worn incorrectly. Furthermore, in the same survey, only 30% of Irish GPs provided regular advice to all pregnant women, less than 50% indicated they were aware of the correct advice to give, and 75% thought it was important for women in the third trimester to wear seat belts.

Women should be educated that it is important to wear a seat belt during pregnancy and in the correct method of doing so. A recent survey found that fewer than half of the maternity units surveyed taught women about the use of seat belts during pregnancy, although all felt able to give advice[5].

The commonest reason for not wearing a seat belt is fear of risk of injury to the fetus[6]. The most important factor in fetal injury is deceleration, followed by forced flexion of the maternal body over the lap belt with subsequent uterine compression and distortion. Seat belts can prevent flexion, but deceleration may cause placental abruption. This is estimated to occur in 1-5% of minor injuries and 20-50% of major injuries[5], with the lower figures coming from women who were wearing seat belts. Lap belt restraint alone used to be considered appropriate, but although it helped to prevent fatal injuries to some mothers, it was associated with an increased fetal loss[2-5] due to placental abruption. Therefore both maternal and fetal mortality are significantly reduced when a three-point seat belt is worn.

The correct use is to place the lap strap as low as possible beneath the bump, lying on the upper thighs, with the diagonal shoulder strap above the bump, lying between the breasts, see Figure 1.

Figure 1. The corect and incorrect use of a seat belt in pregnancy

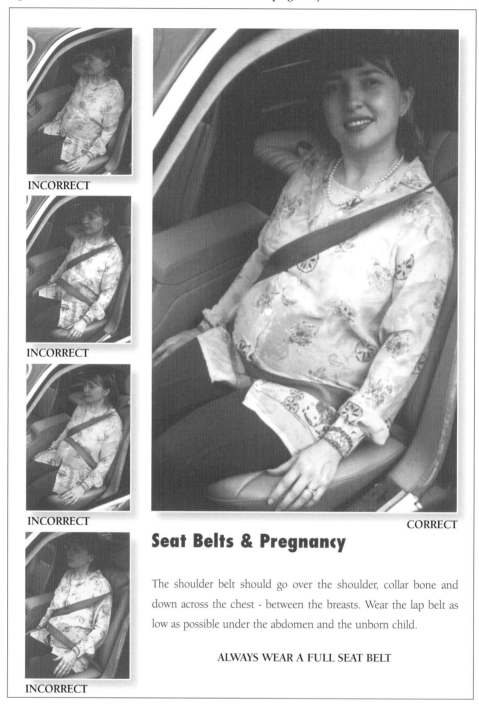

INCORRECT

INCORRECT

INCORRECT

INCORRECT

CORRECT

Seat Belts & Pregnancy

The shoulder belt should go over the shoulder, collar bone and down across the chest - between the breasts. Wear the lap belt as low as possible under the abdomen and the unborn child.

ALWAYS WEAR A FULL SEAT BELT

Recommendation

"Above and below the bump, not over it"[3].

All pregnant women should be given advice about the correct use of seat belts as soon as their pregnancy is confirmed. Three-point seat belts should be worn throughout pregnancy with the lap strap placed as low as possible beneath the bump, lying across the thighs with the diagonal shoulder strap above the bump lying between the breasts. The seat belt should be adjusted to fit as snugly as comfortably possible, and if necessary the seat should be adjusted to enable the seat belt to be worn properly.

REPORT ON CONFIDENTIAL ENQUIRIES INTO MATERNAL DEATHS IN THE UNITED KINGDOM

References

1. Pearlman, M., Tinitinalli, J.E. & Lorenz, R.P. A prospective controlled study of outcome after trauma during pregnancy. *Am J Obstet Gynecol* 1990; **162**: 1502-10.

2. Williams, J., McClain, L., Rosemergy, A.S. & Colorado, N.T. Evaluation of blunt abdominal trauma in the third trimester of pregnancy: Maternal and Fetal considerations. *Obstetrics and Gynecology* 1990; **75**: 33-7.

3. Pearce, M. Seat belts in pregnancy. *BMJ* 1990; **304**: 586-9.

4. Wallace, C. General Practitioners' knowledge of and attitudes to the use of seat belts in pregnancy. *Irish Medical Journal*. March 1997; **90**: No2.

5. Griffiths, M., Usherwood, MmcD, & Reginald, P.W. Antenatal teaching of the use of seat belts in pregnancy. *BMJ* 1992; **304**: 614.

6. Hammond, T., Mickens-Powers, B.F., Strickland, K. & Hamkins, D.V. The use of automobile safety restraint systems during pregnancy. *J Obstet Gynaecol Neonat Nursing* 1990; **19**: 339-43.

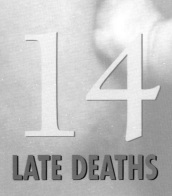

14

LATE DEATHS

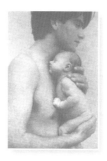

CHAPTER 14
LATE DEATHS

Summary

Deaths occurring in women more than 42 days, but less than one year, after miscarriage, abortion, or delivery are defined as *Late* deaths. The International Classification of Maternal Deaths (ICD9) used in coding this Report excludes such deaths but during the collation of earlier Reports it became apparent that strict adherence to an upper limit of 42 days led to the omission of a number of *Late* deaths which were related to pregnancy. For this reason *Late* deaths reported to the Enquiry for 1994-96 are discussed in this Chapter, but are not included in the overall maternal mortality rate. For the next triennium the tenth revision of the International Classification of Maternal Deaths (ICD10) will be used, which recognises that some maternal deaths occur after 42 days following pregnancy or delivery, and defines *Late* deaths as "those deaths occurring between 42 days and one year after abortion, miscarriage or delivery that are due to *Direct* or *Indirect* maternal causes".

With the increasing sophistication and skill of intensive care support, more women are now surviving the initial pregnancy-related event and are being actively treated for several weeks or months after delivery. However, because the immediate cause of death, as given on the death certificate, is not usually directly related to pregnancy, it is likely that a number of *Late Direct* maternal deaths are being excluded from the Enquiry as they are not picked up on death certificate data or notified by intensive care unit (ICU) staff who may be unaware of this Report.

A total of 72 *Late* deaths were reported in this triennium compared with 46 in the last Report. This again reflects the greater degree of case ascertainment seen elsewhere in this Report. Completed reports were available for all but seven cases. *Late* deaths are further classified as *Direct*, *Indirect* or *Fortuitous*, although for statistical purposes none is included in the numerators for determining standard mortality rates.

The interval between delivery and death for all *Late* deaths is shown in Table 14.1.

Table 14.1

Interval between delivery or abortion and death - *Late* cases; United Kingdom 1994-96.				
Days after delivery	Direct	Indirect	Fortuitous	Total
43-91	1	7	10	18
92-182	2	11	17	30
183-273		10	5	15
274-365	1	4	4	9
Total	4	32	36	72

Direct causes

Four of the 72 *Late* deaths were considered to be directly related to maternal causes and are discussed in the relevant Chapters but counted here:

Amniotic fluid embolism

> This case is discussed in Chapter 5. A parous woman had an uneventful pregnancy and a planned home delivery. During the second stage she became cyanosed and collapsed. The midwives resuscitated her and she was immediately transferred to hospital where all measures were taken. Despite this she remained in a coma and died some months later. The clinical features of her collapse are considered consistent with amniotic fluid embolism.

Her care at all times appears to have been excellent. This case demonstrates the unexpected nature of this, fortunately rare, cause of maternal death.

Pulmonary embolus

> In one case, discussed in Chapter 2, an obese woman with a history of a previous deep vein thrombosis in a previous pregnancy was given aspirin during her pregnancy as it was considered she would have difficulty in complying with self-administered heparin. It was written in her case notes that she should be anticoagulated following delivery. She developed thrombophlebitis shortly before delivery and heparin was commenced. Following a spontaneous vaginal delivery her thrombophlebitis settled and the heparin was discontinued by the Specialist Registrar. The patient was discharged with no anticoagulation and in particular, she did not receive the warfarin which had been prescribed by the consultant and recorded in the case notes and in the letter to the GP. Several months later she complained of increasing dyspnoea and was referred to a consultant physician. A diagnosis of hyperthyroidism was made. She continued to complain of dyspnoea and was eventually admitted for investigation but collapsed and died of the pulmonary embolus the following day.

The fact that she was not prescribed any anticoagulation in the six-week period following delivery probably represents substandard care. Although she died several months after delivery, her symptoms of increasing dyspnoea could well have been caused by the recurring pulmonary emboli shown at autopsy. Her obesity and chronic asthma added to the difficulty in diagnosis but pulmonary embolism was not considered a possibility by her GP or physicians until the autopsy had been performed.

Cardiomyopathy and thromboembolism

In another case, mentioned in Chapter 10, a very young woman died of extensive thromboembolism with the source of the emboli being the heart. During her pregnancy she had pregnancy-induced hypertension and labour was induced at 39 weeks. Following failure to progress, a caesarean section was performed from which she apparently made an uneventful recovery. Three months later she was admitted, normotensive, with an acute hemiparesis and dysarthria, but she took her own discharge before investigations could be fully performed. She was re-admitted shortly afterwards with further weakness of her arm, and again discharged herself. Several days later she was again admitted, with chest pain, haemoptysis and a swollen leg. A pulmonary embolus was diagnosed although ultrasonography of her leg did not show any deep vein thrombosis. She was anti-coagulated but developed extensive oedema and intermittent eosinophilia. Nephrotic syndrome was diagnosed and it was thought she had an underlying vasculitis with widespread venous thrombosis. She was transferred for renal therapy and intensive care but died of a cardiac arrest. At autopsy it was found that she had a dilated cardiomyopathy with thrombus present in both ventricles. Evidence of infarction was found in the lungs, kidneys, ovaries and brain. The only source of the emboli was from the heart.

Dilated cardiomyopathy is a recognised, though rare, complication of pregnancy and is also a recognised source of thromboemboli.

A case of possible post-partum sepsis

In one case, discussed in Chapter 7, a woman in her thirties who had an uncomplicated pregnancy, delivery and puerperium was admitted some weeks after delivery with flu-like symptoms and with swelling and a purpuric rash on her arms and chest. A diagnosis of group A streptococcal septicaemia was made and she was immediately commenced on appropriate therapy. Despite this she developed disseminated intravascular coagulation (DIC) and multi-organ failure. High vaginal swabs, gynaecological examination and ultrasound were all normal. Despite intensive care she died with a clinical diagnosis of toxic shock syndrome. At autopsy a small amount of pus was found in her fallopian tubes and ureters. The cause of death was given as septicaemia as a consequence of post-partum sepsis.

In the opinion of the Assessors, because of the negative gynaecological examinations prior to death, and the time elapsed between delivery and the development of septicaemia, it is not possible to decide with any degree of certainty if this was a true case of puerperal sepsis.

Indirect causes

There were 32 cases where the pregnancy may have indirectly contributed to the death. They are listed in Table 14.2 and some are discussed further.

Table 14.2

Late Deaths - *Indirect* Causes: United Kingdom 1994-96.	
Cause of Death	**Number**
Neoplastic Diseases	
Carcinoma arising in endometriosis	1
Carcinoma of bladder	1
Carcinoma of colon	1
Unknown primary	1
Carcinoma of the cervix	1
Diseases of the circulatory system	
Myocardial fibrosis	2
Cardiomyopathy	5
Thromboembolism	2
Cerebral thrombosis	1
Other	
Cystic fibrosis	1
SLE	1
Asthma	1
Sudden unnatural deaths	
Suicide	12
Overdose	2
Total	**32**

Neoplastic disease

There were five deaths from carcinoma in which the pregnancy may have masked or affected the diagnosis or outcome. In the opinion of the Assessors the first three cases had pain reported during pregnancy which was not investigated fully. It is recognised that whilst the delay in diagnosis may not have made any difference to the outcome, earlier diagnosis would have made the women more comfortable.

A woman had an "ovarian cyst" identified at her booking scan. She had a history of endometriosis and had been receiving treatment for infertility. The cyst increased in size and was reported to be 10 cm at 30 weeks' gestation. During her pregnancy she started to complain of crippling abdominal pain and backache which was ascribed to an "exaggerated form of pelvic pain associated with pregnancy". Two weeks later, following the patient's insistence that she could tolerate the pain no longer, an elective caesarean section was performed at her request and the left ovary was noted to be slightly enlarged. The Pouch of Douglas was also obliterated by adhesions. After delivery the patient went into urinary retention and an X-ray revealed bilateral lytic lesions in her pubic rami with a pathological fracture. Biopsies confirmed widespread metastatic carcinomatosis, which was thought to have been ovarian in origin.

This is substandard care. The fact that she required support to help her move around at home and was brought to later antenatal appointments in a wheelchair clearly demonstrated abnormal pain which should have been investigated further. Such investigations could certainly have included an X-ray of the spine, or better, an MRI.

As well as the clinical substandard care in this case, where the patient was clearly suffering intolerable pain, there were also deficiencies in the pathological investigation of the tumour. No autopsy was performed and several opportunities were lost to convert speculation about the cause into fact. The disease was centred on the pelvis, and therefore probably genital in origin, especially since the bladder was clear; the cervix and vagina were not the primary source; the carcinoma was squamous and she had a history of endometriosis, with the ovarian cyst having been originally diagnosed as an endometrioma. In the opinion of the Central Pathology Assessor it was most likely to be a carcinoma arising in endometriosis. These can occasionally be pure squamous neoplasms[1].

In the second case a multiparous woman who had been complaining of severe backache in the final weeks of pregnancy was found to have metastatic bone disease in her spine shortly after delivery and she died several months later. She also had not been X-rayed whilst pregnant. The primary site was never identified, but although an autopsy had not been performed, a review of the histology suggested the appearance was in keeping with, but not diagnostic of, metastatic breast cancer.

There was no suggestion of substandard care in this case although it does emphasise the need to investigate other possible causes of severe backache in pregnancy, as with the preceding case.

In the third case a small (2 cm) mass at the side of the uterus was found in a primipara who attended a gynaecological clinic very early in pregnancy. It was not detected on two later routine ultrasound scans. She then presented at about 24 weeks' gestation with right iliac fossa pain which was presumed to be due to a urinary tract infection. Some weeks later a further scan showed a bladder mass and hydronephrosis. Investigations revealed widespread dissemination of a poorly differentiated carcinoma. An elective caesarean section was performed at 32 weeks' gestation and appropriate surgery and chemotherapy were commenced. Despite all efforts, this aggressive tumour spread rapidly and the woman died some months later. At autopsy the final diagnosis was considered most likely to be a poorly differentiated carcinoma of the bladder although it was possible that the primary sites could have been the lung, gastrointestinal tract, or breast.

Although it would probably not have altered the subsequent course of events it is possible that a more energetic follow up of the small mass found early in pregnancy might have led to an earlier diagnosis.

> An older multipara was admitted to hospital in the first trimester, before her booking visit, with a very low haemoglobin level (5.5 g/dl) and required transfusion. It would seem, from the limited information available to the Enquiry in this case, that the cause of the anaemia was not sought. What appeared to be a fibroid was subsequently found on a routine ultrasound scan. She then had an unremarkable pregnancy until she delivered some weeks early. Following this, she was referred to the general surgeons and underwent a laparotomy during which carcinoma of the colon was diagnosed. She died two months later.

Because the records were unavailable to the Enquiry it is difficult to assess whether or not there was any substandard care in this case.

> A young grandmultiparous woman died of carcinoma of the cervix some nine months after a termination of pregnancy undertaken to enable appropriate surgery and chemotherapy. She had been found to have a borderline dyskaryotic cervical smear at a postnatal check-up three pregnancies earlier. At that time it was suggested it be repeated in six months' time. However, she was then found to be in the early stages of another pregnancy, and a decision was made to defer the repeat smear until after delivery, which took place without incident within a year of the preceding birth. She was given two appointments to have the smear repeated but she did not attend although she was suffering from intermittent vaginal bleeding. She was a known poor attender and had a history of substance misuse. Three months after delivery of the child her social worker persuaded her to seek help and a frank cervical carcinoma was found on examination. She was also in the early stages of another pregnancy. A Wertheim's hysterectomy was performed at the time of the termination of this pregnancy but, despite treatment, she died several months later.

Cardiac/circulatory disease

There were seven *Indirect* cases of cardiac disease, which are also discussed in Chapter 10, and two cases of thromboembolism.

There were two cases of myocardial fibrosis:

> In the first case of a woman who died suddenly at home, the autopsy gave the cause of death as idiopathic myocardial fibrosis. She had died two months after delivery. In the opinion of the Assessors her death could be considered as *Indirect* as the extent of the fibrosis suggested that she either contracted or already had the condition whilst she was pregnant. There was also a suggestion that during pregnancy she had chicken-pox which is often worse if contracted during pregnancy and may have contributed to the condition.

In the second case, a woman died whilst exercising 11 months after delivery of her second child. The cause of death was given as "acute left ventricular failure due to idiopathic myocardial fibrosis". During both pregnancies she had complained of irregular heartbeats and palpitations but it was not considered necessary to refer her to a cardiologist at that time.

Apart from the case discussed under *Late Direct* deaths, there were five *Indirect* cases of post-partum cardiomyopathy, also mentioned in Chapter 11.

Cerebral haemorrhage

A woman who had recently been discharged from hospital suffered a cerebral haemorrhage. She had had an uneventful pregnancy until near to term when her blood pressure was recorded at 152/100 mmHg and labour was induced. She was discharged home on the third day with a BP of 140/100 mmHg and she had been prescribed methyl dopa. This was not considered to be substandard care. Shortly afterwards she complained of a headache and collapsed. An MRI scan and angiogram showed a subarachnoid haemorrhage and an aneurysm which was subsequently clipped. However, she remained unconscious and died several months later of a cerebral infarction. The standard of care she received at all times was considered excellent.

Thromboembolism

In two cases obese women who were prescribed oral contraception postnatally died of thromboembolism:

In the first case a young primipara with a weight of 86 Kg and a Body Mass Index (BMI) of 29.78 was prescribed "low-dose" oral contraception at her six-week postnatal check. She had not been on contraception for two years prior to the pregnancy. Several months later she collapsed and died at home of a pulmonary embolus.

In the second case, a woman who had developed a postpartum cardiomyopathy, and who was morbidly obese, weighing 102 Kg (and having weighed as much as 119 Kg) with a BMI of 36.72, was prescribed oral contraception by her consultant cardiologist to prevent a further pregnancy complicating her cardiomyopathy. She subsequently suffered a series of strokes which led to her death some months later.

In the second case, not only was the woman at increased risk of thromboembolism due to her weight, but puerperal cardiomyopathy is a known risk factor for cerebral thrombosis. To have prescribed the oral contraceptive pill to such an obese woman with puerperal cardiomyopathy represents substandard care.

The Handbook of Family Planning and Reproductive Health Care[2] states that "a body weight of more than 50% above the ideal weight for height (BMI>35) is an absolute contraindication for the combined pill and excess weight 20-50% above the ideal for weight and height (BMI 30-35) is a relative contraindication".

A key message is that a woman's weight may remain higher after pregnancy and account should be taken of this when considering oral contraception. In addition, puerperal cardiomyopathy is a known risk factor for cerebral thrombosis and women with this condition should not be prescribed oral contraception.

REPORT ON CONFIDENTIAL ENQUIRIES INTO MATERNAL DEATHS IN THE UNITED KINGDOM

Cystic Fibrosis

There were one *Late* and two *Indirect* deaths from cystic fibrosis reported in this triennium. These cases are discussed together in Chapter 11.

> The *Late* death occurred in a young primiparous woman with severe cystic fibrosis, who was reluctant to comply with the treatment offered to her during her pregnancy. At seven months' gestation her health was severely compromised due to increasing respiratory distress and she underwent an emergency caesarean section with a live birth. She then rapidly developed respiratory failure requiring intensive care support, and despite this being of the highest possible standard, she died six weeks after her admission to ICU.

Systemic Lupus Erythematosus (SLE)

> A young primipara was admitted late in the second trimester with dyspnoea and a working diagnosis of SLE. Shortly afterwards she had an intrauterine death and labour was induced with prostaglandin pessaries. After delivery she became acutely short of breath and was transferred to the ICU, where she made an initial recovery. She was moved back to the postnatal ward but required readmission to the ICU after a further week when she developed pneumonia and ARDS. She then suffered a cardiac arrest from which she did not regain consciousness. She was transferred to the regional ICU with respiratory failure but died after three months' intensive support.

The details of this case were inadequate, particularly in relation to the care she received in the ICUs and the eventual underlying cause of death. It is not possible to assess if there was any substandard care.

Asthma

> A morbidly obese woman with chronic asthma and other medical problems, and who was suffering from post-traumatic stress disorder and depression following a stillbirth after an undiagnosed pregnancy, became pregnant again. Her pregnancy was treated as high risk and she received appropriate consultant-led support and treatment. Her GP was also very supportive. Her asthma caused severe problems during pregnancy and she was admitted several times. Eventually she required an elective caesarean section from which, following a short stay in the ICU, she recovered well. She was discharged home but her asthma continued to cause problems requiring further admissions. During her last admission she suffered an irreversible respiratory arrest and died.

Although this woman died from complications of her asthma, possibly linked to smoking and weight, these problems were probably linked to her continuing depression and bereavement reaction to the loss of her earlier child. She had received counselling before, during and after the birth of her second child and antidepressant medication following the birth.

Suicide and overdose

All deaths from suicide, substance misuse and other psychiatric causes are discussed in Chapter 12, which also makes recommendations regarding the early identification of cases of possible postnatal depression, and regarding the subsequent care for these women as well as those with other psychiatric conditions or involved in substance misuse. There were twelve *Late* deaths due to suicide and two ascribed to an overdose with an open verdict.

Fortuitous

There were 36 such incidental deaths which are listed in Table 14.3, some of which are described further.

Table 14.3

Fortuitous Late deaths ; United Kingdom 1994-96.	
Cause of Death	**Number**
Diseases of the Circulatory System	
Myocardial infarction	3
Cardiac arrhythmia	1
Diseases of the Nervous System	
Epilepsy	2
Diseases of the Respiratory System	
Pneumonia	1
Asthma	2
Diseases of the Endocrine System	
Diabetic ketoacidosis	2
Neoplastic disease	
Thymoma /lymphoma/Hodgkins	3
Carcinoma of the pancreas	2
Cholangiocarcinoma	1
Malignant melanoma	1
Rhabdomyosarcoma	1
Carcinoma of the kidney	1
Acute myeloid leukaemia	1
Carcinoma of the ovary	1
Carcinoma of the breast	1

(continued)

Table 14.3 (continued)

Fortuitous Late deaths; United Kingdom 1994-96	
Cause of Death	**Number**
Infectious diseases	
Meningitis/ septicaemia	2
Sub-acute bacterial endocarditis	1
Other	
Anaphylactic shock	1
Pancreatitis	1
Liver/multi-organ failure due to pre-existing disease	2
Sudden Unnatural Deaths	
Substance abuse	3
Murder	3
Total	**36**

Epilepsy

> A multiparous woman in her twenties died of an epileptic fit many months after delivery. She had a clinical history of repeated abortions associated with antiphospholipid syndrome and had also had multiple hospital admissions for abdominal pain. The pains grew worse with her pregnancies and she also attended a pain clinic. She took oral pethidine and amitryptyline.

The late onset of her epilepsy, some seven months after delivery, is considered to be unrelated to pregnancy, although it may have related to the antiphospholipid syndrome, or excess pethidine use.

Neoplastic disease

There were 12 cases of neoplastic disease considered to be unrelated to pregnancy. These are shown in full in Table 14.3, but some are discussed further:

> An unusual case of acute myeloid leukaemia was diagnosed on a routine full blood count (FBC) whilst the woman was in labour. After delivery she was immediately transferred to a specialist unit for treatment, but despite intensive efforts, she died a few months later. Unfortunately her antenatal card was not available to the Enquiry and it was not possible to ascertain whether an FBC was carried out at booking. It seems an FBC a few weeks prior to delivery was reported as normal, but given the short interval between delivery and death, it would have been unlikely that an earlier diagnosis would have affected the outcome.

A multiparous woman who had a biopsy of a breast lump, reported as benign, one year prior to her next pregnancy complained of a lump and pain in the breast shortly following her booking appointment. A routine breast examination had not been performed at that time. On presentation with breast symptoms she was found to have metastatic breast cancer and, after much discussion, opted for a termination of pregnancy to enable chemotherapy to commence. The aggressive nature of the tumour meant it did not respond to treatment and she died a few months later.

Sudden unnatural deaths

Three women were murdered, and appear to have suffered domestic violence in the past. In one of these cases, a woman with a history of being physically abused died of multiple stab wounds some months after delivery. The full details of this case are not known to the Enquiry, but it is noted that the management of the pregnancy was problematic as it appears to have been made difficult for her to travel to, or attend, antenatal clinic appointments. The Enquiry also received two other reports, one of a woman shot by her estranged husband who then killed himself, and another where further details were not available. These cases could not be investigated further.

Lessons from all such difficult cases are discussed in the section on Domestic Violence in Chapter 13, in which key recommendations are made.

References

1.	Macko *et al*. Primary squamous ovarian carcinoma . *Cancer* 1983; **52**: 1117-180.

2.	Guillebaud, J. Combined hormonal contraception. In; Loudon, N., Glasier, A. & Gebbie, A. (eds). *Handbook of Family Planning and Reproductive Health Care (3rd edn)*. Edinburgh: Churchill Livingstone, 1995: pp. 37-89.

15
MIDWIFERY

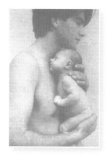

CHAPTER 15
MIDWIFERY

Introduction

This new Chapter marks a milestone in the history of the Confidential Enquiries into Maternal Deaths and describes how midwives may, directly and indirectly, affect the safe outcome of pregnancy and how they can develop their wider public health role. Midwives should read this Chapter in conjunction with the main body of this Report and cross reference is made to the appropriate more specialised sections.

This Chapter has the following sections:

> The developing role of the midwife
> Regional Midwifery Assessors
> Improving health in pregnancy
> General risk factors
> Specific conditions
> Recommendations

As with previous Confidential Enquires, there are important lessons to be learnt by the different professionals contributing to the care of women and their babies. Putting these lessons into practice, however, has proved to be more difficult than most would expect. Midwives must play an active role in challenging poor practice and ensuring that recommendations from this Report are incorporated into local policies and procedures.

Summary of key recommendations: midwives

Midwives should:

- Help provide accessible services for all pregnant women, recognising that some women still feel unable to seek help during their pregnancy and some, particularly the socially excluded and/or from minority ethnic groups, do not appear to have their specific concerns understood during their care. Efforts should be made to allow those least likely to utilise services the opportunity to gain professional and social support during their pregnancies.

- Provide advice and support on healthy life-styles to include:
  diet and exercise,
  smoking, alcohol and substance misuse,
  safety in the home and workplace,
  basic first aid measures especially for women with existing conditions such as epilepsy,
  safety and car travel, and
  guidance on the warning signs of obstetric complications such as pre-eclampsia.

- Take a clear history of current or past psychological, social and physical problems of women, including violence from their partner.

- Feel confident to challenge current practice in a proactive and assertive manner if concerned.

- Work in partnership with women and other professional groups to ensure the provision of timely, relevant information which highlights possible complications during pregnancy and the postnatal period, thereby enabling women to access appropriate care when concerns are raised.

- Utilise existing systems of midwifery supervision to ensure continuing professional development and actively demonstrate evidence-based care.

- Acknowledge that as members of a multi-disciplinary team, midwives have an equal responsibility in ensuring high standards of care and positive outcomes of pregnancy.

The developing role of the midwife

In the past, the Confidential Enquiry has produced a predominately medical report. This may be understandable as maternal deaths are often seen as the results of medical complications of pregnancy. However, it may have resulted in a systematic bias in case assessments, leading to under representation of the potential contribution of a different professional group. The position has now started to change through the introduction of Regional Midwifery Assessors whose role is described later.

REPORT ON CONFIDENTIAL ENQUIRIES INTO MATERNAL DEATHS IN THE UNITED KINGDOM

The midwife's role in the provision of maternity care has long been established and even through an age of medicalisation, midwives have maintained their place as the most senior professional present at the majority of deliveries within the UK. They provide the professional lead at approximately 70% of all births and are present at around 99% of the remaining births.

Midwives provide or play a key role in maternity care provision and with a greater emphasis on continuity of care and carer, they may be able to provide a more holistic approach to care. Their knowledge and influence can greatly affect the outcome of pregnancy for mother and baby, and their role in health surveillance, education and promotion is invaluable.

With this in mind, it is important to discuss the effects and benefits of midwifery care when considering maternal mortality and morbidity, whether or not underlying medical conditions or pregnancy-related complications are present.

Recent developments in the philosophy underpinning maternity care, supported by national strategies[1-3] and, in England, Government policy, have resulted in changing patterns of care delivery. Women should now be receiving appropriate and timely information concerning access to available services, health education and possible complications during and after pregnancy. They should also be the focus of care with midwives, GPs and obstetricians working in a collaborative and cohesive manner.

These changes have called for a re-assessment of clinical roles and re-examination of professional boundaries. Although during this century, the shifts in models of maternity care have been marked, the midwife's role and responsibilities in law have remained unchanged. The midwife still maintains absolute accountability for the care she/he delivers.

Regional Midwifery Assessors

In 1993 the first Regional Midwifery Assessors (RMA's) were appointed to this Enquiry to contribute to the professional assessment of maternal mortalities in their geographical area. It is apparent from case reviews that at the start of the triennium the RMAs' expertise was not always called upon. This was due to several factors, such as *Indirect* deaths not being considered appropriate for referral for midwifery assessment, slow implementation of the new system and the lack of understanding of reporting mechanisms. Although towards the end of the triennium this situation improved, further effort is required to ensure a midwifery perspective is gained in the majority of case reviews.

Improving health in pregnancy

It has long been recognised that the better a woman's health directly before and during pregnancy, the better the outcome for mother and baby. The fall in maternal deaths over the last century has partly been due to changes in social and economic conditions. Although in comparison to developing countries, the UK enjoys low maternal mortality rates, it is apparent that socially deprived women living in the UK are likely to have an increased risk of maternal mortality.

This has also been found to be the case in other developed countries such as the USA. In a recent World Health Organisation publication[4] comparisons in maternal mortality rates in the USA were made between those women who were economically and socially supported and those who were not. A stark contrast was demonstrated, with the most vulnerable women experiencing mortality rates as high as 100 deaths per 100,000 live births, compared to the overall US rate of under 10. Vulnerability can be classed as having insufficient financial and social support, poor diet and/or housing, substance misuse, poor access to health care and, in some instances, belonging to a minority ethnic group.

Most midwives would acknowledge these facts but relatively few midwives work in a way that targets care to those women most in need. Midwives have a unique role in improving access to and availability of good antenatal care, ensuring sound health promotion messages, and working in partnership with other professional groups and outside agencies.

Several cases in this Report highlight the need for accurate non-judgmental antenatal care. Some women died without having sought any help during their pregnancy and some, particularly from minority ethnic groups, did not appear to understand or be understood during their care.

Antenatal care should be accessible to all, and every effort needs to be made to allow those least likely to utilise services, owing to disempowerment, the opportunity to gain professional and social support during their pregnancies.

The planning and delivery of maternity services should focus on these areas, and should not view pregnancy in isolation from other important factors that influence the health of the individual and her developing baby.

General risk factors

Obesity

Many women who died were classified as obese. Although this may be impossible to rectify in pregnancy, midwives are well placed to offer advice about healthy diet before and during pregnancy and to provide support through effective health promotion models. While advice on not eating for two is necessary, seriously overweight women also need to be aware of the increased risks they are exposed to during and after pregnancy, and need to be able to recognise early warning signs of complications. Thus midwives can work in partnership with these woman to minimise risk and act swiftly should complications present. Sadly some of these women were also disabled. One in particular used a wheelchair due to spina bifida. There appeared to have been little advice or support given concerning the increased risk of deep vein thrombosis in the postnatal period and she later died from an embolism. Midwives must acknowledge their specific duty to ensure such women receive the required prophylaxis, advice and support to minimise such risks.

Smoking

Although not cited as a specific cause of maternal mortality in this Report, the dangers of smoking to a woman's health and that of her developing baby are well recognised. There are a growing number of examples of good practice where midwives are taking the lead in cessation of smoking programmes, in which pregnant women are given advice and support based on effective health promotion methods.

Ethnicity

Data in this Report suggest that the rate of mortality amongst some minority ethnic groups may be higher than that in the general population (Chapter 1). More research is needed to confirm or refute this suggestion but midwives should be alert to these issues and ensure individualised care to women from different cultural backgrounds, especially if the expectant mothers have difficulty in communicating in English. This will require the translation of appropriate information, whether written or spoken, and a greater awareness of cultural and religious differences. Midwives should also be aware of the effects of racial prejudice, overt and covert, and must ensure that the lives of all women and their babies are equally valued by all professional groups involved in their care

Road traffic accidents and the use of seat belts

Deaths following road traffic accidents may appear to be outside the midwife's remit but women often seek advice about driving in pregnancy and positioning of seat belts. It would appear that greater efforts have been directed to advice and information on child safety postnatally rather than antenatally. Midwives should provide up to date, evidence-based information to women concerning the wearing of seat belts, driving in pregnancy, road safety and baby car seats. Further information and advice are given in Chapter 13. An illustration of the correct positioning of a car seat belt during pregnancy is seen in Fig 15.1, and further pictures in Figure 1 on page 170.

Figure 15.1

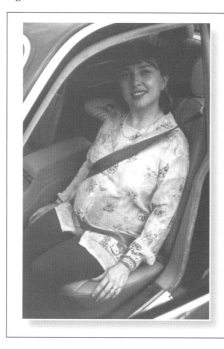

The Correct Use of Seat Belts in Pregnancy

The shoulder belt should go over the shoulder, collar bone and down across the chest - between the breasts. Wear the lap belt as low as possible under the abdomen and the unborn child.

ALWAYS WEAR A FULL SEAT BELT

Professional decision-making

In some reported cases the level of professional decision-making was criticised. Midwives must be able to assert their views on an individual's care if inappropriate decisions are being made. Local policies and procedures should support effective reporting of incidents, and ensure bypass mechanisms are in place to enable midwives to access advice and support from an appropriate professional at a senior level. Midwives should be aware of their professional responsibilities in the protection of the patient or client's interest as stated in the UKCC Code of Practice[5].

Postnatal depression

The effects of postnatal depression for some women remain a concern and although midwives have relatively brief contact in the postnatal period it is essential that they can detect any deterioration of a woman's mental health, directing care to the appropriate professional group. In some instances it is possible to identify women at particular visits in the antenatal period. Chapter 12 recommends that midwives ask for a brief psychiatric history during the booking visit. They can help also by providing women and their families with relevant information about postnatal depression and whom to contact if signs and symptoms present. Midwives should strengthen their links with mental health services and in particular community psychiatric nurses. Psychiatric disorders during pregnancy are discussed later in this Chapter.

Rare conditions in pregnancy

Some women with serious medical conditions, such as cancer, were not provided with appropriate support or care due to professionals' failure to recognise the severity of their symptoms. Although backache and pelvic pain are commonly experienced in pregnancy it is reasonable to arrange investigations if pain and disability are exceptional. In one such case, a woman required a Zimmer frame to get to the clinic but no investigations were initiated. She later died of metastatic cancer. Midwives are well placed to recognise when these rare events deviate from the normal symptoms of pregnancy and, even though diagnosis may not influence the eventual outcome, midwives can ensure appropriate supportive care.

Domestic violence

There is a growing awareness of violence in the home situation and emerging evidence suggests that it may start or become more pronounced during pregnancy. Violence of this nature can involve physical, sexual, verbal and psychological elements which may be difficult to detect due to the woman's fear of reprisal. However, there are indicators which midwives are well placed to identify, such as repeated contact with health care professionals and hospitals for minor injuries or non-existent complaints, the constant presence of a partner at examinations who may not allow the woman to answer enquiries herself, and minimalisaton of bruising. On the other hand, these women may show a reluctance in attending antenatal clinics due to restrictions dictated in the home or may not comply with advice and prescribed treatment.

Midwives need to be alert to these signs and know how to provide the best support to women in these circumstances. This will require midwives to work closely with other professionals and outside agencies. Chapter 13 refers to guidance on these issues, including those produced by the Royal College of Midwives. There is a need for midwives to incorporate this guidance into their daily practice.

Specific conditions

Pulmonary Embolism (Chapter 2)

In this triennium not only does pulmonary embolism remain the major direct cause of maternal death but also there appears to be a marked increase in incidence.

Chapter 2 highlights the fact that many of the women who died had recognised risk factors for venous thromboembolism. Appropriate prophylaxis or prompt clinical diagnosis may have avoided these tragic outcomes.

Recurring risk factors in these cases included women who required bed rest before and after delivery, women who were classified as obese and those who had a previous or family history of thromboembolism.

Midwives have an important role in screening for family history during the antenatal period and identifying relevant risk factors which require preventive action. This will include appropriate and timely information to women, ensuring that prophylactic measures such as the use of thromboembolic stockings and anticoagulation are initiated in accordance with published guidelines[7].

Although prevention of pulmonary embolism is paramount, midwives must also be able to recognise early warning signs of this and other vascular abnormalities and initiate urgent referral. It is of great concern that on several occasions the diagnosis was not considered when women presented with classic symptoms such as breathlessness, chest pain, or calf pain.

As the majority of the postnatal deaths from this cause occurred between 15 and 28 days after delivery midwives need to consider the knowledge women require concerning these complications, how rapidly they can access appropriate care and the availability of midwifery advice during this period.

Hypertensive disorders in pregnancy (Chapter 3)

Although a fall in rates of death due to hypertensive disorder is welcome, nevertheless substandard care contributed to the deaths of several of these women.

Midwives have a key role to play in antenatal surveillance by monitoring blood pressure and proteinuria at every antenatal contact. Owing to the unpredictable nature of the disease and variations in signs and symptoms, midwives should ensure that women are provided with sufficient information to judge their own well-being and to contact professionals when concern arises. Such information is produced by the voluntary organisation Action on Pre-eclampsia (APEC).

Midwives with responsibility for managing maternity services, should ensure easy access to antenatal care for all women and good communication between professionals involved in care. They should also review what information on the warning signs of pre-eclampsia is available to women and ensure it is updated and made available as a matter of routine.

All midwives have a responsibility to ensure that appropriate care is given by a professional with the right level of experience and to respond rapidly if there is a compromise to safe practice. This applies to midwives with limited experience but is equally important when junior medical staff are left to make decisions beyond their current ability. Guidelines on the management of severe hypertension in pregnancy produced by the Royal College of Obstetricians and Gynaecologists[8] should be implemented in all maternity services.

Haemorrhage (Chapter 4)

Deaths from severe haemorrhage remain a concern although there has been a slight reduction in cases compared with the last triennium. Considering the speed with which severe obstetric haemorrhage can occur and kill, it is essential that effective protocols are in place which are reviewed and tested at regular intervals. Midwives should organise emergency rehearsals to test out current policy and procedures and to ensure staff have maintained their knowledge and skills. These rehearsals should be multidisciplinary, based in hospital and community settings, and with particular attention given to the orientation of all new staff.

Amniotic fluid embolism (Chapter 5)

There has been an increase in deaths reported as due to amniotic fluid embolism during this triennium. Although there appear to be links with maternal age, overstimulation of the uterus and obstructed labour, it is difficult to predict and prepare for this catastrophic complication.

Five of the 17 deaths from amniotic fluid embolism were associated with substandard care. Midwifery care is viewed as a contributory factor in two cases in which substandard care involved the management of labour. One related to the use of prostaglandins and in the other there was exceptional delay in the second stage of labour in a multiparous woman.

Midwives should take note of these cases and during labour and delivery they should take into account any risk factors present. They should also play an active role in ensuring that they can respond effectively in such cases and that communications with emergency services are well established.

Genital tract sepsis (Chapter 7)

Sepsis around the time of childbirth is often considered a thing of the past owing to the availability of antibiotics, improved socioeconomic circumstances and better general health of women. However, midwives should always be vigilant in their observations for those conditions which now appear rare.

Such infections can quickly develop into fulminating septicaemia and therefore rapid assessment, investigation and treatment are necessary. Midwives should be aware of current research regarding the use of prophylactic antibiotics for caesarean sections and should contribute to local guidelines on the prevention and management of infection.

Chapter 7 includes three cases where midwifery care during the postnatal period was discussed. Although the midwives had involved GPs in the care of these women, it appears that appropriate action and investigations were not carried out.

Any woman presenting with pyrexia, flu-like symptoms, offensive vaginal discharge or diarrhoea and vomiting in the postnatal period should be observed closely. If symptoms are persistent, urgent investigations should be initiated or direct referral made for obstetric care.

Cardiac disease (Chapter 10)

Women with known cardiac disease carry an increased risk of mortality. Midwives have a responsibility to ensure that these women have, and understand, appropriate information regarding these risks. Midwives should also provide support in decision-making and monitor their progress during pregnancy and the postnatal period.

Chapter 10 provides several medically related recommendations related to cardiac disease and also provides useful pointers for midwives to consider. For example, of seven women reported as dying from myocardial infarction, six smoked, one abused various substances including alcohol, and obesity was a feature in one case. Sudden, severe chest pain and numbness or pain radiating into the left arm should always be considered as serious in pregnancy and the postnatal period, requiring urgent referral to expert medical opinion and investigation.

Familial history was a factor in one reported case where two of the woman's immediate family had died from dissecting aneurysm. However, when she presented with severe epigastric pain other differential diagnoses were considered, none of which was cardiac related.

Midwives should be vigilant in their history taking and observations. They should be aware of cardiac conditions and their presentation during pregnancy and the postnatal period. Any woman reporting non-specific illness, chest pain and breathlessness should receive immediate attention.

Epilepsy (Chapter 11)

The increase of deaths from epilepsy gives cause for concern and highlights the importance of appropriate care and support during pregnancy and the postnatal period.

Midwives should have a sound basic knowledge of the condition itself and understand the practicalities of pregnant women living with the condition. Advice should be available on additional risks to which the woman might be exposed and how these can be managed. Where possible women at risk of an epileptic fit should not bathe alone or should use a shower instead. Midwives should be able to provide instruction for women and their families in basic first aid measures, such as clearing the airway and placing the woman in the recovery position, which improve survival following seizures. Ensuring appropriate medical input and patient compliance with taking prescribed drugs is also important.

REPORT ON CONFIDENTIAL ENQUIRIES INTO MATERNAL DEATHS IN THE UNITED KINGDOM

It is interesting to note that five of the 19 women who died were obese and four had major social problems. As stated previously, midwives should target their care and health promotion activities to those most in need.

Deaths from psychiatric causes (Chapter 12)

Midwives are well placed to assess the physical and mental health of women during pregnancy and to provide appropriate support. With the high levels of stress and mental illness in the general population, it is not surprising to find many more women starting pregnancy with histories of depression, or receiving treatment for mental health problems. Midwives should have a sound knowledge and understanding of these conditions and of how best to support women in such circumstances. To provide effective care, midwives must work in collaboration with other professional groups and agencies, paying particular attention to the development of effective communication links.

Midwives should evaluate screening methods for postnatal depression during the antenatal and postnatal period and adopt systems which are shown to be effective.

Recommendations

In most of these cases, midwives were involved at some stage, with the exception of those in very early pregnancy. Although they were not directly cited in every case, they would have had some opportunity for influencing care, and therefore outcome, for some of these women.

As with previous Confidential Enquiries, there are important lessons to be learnt by the different professionals contributing to the care of women and their babies. Putting these lessons into practice, however, has proved to be more difficult than most would expect. Midwives must play an active role in challenging poor practice and ensuring that recommendations from this Report are incorporated into local policies and procedures.

To achieve this, midwives must:

- Ensure effective surveillance throughout pregnancy, childbirth and the postnatal period, with services focused on those vulnerable groups at higher risk of poor pregnancy outcomes.

- Provide clear information to all women on the recognition of signs of departure from the normal in respect of the major causes of maternal death and ensure that women have access to expert advice at all times.

- Provide advice and support on healthy lifestyles to include:
  diet and exercise,
  alcohol and substance misuse,
  safety in the home and workplace,
  basic first aid measures, and
  safety and car travel.

- Ensure screening for mental, social and physical well-being of women during and after pregnancy with, where available, effective assessment tools. Where these are not available midwives should provide active involvement in the development of them.

- Challenge current practice in a proactive and assertive manner if concerns are raised.

- Work in partnership with women and other professional groups to ensure the provision of timely, relevant information which highlights possible complications during pregnancy and the postnatal period, thereby enabling women to access appropriate care when concerns are raised.

- Fully utilise existing systems of midwifery supervision to ensure continuing professional development and actively demonstrate evidence-based care.

- Acknowledge that as members of a multi-disciplinary team, midwives have an equal responsibility in ensuring high standards of care and positive outcomes of pregnancy.

- Ensure that continuing professional development is accepted as the responsibility of the individual practitioner and that proactive updating of knowledge and skills using current research evidence becomes the norm.

References

1. *Changing Childbirth*. Report of the Expert Maternity Group. Department of Health. 1994.

2. *The Protocol for Investment in Health Gain*. Maternal Health. The Welsh Office. 1991.

3. *Provision of Maternity Services in Scotland - a Policy Review*. The Scottish Office Home and Health Department. Scotland. HMSO. 1993. ISBN 0-11-495169-1

4. Northern Ireland. *Delivering choice – Midwifery and General Practitioner led Maternity Units*. Report of the Northern Ireland maternity Unit Study Group – DHSS (NI). August. 1994.

5. WHO(1998) *World Health, 51ˢᵗ year*. Number 1, Feb - Jan 1998. IX (ISSN 0043- 8502).

6. United Kingdom Central Council for Nursing Midwifery and Health Visiting. *Code of Professional Conduct*, paragraph 11. 1992. London: UKCC.

7. Royal College of Midwives. *Domestic Abuse in Pregnancy*. Position Paper 19. London: RCM. 1997.

8. Royal College of Obstetricians and Gynaecologists. *Report of the RCOG Working Party on prophylaxis against thromboembolism in Gynaecology and Obstetrics*. London: RCOG. 1995.

9. Royal College of Obstetricians and Gynaecologists. *Management of Eclampsia. Guidelines Number 10*. London: RCOG. 1996.

16
PATHOLOGY

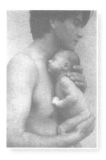

CHAPTER 16
PATHOLOGY

This Chapter differs from the others in that it is designed to stand alone and be used by pathologists without the need to read the entire Report.

The quality of the autopsy

The quality of the maternal autopsy has been adversely commented upon in previous Reports and it is disappointing that the standard of so many autopsies remains inadequate when judged against criteria defined by the Royal College of Pathologists' Bulletin (1993)[1]. Some autopsies were technically deficient in one or more ways - no clinical history, inadequate descriptions of organs, no organ weights, or no histology. For example:

> A woman had a tricuspid valve replacement some years ago. During her uneventful pregnancy she had been reviewed by cardiologists who recommended prophylactic antibiotics in labour. Prophylactic anticoagulation was not considered necessary. She was admitted at term with prolonged rupture of membranes and whilst in labour developed pyrexia and tachycardia, for which she received intravenous antibiotics. Poor fetal progress resulted in a caesarean section, following which the patient made a good recovery and was discharged home. She was found dead at home about three weeks postpartum.

The cause of death at autopsy was given as cardiac failure due to tricuspid incompetence. The lungs were described as grossly oedematous but neither the lungs nor the heart were weighed. The right ventricle was described as hypertrophied, but neither ventricle was either measured or weighed. The tricuspid valve showed extensive nodular calcification of the undersurface adjacent to the valve ring but there was no attempt to culture the valve. There was no attempt to explain how tricuspid incompetence gave rise to severe pulmonary oedema, particularly when the strain of pregnancy had not produced any clinical cardiovascular deterioration. Apart from acute congestion of the liver all other organs were described as normal but there were no weights and the descriptions of the organs were minimal. No histology was performed.

> An older woman was eight weeks pregnant and suddenly collapsed at home. Emergency laparotomy showed extensive right-sided retroperitoneal bleeding but she was moribund and could not be resuscitated.

At autopsy, ruptured iliac veins were given as the cause of the extensive retroperitoneal bleeding, but there were no details with regard to its site, pathological appearance or relation to the uterus and pelvic organs. There was no description of the uterus or the conceptus.

Although thrombus in the inferior vena cava was identified, its extent and location were not described. Despite the very unusual nature of this case, no histology was taken.

Whilst some autopsies are technically deficient, in many the cause of an unexpected death is clearly identified from the autopsy, but there is failure to address other clinical problems relating to the case:

> An obese multiparous woman suddenly died at 12 weeks of pregnancy. She had a history of myocarditis and at 10 weeks gestation had had chorionic villus sampling.

The autopsy clearly identified death as due to pulmonary embolus with an iliac vein thrombosis. However, there was no mention of some organs in the report - pancreas, bladder and ovaries. There was no description of the placental bed site and the descriptions of the pulmonary artery emboli and of the venous tree were very simple. As no histology was performed, confirmatory evidence of the previous myocarditis was not obtained and alternative cardiac pathologies were not excluded. Also there was no search for any evidence of pulmonary hypertension or previous pulmonary emboli as an alternative explanation of her previous 'myocarditis'.

> An obese multiparous woman had a history of severe asthma and was a heavy smoker. Her current pregnancy was complicated by a placental cord tumour with polyhydramnios, and elective caesarean section was planned. Bronchodilators were given, together with preoperative hydrocortisone. The patient collapsed immediately after delivery of the placenta, severe disseminated intravascular coagulation supervened and she quickly died. A clinical diagnosis of amniotic fluid embolus was made.

No clinical history was given in the post-mortem report, which recorded an abnormal heart weighing 500 g. The ventricles were not separately weighed, and there was no attempt to identify the cause of this abnormality. No cardiac pathologist's opinion was sought. Clots and remnants of amniotic membranes adherent to the uterine wall were identified, but there was no documentation of any uterine wall tears or damage. The liver, at twice the normal weight, was described as fatty. There was no reference to the pathological changes of asthma within the lungs. Histologically, only the lungs were examined and there was no reference to the changes of asthma nor was there any indication of any special search for amniotic fluid embolus. There was no histological examination of the heart, the placental bed site, or any other organ.

> A primipara in her twenties had a normal pregnancy up to 37 weeks, when she became breathless. She was admitted the following day and a cardiologist diagnosed cardiomyopathy. She was anticoagulated and labour was induced. After delivery she was transferred to the Intensive Care Unit and made rapid recovery. Massive pulmonary embolus clinically occurred on the 16th postpartum day.

In the autopsy report there was no review of the clinical history and only the heart was weighed. Description of the heart identified right ventricular hypertrophy, without detail, and up to 40% narrowing of the left anterior descending coronary artery. Pulmonary emboli within the pulmonary trunk and major arteries were confirmed as the immediate cause of death but there was no attempt to identify any previous episode of thromboembolisation. Despite the discrepancies in the pathological findings and with the clinical diagnosis of cardiomyopathy, there was no histology performed on the heart or any of the other organs, nor was specialist cardiac pathological opinion sought.

The inadequacy of the autopsy does not necessarily relate to failure to address specific pathological features of *Direct* maternal deaths:

> A primigravida had suffered from epilepsy for many years. Her therapy was changed from phenytoin to carbamazepine during her pregnancy. Her drug levels were subsequently monitored and were within the therapeutic range three weeks before death. When 36 weeks pregnant, she had a 'stomach upset' and she was found dead in bed the following day. There was a previous medical history of depression with five suicide attempts.

None of the previous medical history or features of drug therapy were identified in the post-mortem report and, although histology was performed on the heart, lungs, liver and kidneys, there was no histology on the placental bed or placenta. More particularly, even though death was attributed to epilepsy, no drug levels were obtained either to establish therapeutic levels at the time of death or to exclude overdose as an alternative cause of death.

Good autopsies

Conversely, a good autopsy contributes significantly to the assessment:

> A woman in her thirties had a spontaneous vaginal delivery at 41 weeks' gestation. Within minutes of delivery there was sudden collapse with rapid demise. Clinically, amniotic fluid embolus was diagnosed.

At autopsy, massive haemoperitoneum with a ruptured aneurysm of the splenic artery was identified. There was detailed comprehensive description of all the organs but, more especially, there was detailed histology. Amniotic fluid embolism was carefully excluded and the lack of any systemic arterial pathology was demonstrated.

> An obese, multiparous woman had had a deep vein thrombosis (DVT) in her first pregnancy. Since then she had been on warfarin, recently changed to aspirin. She was not taking the oral contraceptive. She was a late booking at 26 weeks in her second pregnancy and was a poor attender at antenatal clinic. It was considered that heparin self-administration would be unreliable and that she should be anticoagulated with warfarin postpartum. At 39 weeks she presented with a swollen hot, tender, right thigh. Labour was induced. A small postpartum haemorrhage occurred but there were no retained products. She was out of bed after 24 hours, ambulant at 48 hours and discharged at 5 days postpartum. Heparin was given postpartum, but warfarin was not re-started. Four months postpartum she was referred to physicians with recurring breathlessness and weight loss since her pregnancy. A diagnosis of hyperthyroidism was made and she was treated with carbimazole. When seen again six weeks later she still had distressing shortness of breath and was admitted for investigation. She collapsed and died the following day.

The autopsy included a detailed review of the clinical history and documented the height and weight of the body. At the autopsy, pulmonary emboli of varying ages were identified, there was a detailed search of the venous tree and right ventricular hypertrophy was documented as the major abnormality in the enlarged heart. There was detailed histology of all organs and recanalised pulmonary emboli, plexiform lesions and pulmonary hypertension were identified in the lungs. The thyroid was histologically normal.

Autopsies by Chapter

Chapter 2: Thromboembolism:

Of the 48 deaths attributed to thromboembolism in this Report several did not have a post-mortem and in some further cases no autopsy report was available. Of the remainder, only eight could be described as model (five) or good (three). These reports not only established the cause of death and searched for the source, but also specifically searched for pathological changes that would contribute to understanding other significant episodes in the clinical history.

> An obese woman, whose mother had had multiple pulmonary emboli, developed proteinuria at 41 weeks of her pregnancy. Labour was induced and a large baby was delivered by ventouse and forceps. She was immobile after delivery. Two weeks postpartum she had an episode of pleuritic chest pain treated conservatively but without anticoagulation. Some weeks later she became suddenly short of breath and the following day she collapsed and died.

Autopsy demonstrated a large saddle embolus in the pulmonary trunk with widespread embolism of small pulmonary arteries throughout both lungs (which also showed infarction). Thrombus was identified in the right external iliac vein and there was a detailed description of the patent veins of the abdomen, pelvis and legs. Extensive histology confirmed that there was fresh embolization of the lungs, but also showed organisation of some thrombi to pulmonary arterial walls, indicating a previous episode of embolization, entirely consistent with the clinical episode two weeks prior to death.

Sadly, not all cases reach this standard. Many have been classified as adequate because the autopsy findings satisfactorily explained the clinical history, even if no histology was performed and the College Guidelines were not met.

Ten reports would be considered inadequate/poor even by these relaxed criteria, the following being typical examples:

> A parous woman in her thirties was admitted to hospital in early pregnancy with hyperemesis gravidarum. She was rehydrated, treated with pyridoxine and given TED stockings to wear, but a week later she collapsed and died with chest pain, severe shortness of breath and cyanosis. She had a history of severe headaches with left-sided weakness which had been diagnosed on CT scan as infarction adjacent to the anterior horn of the left ventricle.

The autopsy report, including patient details and cause of death, was limited to one side of A4 paper. There was no history, and there were no organ weights. The brain was described as "normal external and cut surfaces" . Emboli were identified in the lungs, but the venous source was not identified. No search of pelvic veins was made. Histology of the brain, liver, kidneys and lungs was not undertaken. The brain, liver and kidneys were described as normal. There was no attempt to identify the area of radiologically diagnosed cerebral infarction, there was no description of the hypothalamus or mamilliary bodies to exclude acute Wernicke's encephalopathy, and the search for the source of the pulmonary emboli was inadequate.

> A known multiparous asthmatic had an uneventful pregnancy until term, when failure to progress in labour resulted in a caesarean section under spinal anaesthesia. Postoperatively she had puerperal sepsis with positive high vaginal swabs and blood cultures. This was vigorously treated with intravenous antibiotics. She was discharged after a week on penicillin, metronidazole and ciprofloxacin. She had complained of pain in her calf postoperatively and, although there was no evidence of thrombosis on Doppler ultrasound, TED stockings were prescribed. She had a transient undiagnosed illness 11 days after discharge, but otherwise seemed reasonably well until three weeks postpartum when she complained of feeling very unwell, and then suddenly collapsed and died.

Autopsy macroscopically was very thorough and detailed, identifying the massive pulmonary emboli, a source in the leg veins and patent pelvic veins. However, the clinical history of asthma and puerperal sepsis was not addressed, and no histology was taken. There was no attempt therefore to assess whether previous episodes of embolism had occurred.

Chapter 3: Hypertensive disorders of pregnancy

There were 20 deaths directly attributed to pregnancy-induced hypertension. As has been identified in the Chapter, the mean time between the last antenatal attendance and the development of severe pre-eclampsia or eclampsia was 6.5 days. Many cases also occurred between 26 and 33 weeks of gestation. It is therefore entirely conceivable that fulminating pre-eclampsia, giving rise to unexpected death, may occur *de novo* in the intervals between antenatal assessments.

> A young primigravida developed proteinuria at 31 weeks' gestation but had a normal blood pressure and, therefore, was not referred for assessment. One week later she died at home. She had been complaining of feeling unwell with a swollen face when last seen by friends.

The autopsy was thorough and detailed and clearly demonstrated findings consistent with fulminating pre-eclampsia.

> A multiparous woman had been treated for one month for a microcytic hypochromic anaemia. There was no history of epilepsy and during her pregnancy, blood pressure and urinalysis had been normal. At 31 weeks' gestation she was found drowned in the bath.

A detailed and thorough autopsy showed minimal macroscopic pathology but histology clearly identified changes of pre-eclampsia in the liver, kidneys, placenta and placental bed. A drug screen was negative. Death was attributed to drowning secondary to an eclamptic fit.

> A primigravida was admitted unconscious with hypertension and proteinuria. She had been normotensive 11 days prior to admission. CT scan of the brain showed a large, right parietal haematoma.

A very detailed autopsy with histology confirmed the intracerebral haemorrhage with changes of pre-eclampsia within the brain, liver, kidneys and placenta.

In contrast to the last case there is an increasing tendency for death from cerebral haemorrhage not to come to autopsy. Frequently, therefore, the cause of the cerebral haemorrhage - arteriovenous malformation, berry aneurysm, systemic hypertension, or pregnancy-induced hypertension is not ascertained.

> A multiparous woman had suffered from severe essential hypertension since her teens. She also had asthma for which she used salbutamol. She was under the care of renal physicians. During her pregnancy she was on Isradapine and frusemide. At 28 weeks' gestation she was admitted for an assessment of her blood pressure, which was 160/110 mmHg. One week later she was admitted with signs of a stroke which clinically was diagnosed as subarachnoid haemorrhage. There was no post-mortem.

The lack of post-mortem is surprising as severe essential hypertension from such a young age is unusual in itself. Also, the true nature of the cerebral haemorrhage was not ascertained and pre-eclampsia/eclampsia was not satisfactorily excluded.

> A primigravida with a history of asthma and a family history of hypertension had borderline raised blood pressure during the course of her pregnancy. She was admitted at 36 weeks' gestation with a blood pressure of 140/85 mmHg and digital and ankle oedema. There was no proteinuria. Spontaneous vaginal delivery occurred the next day, following which her blood pressure settled to 110-135 systolic and 80-90 diastolic. She was discharged on day five post-partum, but was re-admitted four days later with headache and vomiting, and a blood pressure of 154/100 mmHg. She was orientated in time, place and person, but two hours later she was drowsy, writhing and moaning. One hour later she had a severe, right hemiplegia. CT scan showed intracerebral haemorrhage and she was declared brain dead.

There was no post-mortem, and the cause of the cerebral haemorrhage remained undetermined.

Even when active treatment has been initiated, death can be due to other causes:

> An older woman was admitted at 35 weeks' gestation with hypertension (150/95 mmHg) and proteinuria. Labour was induced with prostaglandins. Shortly afterwards she started to feel unwell and medical staff were urgently summoned. When they attended, she was cyanosed, foaming at the mouth and unresponsive to commands. Cardiac arrest procedures were performed, but she could not be resuscitated. At autopsy the changes of eclampsia were minimal, but numerous fetal squames were found in the pulmonary capillaries.

REPORT ON CONFIDENTIAL ENQUIRIES INTO MATERNAL DEATHS IN THE UNITED KINGDOM

Chapter 5: Amniotic fluid embolism (AFE)

This condition has a classical clinical presentation - sudden collapse during labour with cyanosis and rapid onset of disseminated intravascular coagulation (DIC) - which is so strongly suggestive that in the last triennial Report cases were included in this category that were not confirmed at autopsy. Similarly in this Report deaths have been attributed to AFE that have not been substantiated at autopsy.

Reasons for this vary. Some autopsy reports are so bad that no reliance can be placed on their findings. In others a search for AFE was apparently made and none found but it is unclear what techniques were used or how diligent was the search. In other instances survival in ICU raises doubts about how long fetal squames persist in the maternal pulmonary circulation. Finally, because AFE can masquerade as intrapartum/postpartum haemorrhage it is rare to encounter an autopsy report where this diagnosis has been carefully excluded from the causes of massive uterine haemorrhage.

> An obese severe asthmatic who weighed over 100 kg had an elective caesarean section at 36 weeks but had a cardiac arrest just after the placenta was delivered. Clinically, amniotic fluid embolus was suspected.

The very brief autopsy report failed to address any of the issues. The heart was enlarged at 500 g but no separate ventricular weights were undertaken and the macroscopic description was terse. No specialist opinion was sought. Clots and remnants of amniotic fluid membranes were identified but there was no documentation of any damage or tears in the uterus. There was no histological examination of any organs apart from the lungs. Although it was stated that there were no fetal squames in the maternal circulation, no special techniques were employed and there was no evaluation of the changes of asthma in her lungs, nor was any search for DIC made. These factors create a lack of confidence that AFE has been satisfactorily excluded.

> An older woman with known uterine fibroids was admitted at 24 weeks with severe right iliac fossa pain, thought to be due to infarction of her fibroids. After two days the pain had settled and she was discharged, only to be quickly readmitted the same day with increasing pain. The following day she collapsed, became cyanosed and developed coagulopathy. She had a spontaneous abortion and died 24 hours later in Intensive Care .

Autopsy showed evidence of DIC macroscopically and the lungs were oedematous and congested. The infarcted uterine fibroid was confirmed and some tears were noted in the cervix. Histology confirmed DIC and 'probable' fetal squames were found in occasional pulmonary capillaries. Given the gestation and the unusual clinical presentation it would have been appropriate to confirm the fetal squames in the maternal circulation immunocytochemically.

> A parous woman was admitted at term + 10 days for induction of labour. Following rupture of membranes fetal distress was noted and emergency caesarean section was performed. The fetal head was jammed in the pelvis. During the section blood came out of the urinary catheter and there was vaginal bleeding but initially it was not certain whether this was due to trauma to the

urogenital tract or to DIC. The bleeding could not be controlled so eventually total hysterectomy was performed. After this the patient was transferred to Intensive Care where DIC was confirmed but despite supportive measures, she died the following day.

A detailed autopsy was performed which included detailed comment on the absence of surgical trauma, review of the resected uterus and extensive histology on a wide range of organs. Histology confirmed the widespread DIC and confirmed the clinical diagnosis of AFE.

Modern immunocytochemical techniques are more sensitive than the standard histochemical methods. It is therefore recommended that unless fetal squames are easily found on standard histology, any search for AFE should incorporate probing the maternal lung sections with cytokeratin markers. Whilst CAM 5.2 is the most commonly used cytokeratin probe, LP34 gives stronger marking of fetal squames and a cleaner pulmonary background.

Such findings need to be interpreted against a background of knowledge about the frequency with which fetal squames can be detected in maternal lungs without the clinical syndrome normally associated with AFE. We also need to have information about the survival time of fetal squames in the lung, now that putative clinical cases are surviving.

Chapter 6: Deaths in early pregnancy

These are most commonly due to ectopic pregnancy but also include deaths from abortion before 24 weeks. Deaths from ruptured ectopic pregnancy are usually due to hypovolaemic shock from massive haemorrhage, or DIC supervening after successful resuscitation. The cause of death is therefore usually obvious at autopsy if clinically undiagnosed, or clinically apparent if resuscitation has been attempted. However, neither of these reasons excuses inadequate documentation of findings. Adequate documentation would become even more important if conservative treatment for ectopic pregnancies of less than 4 cm diameter becomes the established norm.

> A multiparous woman presented to A&E in a collapsed state, and asystole rapidly supervened. She had not been to her GP about her early pregnancy.

At autopsy there was fresh massive haemoperitoneum and a ruptured left fallopian tube. The rupture measured over 1cm in diameter and spongy placental tissue was present in the pelvis near the tube.

There are occasions when complications, particularly after abortion, demand a more detailed autopsy:

> A young mother had several episodes of threatened miscarriage and re-presented to the hospital at 17 weeks with further bleeding. She miscarried 9 hours later and a foul smelling discharge was noted. At this stage she was tachycardic, jaundiced, oliguric and anaemic. Treatment for DIC was initiated and evacuation of putrid placental tissue was undertaken but death occurred some hours later.

Autopsy included detailed histology and microbiology. There was no histological evidence of DIC. Swabs taken from the uterine cavity, and tissue taken from several organs grew *Escherichia coli*.

Unfortunately this is not always the standard provided:

> A multiparous woman had retained products evacuated after an incomplete miscarriage at 10 weeks. Four days later she was re-admitted with a three-day history of shortness of breath and leg swelling. She was hypotensive with a tachycardia but her temperature was normal. Intravenous antibiotics were started. She was noted to be jaundiced with a falling platelet count. Subtotal hysterectomy for suspected gangrene was undertaken and the patient was transferred to ICU but she died the next day.

At autopsy the lungs were heavy and airless and the liver and spleen were grossly enlarged. Despite the clinical history there was no attempt to culture any tissues. Histology confirmed widespread changes of septicaemia in the heart and kidneys and there was liver "necrosis" which was not further defined.

It is necessary to repeat the recommendation from the last Report that it is inadequate not to have taken tissues and swabs for culture and not to have undertaken extensive histology in such cases.

Chapter 7: Genital tract sepsis

There were 16 deaths from genital tract sepsis excluding abortion. Of these, three were post-surgical and 11 occurred after spontaneous delivery.

Streptococcal septicaemia caused 10 deaths. Because of the speed with which it progresses, a high index of clinical suspicion, rapid laboratory responses and vigorous therapy are needed to combat it. This in turn demands careful and thorough autopsy when death does supervene.

> A primigravid patient presented at 37 weeks by ultrasound dates with a "concealed" pregnancy. She was normotensive and fetal movements and heart beat were present. She was admitted next day with abdominal pain and evidence of intrauterine death, which was confirmed by ultrasound. DIC rapidly supervened and labour was induced by ARM and oxytocin. The liquor was blood stained. The patient developed a mottled appearance with an increased respiratory rate and poor urine output. A clinical diagnosis of AFE was made. Because of poor progress in labour an emergency caesarean section was successfully performed with minimal postoperative bleeding and the patient was returned to ICU. Despite further supportive measures her condition inexorably deteriorated and she died that evening.

Autopsy showed features of DIC with extensive petechial haemorrhages throughout all organs. Massive bilateral adrenal haemorrhages were found and the spleen was enlarged. Extensive histology confirmed the DIC with haemorrhagic infarction of adrenals and liver but no amniotic fluid embolus was found in the lungs. However, there were microabscesses in the myocardium with Gram-positive cocci present, and Group B streptococci were grown from a post-mortem intra-uterine swab.

Other infections can be as deadly:

> A woman in her thirties had an intrauterine death after an antepartum haemorrhage at 26 weeks of pregnancy. Overnight she collapsed and was transferred to Intensive Care. She died 24 hours later.

At autopsy there was evidence of a bleeding diathesis but the major abnormality was an enlarged uterus filled with blood and with numerous bubbles of gas throughout the endometrium. Histology confirmed the presence of DIC and there were numerous colonies of Gram-positive cocci throughout the necrotic myometrium, confirming the growth of *Clostridium perfringens* on culture.

Necrotising fasciitis can complicate both surgical and non-surgical genital tract sepsis:

> A woman was admitted to hospital 12 days postpartum with several days' history of pain in the left leg and back. She had had a spontaneous vaginal delivery without complications and had not required an episiotomy. A few days prior to admission there had been an offensive blood-stained vaginal discharge. On examination she was shocked and a diagnosis of pelvic sepsis with septicaemia was made. Further investigation suggested necrotising fasciitis extending down the left thigh associated with ß haemolytic streptococcal infection. Despite aggressive antibiotic therapy combined with hyperbaric oxygen her condition deteriorated with extensive necrotising fasciitis, renal failure and DIC. Five days after admission subtotal hysterectomy was performed. Despite further aggressive treatment her condition relentlessly deteriorated and she died three weeks after delivery.

The autopsy macroscopically confirmed the extensive necrotising fasciitis together with evidence of septicaemia but there was no confirmatory histology or microbiology. Review of the uterus, however, did confirm extensive haemorrhagic infarction with a minimal inflammatory response, thus implicating the genital tract as the source of the infection.

Chapter 8: Genital tract trauma and other *Direct* deaths.

In cases of genital trauma it is important to provide a detailed description of the injuries, to identify the site of the placenta and to exclude amniotic fluid embolus.

> A multiparous woman had a trisomy-13 pregnancy but declined termination. An intrauterine death occurred and labour was induced with prostaglandins at 38 weeks of pregnancy. During labour there was evidence of a ruptured uterus, with DIC rapidly supervening. Emergency hysterectomy was required and large volumes of blood were transfused. She was transferred to an ICU and subsequently required a second laparotomy for ureteric damage. She gradually deteriorated and showed signs of diabetes insipidus before death. Cause of death was given clinically as septicaemia.

Nothing of this complicated history was recorded in the pathology report. The description of the urogenital system was very brief and there was no attempt to either localise or describe the extent of the ureteric damage. Despite the history of diabetes insipidus the pituitary was not described. The liver was twice the normal weight and was described as fatty, but subsequent histology was described as normal. This discrepancy was not explained. No histology of the pituitary was taken. In the description of the cardiovascular system moderate atheroma was identified, but not detailed. Despite the clinical diagnosis of septicaemia, no cultures or attempts to localise the source of infection were made.

A young woman was admitted at 41 weeks for induction of labour. Fetal distress developed and a forceps delivery was attempted. This was unsuccessful and an emergency caesarean section was performed. Following the operation there was blood in the urine and from the vagina. The abdominal incision was reopened and tears were found in the bladder, upper vagina and lower uterine segment. Cardiorespiratory arrest occurred, with successful resuscitation. The tears were repaired but within an hour there were signs of DIC. She was transferred to Intensive Care but over the next few days had an intermittent pyrexia, became increasingly difficult to ventilate and haemodynamically unstable, and died.

Autopsy showed grossly abnormal lungs consistent with adult respiratory distress syndrome, and there were vegetations on the pulmonary valve. However, there was no detailed description of the trauma to the genital tract, no histological confirmation of the macroscopic findings, no exclusion of AFE and no culture of the pulmonary valve vegetations.

Chapter 10: Cardiac *Indirect* deaths

Congenital

There were ten deaths associated with congenital cardiac anomalies. Two were complicated by endocarditis clinically but autopsy was not performed in one. The other autopsy was conducted to a high standard and confirmed the clinical findings. Two deaths were due to pulmonary hypertension complicating Eisenmenger's Syndrome but the autopsy report was available for only one of these. This was very good and detailed, clearly identifying the extensive plexogenic arteriopathy with fibrinoid necrosis in the lungs. The report on the second was not available for assessment though a letter from the consultant obstetrician states that there were no unexpected findings at autopsy. A third death was from primary pulmonary hypertension of long standing, but again no report was available for assessment.

Autopsy was of value in two cases in which sudden unexpected death occurred. In the first case there was a grossly enlarged heart which was histologically confirmed as hypertrophic cardiomyopathy. In the second there were anomalous coronary arteries each of which rapidly subdivided into a leash of very small vessels from a normal ostium.

Acquired

Myocardial Infarction

There were six deaths related to myocardial infarction/ischaemic heart disease. A consistent pattern of heavy smoking in women in their thirties emerges although details of family history and blood lipids are rarely known. All deaths were sudden and unexpected apart from one patient who had central chest pain radiating into the left arm whilst in hospital and died six days later.

A woman in her twenties had a salpingectomy for an ectopic pregnancy. Ten days later at home she suddenly woke up in the early hours of the morning with an apparent panic attack. She died at home shortly afterwards.

Autopsy showed a 0.5 cm long atheromatous plaque producing a 70-80% stenosis of the lumen in the proximal left anterior descending coronary artery. Fresh thrombus occluded the residual lumen and this was histologically confirmed.

Although autopsy clearly demonstrates the cause of death in these cases with thrombotic occlusion or severe atherosclerotic stenosis of an artery, in two instances histology to date the myocardial infarction would have been helpful. One of these has already been described, the other is described below:

> An older woman had a termination of pregnancy at 12 weeks. There were no complications. Five days later she was taken by ambulance to A&E with chest pain and headache but died.

At autopsy there was severe coronary artery atheroma with an occlusive small thrombus in the left anterior descending artery and evidence of myocardial infarction. Histology would have helped date the timing of the infarct.

Other cardiac

There were eight deaths attributed to cardiomyopathy or to myocarditis; half came to autopsy. Of the four available autopsy reports two are inadequate:

> A primipara in her thirties, with a long history of asthma, developed breathlessness and cardiac failure a few days after delivery. She was treated medically for about six weeks, but was then transferred to a cardiac transplant centre for assessment. She arrived shocked with impalpable peripheral pulses and died some three days later.

The autopsy (conducted by a visiting pathologist) made little attempt to correlate findings with the clinical history, and no histology of the organs apart from the heart was taken. Even that histology was not reported on, as the consultant cardiologist commented that "we did not get any opportunity to have further details of the postpartum cardiomyopathy pathology". Perhaps this was because a copy of the autopsy report was only received at the hospital 4½ months after the post-mortem was performed.

> A primipara in her twenties was well until 37 weeks when she became breathless. She was admitted to hospital the next day, and after investigation by a cardiologist, was diagnosed as having cardiomyopathy. She was anticoagulated, labour was induced and ventouse delivery was effected followed by transfer to ICU. She was making good progress when she suddenly collapsed and died two weeks later.

Autopsy showed death to be due to a massive saddle pulmonary embolus, but did not record the presence, or absence, of earlier emboli. The heart was grossly abnormal at 554 g and right ventricular hypertrophy was mentioned but neither ventricle was separately weighed. Atheroma was said to have produced a 40% narrowing of the left anterior descending coronary artery. Despite all this gross pathology, no histology was performed and no cardiac pathology opinion was sought. Whilst it seems likely that this case is a cardiomyopathy decompensating during pregnancy and complicated by a terminal pulmonary embolus, the quality of the autopsy ensures that this will remain speculative.

Aneurysms

Autopsy clearly established the cause of death and its source in the seven cases of ruptured aneurysm. Two were dissecting aneurysms of the aorta, two of the coronary arteries and one each of the splenic, renal and superior mesenteric arteries. However, although histology was apparently often performed on the aneurysm it was rare for this report to be included with the documents, so that identification of any systemic arterial pathology is difficult to assess. Two cases illustrate how it should be done:

> A parous woman in her thirties presented at 39 weeks with severe epigastric pain. Labour was induced and the pain spontaneously resolved only to recur two days postpartum. The patient suddenly collapsed and died shortly afterwards. There was a strong family history of dissecting aortic aneurysm.

The autopsy was detailed and a careful search was made for the stigmata of Marfan's syndrome, which were absent. Haemopericardium from a dissecting aortic aneurysm was found. Cystic medial necrosis of the aorta was identified histologically and the findings were confirmed by a second opinion from a cardiac pathologist.

> A woman who had had a renal transplant but who was still hypertensive, had premature rupture of membranes at 32 weeks and had an emergency caesarean section. She was well until the sixth postpartum day when she developed severe abdominal and back pain needing morphine. Ten hours after onset of the pain she suddenly collapsed and died.

Autopsy was detailed, including identification of a high arched palate, and detailed description of the placental bed site and the renal transplants, as well as the haemopericardium from the ruptured dissecting aortic aneurysm. Histology, which was extensive, confirmed the myxoid degeneration of the aortic wall, and fibroblast culture was attempted.

Chapter 11: Other *Indirect* deaths

These cover a miscellany of diseases, and in many of these the relationship and interaction of the disease with pregnancy is uncertain.

Epilepsy

The highest proportion (10) of the 19 deaths from epilepsy recorded in this Report occurred in the last trimester: almost all were unwitnessed sudden deaths with the diagnosis made at autopsy. Although there was usually a strong clinical history of epilepsy, two patients had not had fits in the previous two years and one other had only had her first minor fits during her pregnancy.

> An epileptic patient who was under the care of her GP only, was having increasing numbers of fits from 30 weeks' gestation onwards. Admission to hospital was sought after one series of fits but was refused. Later that day she was found dead on the floor of her bedroom.

Following autopsy, death was attributed to aspiration of vomit due to epilepsy but there was no toxicology undertaken and there was no histology of any tissues. It is therefore unknown whether or not the patient was taking the prescribed medication, whether or not this produced adequate therapeutic levels and whether or not there was any other potential causes of death.

> A primipara was a known epileptic with a history of depression and multiple attempts at suicide by drug overdose. She had her therapy changed from phenytoin to carbamazepine during her pregnancy. Drug levels were within the therapeutic range three weeks before death. When 36 weeks pregnant she had a stomach upset and she was found dead in bed the next day.

None of the previous medical history or features of drug therapy were identified in the post-mortem report and, although histology was performed on the heart, lungs, liver and kidneys there was no histology on the placental bed or placenta. More particularly, no drug levels were ascertained either to establish therapeutic levels at the time of death or to exclude overdose as a cause of death even though death was attributed to epilepsy.

> Another primipara had been epileptic from a very early age and averaged one grand mal fit a month. When she became pregnant she halved her dose of anticonvulsants with the agreement of her GP. Even on this reduced regime she was having fewer fits whilst pregnant. She was found dead in the bath one day when her husband returned from work.

Autopsy confirmed features consistent with death by drowning. There was no trace of any anticonvulsant in the post-mortem toxicological analysis, suggesting that the patient had inadvertently, or deliberately, not taken her medication. Detailed neuropathological examination of the brain failed to demonstrate any specific seizure-related pathology and there was no evidence of any other specific pathological process on histological examination of many organs.

> A known poorly controlled insulin-dependent diabetic who also had epilepsy was found dead in bed at 12 weeks' gestation. Epilepsy was suspected as the cause of death.

At autopsy, post-mortem blood levels of valproate (37.3 μg) were only marginally below the therapeutic range (40-100 μg) whereas vitreous humour glucose was significantly reduced, being less than 1 mmol/l. Hypoglycaemia was therefore clearly incriminated in the cause of death.

Obviously the role of the autopsy is crucial in establishing the cause of death in these patients. It must therefore be considered an essential part of the autopsy to exclude other causes of fits, such as eclampsia, and to establish the therapeutic drug levels in the body at the time of death.

Phaeochromocytoma

Phaeochromocytoma must be considered here, particularly as some of these deaths presented as other obstetric catastrophes. There were five deaths from phaeochromocytoma and these were almost invariably autopsy-based diagnoses:

A woman who had been normotensive during her pregnancy had an elective caesarean section at term, but shortly afterwards had a cardiorespiratory arrest. Pulmonary embolus from DVT or amniotic fluid was suspected.

At autopsy an infarcted tumour of the right adrenal was found. Viable portions of the tumour were histologically identifiable as a phaeochromocytoma.

Another woman had an episode of sudden, severe headache lasting about two hours during spontaneous vaginal delivery of a full-term infant. Eight days later she was admitted with a 12-24-hour history of very severe, sudden onset headache. She was normotensive and investigations were inconclusive. Another four days later she had another episode of severe headache, and some hours after this she had a witnessed tonic convulsion and went into a deep coma. Evidence of DIC and renal failure developed and she died in Intensive Care a day later.

A thorough, detailed autopsy showed changes consistent with DIC and revealed a 3 cm diameter infarcted left adrenal tumour. Neuropathological examination of the brain showed acute hypoxic/ischaemic changes consistent with an episode of severe hypertensive encephalopathy.

Other causes

There were a small number of deaths from infections that may be regarded as opportunistic. Some complicated diseases which are known to reduce immunocompetence but in other instances the fulminating infection may have been the result of the pregnancy.

A woman suffered from diabetes and renal failure with nephrotic syndrome. She also had cataracts, peripheral neuropathy and asthma. During the last trimester she was investigated for anaemia, tachycardia, pericardial effusions and a peripheral blood eosinophilia: a diagnosis of Churg-Strauss syndrome had been made. At 34 weeks she went into spontaneous labour and had a normal vaginal delivery. Eight days postpartum she collapsed with abdominal pain and then had a cardiac arrest. She was transferred to ICU and a subarachnoid haemorrhage was found on CT scan. She developed peritonitis through her peritoneal dialysis and died 27 days postpartum.

There was an excellent and very detailed autopsy with macroscopic evidence of peritonitis and an abscess in the myocardium. Papillary necrosis of the kidneys was also present. There was no growth on culture of swabs and tissues but hyphae of *Candida* were found in the heart and peritoneum on histology. There were extensive diabetic complications but no evidence of a vasculitis was found.

A young primipara was in the last trimester of her pregnancy when she presented to A&E with fever, a distressing cough and a three-day rash. A diagnosis of varicella pneumonitis was made. Intravenous acyclovir was started together with broad spectrum antibiotics. Evidence of DIC rapidly developed, she continued to deteriorate and emergency caesarean section was undertaken. Cardiac arrest occurred during the procedure and attempts at resuscitation were unsuccessful.

An excellent detailed autopsy confirming the disseminated lesions of varicella virus was supplemented by extensive microbiological and virological culture of tissues as well as histology. Varicella virus was confirmed by immunocytochemistry and by PCR techniques on the histological samples. Lymphoid tissues were reactive with no evidence of any underlying immunodeficiency.

These cases illustrate the positive contribution of an autopsy to assessing the circumstances giving rise to a maternal death.

Chapter 13: *Fortuitous* deaths

Whilst many of these deaths are of no consequence to the Enquiry, it is important that the survey is comprehensive. The difficult "borderline *Indirect*" cases, particularly infections and tumours, have already been highlighted. Even when death is *Fortuitous*, useful information relevant to pregnancy may be available for analysis. Deaths by suicide are an obvious problem area as puerperal depression may have been a factor. There are also several deaths from road traffic accidents in this report and many of these are from acceleration/deceleration injuries. What is often not known is whether or not a seat belt was being worn and whether some of the injuries, particularly to the large gravid uterus, were seat belt-associated or not.

As the circumstances of these *Fortuitous* deaths are so varied it is difficult to formulate precise recommendations, except to re-emphasise the importance of the College Guidelines in the conducting and reporting of autopsies.

For this Report, however, we would recommend that the information on the use of seat belts is recorded as accurately as possible.

Reference

1.   Guidelines for Post Mortem Reports, 1993. Royal College of Pathologists, London.

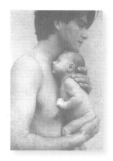

ANNEX 1 TO CHAPTER 16
RECOMMENDATIONS FOR PATHOLOGISTS

The following abbreviated guide to the requirements for a maternal death autopsy should be regarded as **supplementing**, and **not** replacing the Guidelines issued by the Royal College of Pathologists[1]. If in doubt, advice and help should be sought from the local CEMD Regional Pathology Assessor : the current list of Assessors can be found at the end of this Report.

In general:

Maternal deaths are still under-reported and pathologists performing autopsies on women who are pregnant or are known have been pregnant within a year of their death should contact their local Director of Public Health (DPH) to check that the case has been reported.

Clinical information for the Enquiry is sometimes incomplete and pathologists should provide a review of the clinical history in autopsy reports, including height and weight of the woman.

Specific disorders

Hypertensive diseases

Check and note existence of local guidelines for the management of hypertensive disorders of pregnancy.

Identify fluid balance; minimum histology of lungs, liver, kidney, brain, placental site; exclude previous hypertension.

Thromboembolism

Identify any local risk factors protocol, note family history, significance of chest symptoms, heparin prophylaxis.

Describe the nature and distribution of emboli; site of origin; evidence of previous episodes; histology.

Haemorrhage: APH and PPH

Macroscopic: Identify the site and severity of bleeding; location of placenta; detail genital tract trauma.

Histology: placental histology; search for DIC; exclude AFE; review other tissues resected.

Early pregnancy

Ectopics: diagnostic awareness, ultrasound monitoring and diagnosis; Location and size of ectopic; estimate blood loss; review other tissues resected.

Abortions: sites and locations of bowel perforations; culture of tissues.

Amniotic fluid embolism

Macroscopic: detailed examination of genital tract for trauma.

Histology: detailed histology of both lungs; immunocytochemistry for cytokeratins if in doubt.

Women dying after labour **of causes other than suspected amniotic fluid embolism** should have their lungs examined for amniotic squames to check whether amniotic fluid can enter the circulation without a fatal outcome.

Hyperemesis

Exclude acute Wernicke's encephalopathy.

Epilepsy

Macroscopic: exclude specific brain pathology; establish anticonvulsant drug levels.

Histology: exclude eclampsia as cause of fits.

Cardiac deaths

Macroscopic: full description of heart; weigh/measure ventricles separately.

Histology: both ventricles; assess conducting system; seek cardiac pathology opinion if in doubt.

Aneurysms

Macroscopic: nature and site of aneurysm.

Histology: distribution of arterial pathology.

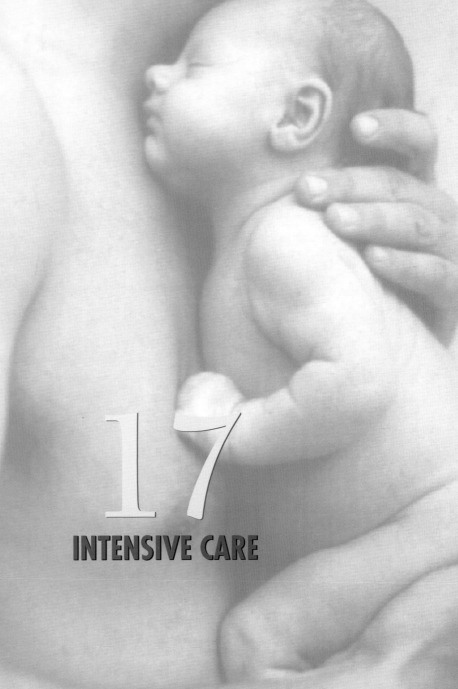

17

INTENSIVE CARE

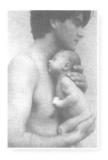

CHAPTER 17
INTENSIVE CARE

There were 107 maternal deaths, including seven *Fortuitous* and six *Late,* in which there was a recorded need for intensive care in this triennium. These are shown in Table 17.1. Due to the incomplete forms for some other cases it is likely that the total number is actually higher.

Intensive care services were required for a range of reasons, from resuscitation for a few hours only to over 40 days of treatment for multiple organ failure, often following acute respiratory distress syndrome (ARDS).

There is a discrepancy between the types of condition causing mortality and those causing ICU admission. This is because fatal conditions may cause rapid death before admission to the ICU and because *Late* maternal deaths are often not reported to this Enquiry. In addition women with some specific disorders are cared for on specialist units, and those with medical disorders are often managed on medical wards.

Direct causes of death

Among the *Direct* deaths, 75% (9) of the women who suffered a haemorrhage required intensive care and 50% (7) of those with sepsis; 35% (7) of women with pregnancy-induced hypertension and 35% (6) of those with amniotic fluid embolism survived long enough to be transferred to an ICU. Not surprisingly, given the speed of collapse following pulmonary embolism, only 19% (9) of these women were admitted to an ICU. Half of the women who died in early pregnancy also required such support. Many of these women died from ARDS, which is still associated with an adverse outcome.

Indirect causes of death

Of the 42 women who had an *Indirect* death on an ICU, the largest number were due to "other *Indirect*" causes of maternal death, as discussed in Chapter 11. These cover a wide range of medical and surgical conditions.

Fortuitous and Late deaths

Seven deaths on ICU were *Fortuitous*, and six *Late*. The causes of the *Late* deaths included cystic fibrosis, cerebral haemorrhage and neoplastic disease. Some *Indirect, Late* and *Fortuitous* deaths associated with ICU are difficult to identify, as in many cases the medical attendants may have forgotten that the patient had been pregnant within the time defined for *Late* deaths, or are not aware of the need to report a maternal death.

Table 17.1

Number Of *Direct* and *Indirect* cases admitted to ICU by Chapter; United Kingdom 1994-96.			
Principal disorder	Number*	Percentage of cases receiving intensive care	Duration of stay (days)
Thrombosis and thromboembolism	9(48)	19%	0.4-20
Hypertensive disease of pregnancy	7(20)	35%	1-19
Haemorrhage	9(12)	75%	0.5-33
Amniotic fluid embolism	6(17)	35%	0.5-5
Early pregnancy deaths	7(15)	47%	0.5-41
Sepsis	7(14)	50%	0.2-42
Other *Direct*			
Genital tract trauma	3(5)	60%	1-23
Other	(2)		
Anaesthetic	1(1)	100%	0.5
Cardiac	9(39)	23%	3-42
Psychiatric	1(9)	10%	12
Other *Indirect*	32(86)	37%	1-34
Total *Direct* and *Indirect*	**94**	**(35%)**	

* - total number of cases counted in the Chapter are given in parentheses

General discussion

The assessment of these cases and a review of the published literature (see the Annex to this Chapter) allow the following conclusions to be drawn.

The development of multiple organ failure is often preceded by ARDs. Pregnant women are at risk of developing ARDS from obstetric complications such as AFE, sepsis, pre-eclampsia, hypertensive disorders of pregnancy, placental abruption and dead fetus syndrome, as well as being at increased risk from some non-obstetric conditions.

Pregnancy predisposes to other pulmonary insults, such as aspiration of stomach contents, pneumonia, air embolism, massive haemorrhage and non-obstetric infections.

The differential diagnosis of ARDS in pregnancy includes venous thromboembolism, AFE, pulmonary oedema secondary to pre-eclampsia, tocolytic pulmonary oedema, aspiration pneumonitis, peripartum cardiomyopathy, pneumomediastinum, air embolism, asthma, pneumonia and cardiac disease. Asthma is associated with prematurity, low birth weight and increased perinatal mortality, probably due to poor asthma control but pregnancy is not a contraindication to steroid treatment.

Tocolytic-induced pulmonary oedema is due to administration of beta-adrenergic agents especially terbutaline and ritodrine which are used to inhibit uterine contractions and their use in pregnancies may be associated with hypokalaemia, hyperglycaemia, tachyarrythmia and sodium retention as well as pulmonary oedema.

Pregnancy predisposes to infection and its increased severity. These include pneumonias due to viruses such as varicella and herpes simplex.

The consensus remains that provision of good intensive and high-dependency care reduces mortality and that the best chance of success occurs when patients are treated early in their illness.

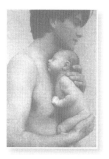

ANNEX TO CHAPTER 17
RECENT REVIEWS OF MATERNAL MORTALITY AND MORBIDITY ASSOCIATED WITH ICU

Since the last triennial Report several centres have reviewed the requirement of pregnant patients for intensive care.

Lapinsky *et al.* reviewed 65 obstetric admissions to an ICU in an academic hospital over a five-year period (0.26% of deliveries)[1]. None of these patients died. Umo-Etuk *et al.* undertook a five-year review and found 39 parturient patients were admitted to their general ICU in a five-year period[2]. The authors suggest from their review that the fall in maternal mortality reflects an improvement in organ support in the ICU but as a result there is an increase in the number of deaths from ARDS. It is recognised that it is much more difficult to measure morbidity (and set standards of care) but admission to the ICU identifies a subset of parturient women at risk of severe morbidity. In this study the majority of patients were admitted to the ICU either as a direct result of pregnancy or because of a medical or surgical problem which was aggravated by the physiological problems of pregnancy.

Bouvier-Colle *et al.* studied 435 obstetric patients admitted to ICU[3] and calculated that the frequency was 36 per 100,000 live births. The mortality was lower with scheduled maternity cases in a teaching hospital and these authors concluded that most obstetric patients with serious diseases were referred for suitable care.

Wheatley *et al.* reviewed admissions to their ICU to see whether admission could have been predicted[4]. They found that 67% of patients had no previous medical or obstetric history. As in other series, the major reasons for admission were hypertensive disorders of pregnancy (66%) and haemorrhage (19%); 79% followed caesarean section and 40% required ventilatory support. The perinatal mortality was 6% and there were three maternal deaths. The need for ICU admission was unpredictable in two-thirds of cases. The authors suggest that a small proportion of women who develop complications of pregnancy (0.1-0.9%) require admission to an ICU. Homerton hospital, from which this survey comes, is in a deprived inner city area. The high rate of ICU obstetric admissions (0.75%) is similar to other inner city areas but for Nottingham during the period 1982-86 it was only 0.1%. A definitive diagnosis of ARDS was only made in two patients both of whom died after amniotic fluid embolism (AFE); a low incidence compared to other published series. There has been a recent trend to increase use of regional techniques for hypertensive disease but, as yet no significant demonstrable difference in fetal or maternal outcome.

A policy of early intervention and treatment on a multidisciplinary basis, which may involve intubation, ventilation, invasive monitoring and vasoactive drugs, was used preventively as well as after the onset of problems. This approach to management by early involvement of all relevant specialties to provide optimal care can alleviate the progression to multiple organ failure, and improve prognosis. They admit that high-dependency unit (HDU) care may have been just as effective for patients who are conscious and have single organ dysfunction.

Stephens reviewed hospital records of obstetric patients from a nearby hospital admitted to ICU for respiratory support after an anaesthetic complication[5]. In a 10-year period there were 126 obstetric admission to the ICU from 61,435 deliveries, of which 16 were due to anaesthetic complications, 12 after general and four after regional anaesthesia. Complications included anaphylaxis, high spinal block and failure of endotracheal intubation. The incidence of major complication causing admission to ICU was 1: 932 after general anaesthesia and for regional anaesthesia 1: 4177 when these were given for delivery. If a complication requiring ICU admission and mechanical ventilation is used as the criterion of safety it appears that regional anaesthesia is safer than general anaesthesia for delivery.

Severe maternal morbidity is easy to underestimate because pregnant women are usually healthy and recover quickly, and are discharged with relatively little follow-up. A review by Bewley & Creighton identified a small but very sick group of pregnant women with high rates of medical intervention, many of whom did not go home with live babies or with their fertility intact[6]. They required a disproportionate amount of resources and skill and are women for whom medical facilities may have been life-saving. The definition of a "near miss" may be identified by severity or by disease - in this case, admission to ICU was chosen as it was easy to measure. The factors Bewley & Creighton associated with increased risk are identified in Table 17.2. It is worrying that nearly half these "near misses" were related to haemorrhage.

Table 17.2

Pre-labour high risk features	Number of Women (%) (n=30)
Hypertension	12/29 (41%)
Age > 35 years	10/30 (33%)
Pre-existing medical problem	8/29 (28%)
Antepartum haemorrhage	7/29 (24%)
Twin pregnancy	2/30 (7%)
Weight > 100 kg	1/26 (4%)
Parity > 4	1/26 (4%)
Low risk (i.e. none of the above)	4/29 (14%)
Peri-post labour high risk features	**n = 28**
Caesarean section	18/28 (64%)
General anaesthetic	12/28 (43%)
Prolonged labour (> 12 h)	6/27 (21%)
Stillbirth or neonatal death	6/28 (21%)
Hysterectomy	5/28 (18%)

High risk features of patients transferred to the Intensive Care Unit; from Bewley (1997). Denominator = 6039 maternities. **Note; this Table is not drawn from data in the main Report.**

Availability of facilities

Cordingley & Rubin carried out a postal survey of all UK obstetric units concerning provision of recovery facilities, HDUs and ICUs in consultant obstetric units[7]. There was an 89% response rate. Only 62% had a designated staffed recovery unit, 41% had specific HDU beds and there were a number of units without consultant anaesthetic sessions or trained anaesthetic assistants around the clock.

Outcome

The outcome for obstetric patients requiring intensive care has been studied by Lewinsohn et al.[8] They found a low standardised mortality ratio (SMR) of 0.416, which is significantly better than that expected. There are various explanations, age alone having been excluded in the analysis - first the subgroup itself may be uniquely different or there may be better care for this subgroup and therefore a better outcome. One explanation offered by Scarpinato & Gerber[9] is that the physiological range of variables considered by APACHE II and the weighting for deviation from normal is for a normal, not a pregnant, population and there are changes in physiological variables for the pregnant state (e.g. tachycardia, pH changes, PCV). Another factor may be that APACHE II does **not** take into account the more serious changes of disease in pregnancy - LFTs, uric acid and platelets. The high emergency caesarean section rate with its significant weighting in the risk equation may have contributed to the findings. Other workers, however, have found that APACHE II, SAPS II & MPMII assess the ICU outcome of critically ill obstetric patients as accurately as non-obstetric patients.

References

1. Lapinsky, S.E., Kruczynski, K. & Slutsky, AS. Critical care in the pregnant patient. *American Journal Respiratory and Critical Care Medicine* 1995; **152**: 427-55.

2. Umo-Etuk, J., Lumley, J. & Holdcroft, A. Critically ill parturient women and admission to intensive care: a 5 year review. *International Journal of Obstetric Anaesthesia* 1996; **5**: 79-84.

3. Bouvier-Colle, M.H., Salanave, B., Ancel, P.Y., Varnoux, N., Fernandez, H., Papiernik, E. & Breart, G. Obstetric patients treated in intensive care units and mortality. *European Journal of Obstetrics, Gynecology and Reproductive Biology* 1996; **65**: 121-5.

4. Wheatley, E., Farkas, A. & Watson, D. Obstetric admissions to an intensive therapy unit. *International Journal of Obstetric Anaesthesia* 1995; **5**:221-4.

5. Stephens, I.D. ICU admissions from an obstetric hospital. *Canadian Journal Anaesthesia* 1991; **38**: 677-81.

6. Bewley, S. & Creighton, S. 'Near-miss' obstetric enquiry. *Journal of Obstetrics and Gynaecology* 1997; **17**: 26-9.

7. Cordingley, J.J. & Rubin, A.P. A survey of facilities for high risk women in consultant obstetric units. *International Journal of Obstetric Anaesthesia* 1997; **6**: 56-160.

8. Lewinsohn, G., Herman, A., Leonov, Y. & Klinowski, E. Critically ill obstetrical patients: outcome and predictability. *Critical Care Medicine* 1994; **22**: 1412-14.

9. Scarpinato, L. & Gerber, D. Critically ill obstetrical patients: Outcome and predictability. *Critical Care Medicine* 1995: **23**: 1449-50.

El-Solh, A.A. & Grant B.J.B. A comparison of severity of illness scoring systems for critically ill obstetric patients. *Chest* 1996; **110**: 1299-304.

Lapinsky SE. Critical care management of the obstetric patient. *Canadian Journal of Anaesthesia* 1997; **44**: 325-9.

Lapinsky, S.E. Respiratory care of the critically ill pregnant patient. *Current Opinion in Critical Care* 1996; **3**: 1-6.

Platteau, P., Engelhardt, T., Moodley, J. & Muckart, D.J.J. Obstetric and gynaecological patients in an intensive care unit: A 1 year review. *Tropical Doctor* 1997; **27**: 202-6.

Royal College of Anaesthetists. *Guidelines for Purchasers of Obstetric Anaesthetic and Intensive Care Facilities.* Revised 1998. London: RCA; 1998.

18
AUDIT OF PREVIOUS RECOMMENDATIONS

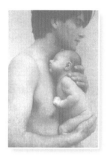

CHAPTER 18
AUDIT OF PREVIOUS RECOMMENDATIONS

Angie Benbow, Research Midwife, the RCOG Clinical Audit Unit.
Michael Maresh, Honorary Director of the RCOG Clinical Audit Unit.

This Chapter describes two recent surveys undertaken by the RCOG Clinical Audit Unit. The aim of these studies was to determine if key recommendations published in the Reports on Confidential Enquiries into Maternal Deaths were being implemented. They were conducted by means of a detailed assessment of a random 10% sample of consultant maternity units throughout the UK and, in addition, by a postal questionnaire to all maternity units.

Introduction

Over the last 10 years there has been an increasing emphasis on clinical audit and the development of evidence-based effective clinical practice. This has recently been reaffirmed by the Department of Health's' publication *A First Class Service; Quality in the NHS*.[1] This not only recognises the requirement for all clinical staff to ensure they undertake audit and base their treatments on evidence but also highlights the key role of the Confidential Enquiries. The Confidential Enquiries into Maternal Deaths (CEMD), referred to as "the Report" throughout this Chapter, have long been recognised as a leading example of professional self-audit. It has not been possible, to date, to investigate systematically whether the recommendations for improving care, made in all Reports, are actually being implemented across the UK. That many of the recommendations were having to be made repeatedly from Report to Report suggested that they were not.

An earlier survey undertaken in 1993[2] supported this conclusion and identified that recommendations from the previous Reports were still not being universally implemented. In particular, the authors found that guidelines for the management of serious maternal complications were still not available in all hospitals. It also showed that there were still split-site hospitals providing maternity services and that some maternity units did not have access to blood transfusion facilities on site. In view of these findings, and in conjunction with the publication *Maternal Mortality: the Way Forward*[3] and the RCOG's pamphlet *Deriving Standards from the Maternal Mortality Reports*[4], a reaudit was considered necessary to ensure that the recommendations were being put into practice.

Method

This study involved (i) a postal survey of all maternity units in the UK and (ii) interviews at selected sites with key members of staff involved in the management of maternal complications.

(i) The postal survey

A questionnaire was sent to the head of midwifery at all maternity units in the UK during November 1996. By May 1997 a 100% response rate was achieved, following one reminder letter or phone call. Two hundred and fifty-nine consultant maternity units were identified and used for this survey. Information collected from Midwifery and GP-led units has not been included in this review as it is incomplete and may not represent the national picture. The questions asked included the siting of the unit in relation to an acute general hospital, and the availability and siting of facilities and services such as an intensive care unit (ICU), a high-dependency unit (HDU) and blood transfusion facilities. All units were asked if they had agreed guidelines for severe hypertensive disorders, eclampsia, massive haemorrhage, thromboembolic disorders and severe genital tract infection and if they would forward a copy to the RCOG Clinical Audit Unit. In addition, they were asked if all staff had access to the Cochrane database and a copy of the CEMD Report and if they found the recommendations useful for developing guidelines. Separate validation of the data on blood transfusion services was obtained by telephoning the laboratory at all units with 1,000 or more deliveries who had reported no blood transfusion facilities on site.

(ii) The interviews

A cross-sectional study of all maternity units in the UK included on the RCOG Clinical Audit Unit database in 1996 (n=325) was conducted between August 1996 and June 1997. Initial stratification identified units that were representative of each of the 11 health Regions in the UK. Further stratification, within each region, identified large and small units. For the purpose of this study, large units are those with more than 3,000 deliveries per annum. A 10% sample was used. The number of units to be included in the study in each health Region was calculated from the number of maternity units and the combined number of deliveries for each of the Regions. Thirty-two consultant maternity units were randomly selected.

In each of the units selected, the clinical director for maternity services, the clinical director for anaesthetics and the head of midwifery were approached for initial agreement to the study and to suggest suitable personnel to be interviewed. Although all units initially agreed, one unit was withdrawn midway through the study due to difficulties with access to key personnel. In total, 149 staff were interviewed in the 31 units. These included 30 consultant obstetricians, 18 Specialist Registrars in obstetrics, 30 consultant anaesthetists, 19 Specialist Registrars in anaesthetics, 31 senior midwives, "G" grade or above, and 21 "E" or "F" grade midwives. A semi-structured questionnaire was developed from the recommendations from previous Reports and RCOG publications[3,4]. The interviews were carried out by the RCOG research midwife.

Results

Provision of services: Availability of facilities for consultant maternity units

The previous Report and the National Confidential Enquiry into Peri-operative Deaths ('1991-92)[5] raised concern that split sites or isolated maternity units may cause deficiencies in the provision of essential services; in particular, access to blood transfusion services and the provision of adequately staffed and equipped facilities such as an iICU, HDU and designated postoperative recovery areas.

Split sites - isolated maternity units

Postal survey

In 1997 91% (235/259) of maternity units were on the site of an acute general hospital. This compares with 86% (213/248) in 1993[2] as shown in Table 18.1. Nine per cent (24/259) of consultant maternity units stated that they were not on the site of an acute general hospital. These are referred to as isolated units. This compares with 14% (35/248) in 1993[2] as shown in Table 18.2. Wales no longer has any split-site consultant units.

Table 18.1

	England		Wales		Northern Ireland		Scotland		UK	
Comparison of 1993 data2 audit data against 1997 reaudit data.										
	No.	%	No.	%	No.	%	No.	%	No.	%
Consultant Maternity Units										
1993	202		17		17		24		260	
1997	203		16		14		26		259	
Units participated										
1993	190	94	17	100	17	100	24	100	248	95
1997	203	100	16	100	14	100	26	100	259	100
Acute site										
1993	168	88	14	82	16	94	15	63	213	86
1997	188	93	16	100	12	86	19	73	235	91
ICU 1993	151	79	13	76	11	65	13	54	188	76
1997	170	84	13	63	10	71	13	46	206	80
Blood Bank on site 1993	167	88	15	88	15	88	19	79	216	87
1997	197	97	16	100	12	86	24	92	249	96
Eclampsia protocol 1993	179	94	17	100	11	65	18	75	225	91
1997	192	95	16	100	12	86	23	88	243	94
Haemorrhage protocol 1993	170	89	15	88	4	24	15	63	204	82
1997	184	91	16	100	13	93	25	96	238	92

Table 18.2

	1993			1997		
Comparision of 1993 with 1997 data for number of isolated maternity units.* The 11 health Regions in the UK.						
	No. of units	No. of isolated units		No. of units	No. of isolated units	
REGIONS		No.	%		No.	%
Northern & Yorkshire	36	5	14	29	4	14
West Midlands	21	1	5	19	1	5
North West	28	5	18	31	5	16
Trent	16	2	13	18	1	6
Anglia & Oxford	18	2	11	20	0	
South & West (inc.Channel Isles)	21	4	19	23	0	
North Thames	30	9	30	31	2	6
South Thames	32	6	19	32	2	6
Wales	17	3	18	16	0	
N.Ireland	17	1	6	14	2	14
Scotland	24	9	53	26	7	27
All UK:	260	47	18	259	24	9

* Isolated units are those not on the site of an acute general hospital.

Ten of these 24 units conduct between 300 and 2,999 deliveries per year, and the rest between 3,000 and 6,500. On-site intensive care facilities were available only in one of these units. For the remaining 23 units the distance to the nearest ICU ranged from 0.5 and 8 miles. 12 units stated that they had HDU facilities on site but the definition clearly differed between units. Seventy-nine per-cent (19/24) had blood transfusion facilities on site.

Provision of an ICU, HDU and postoperative recovery area facilities

The previous three Reports have recommended that facilities for intensive care and for high-dependency care be readily available. In the 1985-87 Report the recommendation was that large maternity units should provide a centralised high-dependency care area with trained staff and appropriate monitoring equipment. This was extended in the 1988-90 Report to include every consultant maternity unit. The last Report recommended that intensive care and high-dependency care facilities must be readily available in the same hospital as the maternity unit. In addition, every maternity unit undertaking caesarean sections should have a designated, staffed and equipped recovery area with staff specifically trained in post-operative care.

Postal survey

In 1997 80% (206/259) of the consultant maternity units had an ICU on site. This compares with 76% (188/248) in 1993[2] as shown in Table 18.1. In 1997 62% (161/259) of units had an HDU on site compared with 41% in 1994[6]. The number of units without an ICU on site are shown in Table 18.3, categorised by the number of births per annum.

Table 18.3

Number of units who do not have an ICU on site by number of deliveries per annum.	
Number of deliveries per annum	Number of units without an ICU on site
< 999	6
1,000 - 1,999	15
2,000 - 2,999	10
3,000 - 3,999	12
4,000 - 4,999	7
> 5,000	3
Total	53

Interviews

All the obstetricians and midwives interviewed (n=100) were asked where women with complications were nursed. The majority, 59%, stated that ill women were nursed in a room within the delivery suite, 33% in a high-dependency area within the maternity unit, mainly on the delivery suite, with 4% stating they were transferred to ICU. The remaining 4% were unsure where ill women were nursed. The responses varied depending on the nature of the complication. For instance women were more likely to go to an ICU with eclampsia (15%) than with severe pre-eclampsia (4%) or if they had had a massive haemorrhage (3%). Asked if there was a designated, fully equipped recovery area, 88% of obstetricians and midwives stated yes; 10% use one of the delivery rooms but stated that equipment was available; and 2% stated that the women went straight back to the ward from theatre.

When anaesthetists' responses were included in the survey (total n=149) 94% of staff interviewed (140/149) stated that a skilled anaesthetic assistant was always available for all maternity theatre cases. When asked if any of the midwives caring for these women had had any further training in critical care, 20% (6/30) of consultant obstetricians, 16% (5/31) of senior midwives and 19% (4/21) of junior midwives stated that some of the midwives had undergone further training; 50% (15/30) of consultant obstetricians, 55% (10/18) of specialist registrar obstetricians, 77% (24/31) of senior midwives and 71% (15/21) of junior midwives said none had. The remaining staff, including all 49 anaesthetists, were unsure.

Discussion

The provision of ICU and HDU facilities has shown an improvement since 1993[2]. Eighty per cent of units had ICU facilities in 1997 compared with 76% in 1993[2]. Similarly, the provision of HDU facilities has improved, with 62% of units having facilities in 1997 compared with only 41% in 1994[6]. It is evident from these interviews that the majority of ill women are cared for within the maternity unit; but, only 15% of obstetricians and midwives considered that the midwives caring for these women had any further training in critical care. This training tended to have occurred before midwifery training and midwives have identified problems with maintaining skills. A study conducted in 1994 stated that the provision of monitoring equipment and training of midwives in its use was "very variable and often suboptimal"[6]. Despite the role anaesthetists have in the clinical management of ill women, none of those interviewed knew if the midwives had had any further training. Whilst senior anaesthetists were very supportive of the midwives' role and capabilities in caring for ill women, many were concerned and identified areas of weakness. Some maternity units have attempted to address this issue by setting up educational packages. The main problems appear to be in relation to identifying the level of training needs, the optimum number to train to maintain the service, the financial cost of training and the maintenance of skills.

Recommendations

- *Units should review their facilities for high-dependency and postoperative care.*
- *Units should review, or implement, training/educational packages for midwives caring. for women requiring high-dependency care and immediate postoperative care.*
- *All maternity units should have a multiprofessional guideline group.*
- *Guidelines should be reviewed regularly to see if they need updating.*
- *Guidelines should be available in all clinical areas.*
- *Multiple methods of disseminating new guidelines are required.*

Staffing

Previous Reports and the National Confidential Enquiry into Perioperative Deaths (NCEPOD)[5] have emphasised the need for 24-hour consultant cover and the discontinuation of inappropriate responsibility being given to, or taken by, by staff not qualified or skilled to do so.

Interviews - obstetricians and midwives

All obstetricians and midwives interviewed ($n=100$) stated that there was always an obstetrician of at least registrar experience readily available on site for consultation, or to attend, in the event of a complication or emergency. When asked what was the usual level of experience of the doctor on call during the day, it ranged from consultant (6%), senior specialist registrar (37%), specialist registrar (54%) and senior house officer (3%). Out of hours, during the night or at weekends, only 2% stated that a consultant was on site, 16% a senior specialist registrar, 78% a specialist registrar and 7% stated that senior house officers would be called to attend.

Specialist registrar obstetricians' duties during the day varied, with 33% stating that they would be on call for maternity only, and 66% covering both maternity and gynaecology units. Out of hours, 11% covered maternity only, with 88% covering both maternity and gynaecology units. In 97% of these hospitals the maternity and gynaecology units were on one site. However, many of these hospital sites are geographically very large, and some specialist registrars in particular highlighted the problem of the time taken going between the maternity and gynaecology departments.

Asked how long it took from the obstetrician being called to arriving on the unit for an emergency, 60% stated the obstetrician would be based on the delivery suite and therefore immediately available. Thirty-nine per cent said they would attend within five minutes providing they were not committed on the gynaecology unit, in which case the attendance time was variable. On further questioning, this did not appear to be a regular problem.

In all units a consultant obstetrician was always on call for consultation or to attend if required. During the day they stated they could attend within 15-20 minutes, often much less. At night and at week-ends, particularly Saturday afternoons, some said they would have difficulty getting in within 30-40 minutes. However, none of their colleagues interviewed highlighted that time was a problem with attendance.

Interviews - anaesthetists

An anaesthetist of at least one year's experience was always available for the maternity unit. They usually had 18 months' anaesthetic experience andwere available when both the senior staff and the trainees themselves had agreed they were competent to practise in maternity.

In 58% (18/31) of the units there was a dedicated anaesthetist, covering the maternity unit only, during the day. In 19% (6/31) the anaesthetist also covered the ICU and in a further 23% (7/31) the anaesthetist covered maternity and the general hospital as well. When asked what level of anaesthetist was most likely to attend to deal with a complication, 17% of all staff interviewed (n=149) stated that it would be the consultant, 71% said a senior specialist registrar and 9% a specialist registrar or the SHO during the day. At night or at the weekend, however, only 3% indicated that the consultant would attend whilst 70% said a specialist registrar and 23% an SHO. All staff interviewed stated that in an emergency, the anaesthetist on call would attend within 10-15 minutes and 86% stated that, if called, a consultant would attend within, at most, 15-20 minutes during the day and 30-40 minutes during the night and at week-ends.

All 31 units had 24-hour consultant anaesthetist cover for maternity. In 27 of these units there were dedicated consultant maternity sessions. These varied between two and eight sessions per week. When asked, 24 (80%) consultants stated that they were based on the delivery suite during these sessions. All units had a consultant lead for obstetric anaesthesia.

Discussion

An obstetrician and anaesthetist of specialist registrar grade, or equivalent, were always available to attend for emergencies. All the staff interviewed were satisfied that the response time was adequate and no-one highlighted any serious deficiencies in the service. However, anecdotally, there was occasionally some disquiet as to the level of skills and competencies of some staff caring for ill women. These concerns were raised by, and about, each group interviewed. There was 24-hour cover of consultant obstetricians and anaesthetists and there was general agreement about the accessibility to consultant staff both for advice and to attend in an emergency. No problems were highlighted in consultant staff attending for an emergency and they would attend within 30 minutes, usually less. It was reassuring to note that all units had a consultant lead for obstetric anaesthesia.

Recommendation

- *Units should consider monitoring the response times for all levels of staff. This will assist in early identification of any problems - organisational, structural, personnel - and early rectification.*

Dealing with maternal emergencies

It is important that all practitioners know how to deal with emergencies. The 1988-90 Report emphasised that new medical and midwifery staff should have an induction course and that their continuing education programme should include regular rehearsals of emergency procedures, especially in cardio-pulmonary resuscitation.

Interviews

All obstetricians were asked if junior doctors were instructed in how to deal with maternal emergencies and whether this instruction was formal or informal. Ninety-three per cent (28/30) of consultants and 89% (16/18) of specialist registrars said that junior doctors were instructed in maternal emergencies, with over 50% of both consultants and specialist registrars stating that this instruction was formal. In addition, all obstetricians were asked if senior obstetricians updated their skills in dealing with obstetric emergencies, for example undertaking basic life support or an advanced life support in obstetrics course. Fifty-three per cent of consultants and 39% of specialist registrars stated that senior obstetricians did update. When midwives were asked if they were instructed in how to deal with maternal emergencies, 68% (21/31) of senior midwives and 57% (12/21) of junior midwives stated that they were, with 42% of senior midwives and 33% of junior midwives stating that this instruction was formal. All anaesthetists were asked if there were any training sessions in dealing with emergency situations for obstetric and midwifery staff. Forty-seven per cent (14/30) of consultant anaesthetists and 37% (7/19) of specialist registrar anaesthetists stated that training sessions took place.

Discussion

In many Trusts the statutory cardio-pulmonary resuscitation lectures were mainly undertaken by resuscitation officers employed by the local Trusts. While the interviews were being conducted, several resuscitation officers were contacted, and they stated that they had very few consultants of any discipline attending the sessions.

Collaborative, multidisciplinary practice sessions or "drills" for dealing with emergency situations are undertaken by all the emergency services and many A&E departments. This allows all members of staff, and especially new and junior staff, to know and understand their specific roles and responsibilities in an emergency. The domestic, portering and clerical staff must also be included as they are important members of any emergency team. All obstetricians, anaesthetists and midwives were asked if they undertook any practice sessions. No practice or drills occurred in any of the units involved in the interviews. However, a few consultant obstetricians and consultant anaesthetists were hoping to address this issue.

REPORT ON CONFIDENTIAL ENQUIRIES INTO MATERNAL DEATHS IN THE UNITED KINGDOM

Recommendations

- *All clinical staff, including consultants, should attend local resuscitation courses.*
- *Units should consider the possibility of undertaking mutlidisciplinary practice sessions.*

Clinical guidelines for the management of severe maternal complications

The use of evidence-based, interdisciplinary, clinical management guidelines is essential. Successive Reports and publications have recommended that such guidelines are introduced and disseminated[3,4,7,8]. These should be regularly reviewed and updated by an interdisciplinary team and drawn to the attention of all staff, including community midwives, ambulance personnel and staff in A&E Departments. The guidelines should also be displayed in a prominent place and immediately accessible to all staff.

Postal survey

All consultant-led units were asked if they had clinical guidelines for the management of; severe preeclampsia, eclampsia, massive haemorrhage, thromboprophylaxis and severe genital tract infection, see Table 18.4. They were asked to forward a copy of these guidelines to the RCOG Clinical Audit Unit.

Table 18.4

Availability of clinical guidelines for the management of major complications - by 11 health Regions in the UK - 1997.										
	No. of units	Severe hypertensive disorders		Eclampsia		Major haemorrhage		Thrombo-embolic disorders		Severe genital tract infection	
		No.	%	No.	%	No.	%	No.	%	No.	%
Northern & Yorkshire	29	27	93	28	96	29	100	18	62	6	21
West Midlands	19	17	89	17	89	17	89	13	68	4	21
North West	31	28	90	29	93	29	93	19	61	7	23
Trent	18	16	89	17	94	16	89	10	56	4	22
Anglia & Oxford	20	16	80	20	100	20	100	13	65	6	30
South & West (inc.Channel Isles)	23	23	100	23	100	21	91	14	61	5	22
North Thames	31	25	81	28	90	26	84	21	68	9	29
South Thames	32	30	94	30	94	28	87	20	62	4	12
Wales	16	16	100	16	100	16	100	12	75	3	19
N.Ireland	14	10	71	12	86	13	93	9	64	2	14
Scotland	26	22	85	23	88	25	96	22	85	3	12
All UK	259	230	89	243	94	240	93	171	66	53	20

Interviews

All of the units whose staff were interviewed had some of the guidelines under review. From the staff interviewed, 75% (36/48) of obstetricians and 83% (43/52) of midwives considered these had been drawn up by a multiprofessional group. Six consultant obstetricians stated that the clinical guidelines in their own unit were developed by medical staff only, mainly obstetricians with anaesthetist input if required. Of these six units, three are large tertiary referral centres and three are large district general hospitals. In total these six units conduct approximately 23,700 deliveries per annum.

Anaesthetists were asked if they were routinely involved in the development of guidelines. Eighty per cent (24/30) of the consultant anaesthetists surveyed, and 58% (11/19) of specialist registrar anaesthetists, stated that they were routinely involved. The six consultant anaesthetists who said they were not involved in the development of guidelines all practised within units that stated that they had a multiprofessional guideline development group.

It is imperative that staff dealing with an emergency are not faced with the dilemma of trying to decide from a multiplicity of guidelines which they should comply with. For instance, the consultant the woman is booked with, or the consultant who is on call that day, may have differing views on the management of a particular condition. Therefore, there should be one set of guidelines agreed on by all the senior staff involved. It was reassuring to note that all those interviewed stated that the guidelines were agreed by all consultant obstetricians and consultant anaesthetists involved in the management of ill pregnant or recently delivered women.

Guidelines need to be readily accessible. All those interviewed stated that the guidelines were kept on the delivery suite, although only 20% (30/149) thought that a copy was also kept on the antenatal and postnatal wards. Making the guidelines available to all clinical areas will help to alert staff to any changes in management, thereby assisting in their implementation.

All staff were asked when their local guidelines were last updated and if there was a fixed schedule for revision. Seventy-two per cent (107/149) of staff thought the guidelines had been updated within the previous 12 months, 5% (7/149) longer than 12 months and 22% (33/149) were unsure. Of the latter, 14 were senior members of staff. Asked if they had a fixed schedule for revision of these guidelines, 23% (34/149) of interviewees thought they were reviewed annually, 42% (63/149) stated that they had no schedule for revision, 4% (6/149) had a rolling programme and 31% (46/149) were unsure. On further enquiry those who stated they did not have a fixed schedule tended to fit into a rolling programme. The term "rolling programme" encompassed a diversity of methods. These ranged from reviewing a different guideline, or a small number of guidelines, on a monthly or three-monthly basis, when new evidence was produced or when requested by a member of staff.

Only 42% (63/149) of those interviewed stated that the units in which they practised had any formal means of dissemination of new or updated guidelines, the most common forum being meetings, mainly perinatal mortality, clinical audit and delivery suite meetings. Dissemination to the medical staff usually took the form of sending a copy to them. In 70% of cases new medical staff were given copies on arrival. As well as these meetings, midwifery staff tended to be informed by ward briefings, notice boards and communication books. It was often stated that they had to sign a "list" confirming that they had read the guideline, but no one was able to explain the purpose of the list or how this assisted in the dissemination of midwives' knowledge of the guidelines. Nevertheless, 87% (27/31) of senior midwives and 38% (8/21) of junior midwives felt they were involved in the development of their local guidelines. The remainder of those interviewed considered that they did not have any formal means of dissemination and tended to be informed by word of mouth or that the guidelines "just arrived one day".

Recommendations

- *All maternity units should have a multiprofessional guideline group.*
- *Guidelines should be reviewed regularly to see if they need updating.*
- *Guidelines should be available in all clinical areas.*
- *Multiple methods of disseminating new guidelines are required.*
- *The implementation of the guidelines should be subject to regular audit.*

The following sections consider specific guidelines in more detail. The clinical guidelines received from the study sites and those in response to the postal questionnaire were evaluated by use of a guideline assessment tool developed for the purpose[9].

Massive haemorrhage

Every Report has featured massive haemorrhage as a cause of death. Although the incidence of death by haemorrhage has decreased, it remains a major complication. Successive Reports have emphasised the need for guidelines for the management of massive haemorrhage and for all those who care for pregnant women to be familiar with them.

Postal survey

Ninety-three per cent (240/259) of consultant maternity units in the UK stated that they have clinical guidelines for the management of massive haemorrhage. This compares with 82% (204/248) in 1993[2] as shown in Table 18.1.

Interviews

All staff interviewed (n=149) in 31 units stated that a guideline for the management of massive haemorrhage was available in their unit.

The RCOG[4] has recommended that uncross-matched blood should be available within 10 minutes and cross-matched blood within 30 minutes. When asked, 95% of staff stated that uncross-matched blood, O RhD-negative, was immediately available, 74% stated that ABO-compatible RhD-negative blood was available within 10 minutes and 50% stated that full cross-matched blood was available within 45 minutes. However, in two large tertiary maternity units, conducting 4,500 and 5,500 deliveries annually, there were difficulties in getting essential services out of normal working hours. In order to overcome any difficulties one of these units has developed a system in collaboration with the laboratory service, for immediate delivery of requests and samples to the laboratory. This ,in combination with a priority coding, ensures rapid attention. This system is audited regularly. The other unit, at the time this study was undertaken, was having problems that were potentially serious.

The RCOG further recommended that for women who have a massive haemorrhage the early involvement of anaesthetists and haematologists is essential[3,4]. All the obstetricians interviewed stated that they can readily get advice from a consultant haematologist, and 78% of all staff interviewed stated that anaesthetists are routinely involved in the management of these cases.

Placenta praevia

The potential problems associated with placenta praevia have been repeatedly emphasised in previous Reports. One of the recommendations has been that an elective or emergency caesarean section for placenta praevia should be performed, or directly supervised, by a consultant obstetrician.

Interviews

Twenty per cent of all staff interviewed (n=149) stated that the consultant obstetrician always performed or assisted at caesarean section for placenta praevia, 13% stated that they did if the case was elective and 61% stated that consultants did not routinely operate for either.

Asked who routinely did perform caesarean section for placenta praevia, 28% of staff stated that a senior registrar would perform both elective and emergency, 36% that a specialist registrar performed both and 15% that the senior specialist registrar operated if surgery was elective and the specialist registrar if it was an emergency. This was apparently irrespective of the degree of placenta praevia, the position of the placenta or any previous caesarean section.

Sixteen (53%) of the consultant obstetricians stated that they routinely performed or assisted at elective caesarean section for placenta praevia. Of these, 11 consultants stated that they also routinely attended for emergency cases. However, none had complete agreement from all their colleagues interviewed in the same unit. In only five of these units was the statement that the consultant obstetrician routinely undertook these cases confrmed by the consultant anaesthetists and senior midwives. The remaining 11 units conduct, in total, over 41,000 deliveries per annum. Six of these units are tertiary referral centres.

The interview also asked about the grade of the anaesthetist attending for caesarean section for placenta praevia. Ten per cent (3/30) of consultant anaesthetists stated that a consultant would attend for both elective and emergency cases, whilst 43% (13/30) said they would attend for elective cases only. The remaining 47% (14/30) stated that a consultant did not routinely attend for either. These figures were confirmed by the specialist registrar anaesthetists who stated that the majority of cases were undertaken by specialist registrars. However, all staff interviewed considered both a consultant obstetrician and a consultant anaesthetist should be able to attend within 15-20 minutes during the day and within 30-40 minutes out of normal working hours.

Refusing a blood transfusion

The problems associated with the management of haemorrhage in women who refuse blood transfusion were highlighted in the last Report, which also contained guidelines for the management of such women. Although there are many women who are fearful of receiving contaminated blood, absolute refusal to have a blood transfusion, irrespective of the outcome, is unlikely in most women, except those who have strong religious beliefs.

Interviews

All obstetricians and midwives were asked if there was any written guidance for the clinical management of such cases. Twenty-two per cent (22/100, involving nine units) stated that there was some form of guidance. The remaining 78% either stated none was available or were unsure. Asked if there was a system in place in which they could get advice on the management of such cases, 34% stated yes and 66% stated no or were unsure.

Nine units stated that they had written "guidance" for the management of these cases, but only one, a district general hospital, had included in its guideline the recommendation from the previous Report. In the remaining ten units, three had disclaimer forms which the women, who were identified on grounds of their stated religion, were asked to sign. The remaining seven units did not have any reference within the guidelines they supplied.

Postal survey

All units were requested to forward a copy of the guidelines under review and 147 (57%) supplied a copy of their guideline for the management of haemorrhage. The need to involve an anaesthetist was mentioned in 69% (101/147) of guidelines and 62% (91/147) mentioned consulting a haematologist. Twelve (8%) of the guidelines were taken directly from the 1991-93 Report.

Only 1.4% (2/147) had any recommendations for the management of women who refuse blood transfusion. These were taken from the previous Report.

Discussion

The number of units with a guideline has improved since 1993[2] although this should be 100%. The interviews have highlighted that there are problems with the access to blood supplies as only 50% of staff stated that cross-matched blood was available within 45 minutes. Guidelines for the management of women who refuse blood products do not appear to be widely available.

Recommendations

- *There still appear to be problems in a few units with regard to the urgent provision of blood. This needs to be audited in all units.*
- *Despite repeated recommendations consultant staff, both obstetricians and anaesthetists, are still not directly involved with either elective or emergency caesarean sections for placenta praevia.*
- *Recommendations for the management of women who refuse a blood transfusion do not appear to be available in most units. This needs to be urgently addressed.*

Severe hypertensive disorders and eclampsia

Previous Reports have highlighted problems with the management of both severe hypertensive disorders and eclampsia. They have repeatedly emphasised that all units should have a lead consultant, clear management guidelines based on current evidence and ready access to a Regional advisory service led by a consultant with special expertise.

Postal survey

Eighty-nine per cent (230/259) of consultant-led maternity units had guidelines for the management of severe hypertensive disorders and 94% (243/259) for the management of eclampsia. This compares with 91% (225/248) for eclampsia in 1993[2]. These figures are shown in Tables 18.1 and 18.4.

Interviews

Ninety-nine per cent (99/100) of obstetricians and midwives interviewed stated that there was a guideline available in their unit for the management of severe hypertensive disorders and eclampsia. All anaesthetists ($n=49$) were asked if they were routinely involved in the management of severe hypertensive disorders and eclampsia. Eighty per cent stated they were routinely involved with cases of severe hypertension and 88% with eclampsia. In addition, 80% of consultant anaesthetists said they were involved with the development of guidelines for the management of these cases.

All obstetricians and midwives ($n=100$) were asked if the guidelines contained details for the management of fluid balance and drug management. In the case of severe hypertensive disorders, 87% stated they contained details for fluid management and 93% for drug management. For eclampsia, 86% thought there were details on fluid management and 87% for drug management. Seventy-nine per cent stated that magnesium sulphate was the drug of choice for eclampsia and 17% used diazepam. Those units who were not using magnesium sulphate stated that this was in the process of being introduced.

In the case of severe hypertensive disorders 70% of consultant obstetricians stated that the management was collaborative. This was confirmed by 71% of senior midwives and 80% of consultant anaesthetists. However, only 44% of specialist registrar obstetricians and 47% of specialist registrar anaesthetists believed this to be the case. There was greater agreement regarding the management of eclampsia, with 85% of all consultants, 73% of all specialist registrars and 81% of all midwives stating that the care was collaborative. Overall, 64% of obstetricians and midwives stated that the consultant obstetrician was more likely to take overall responsibility in the case of severe hypertensive disorders, but with the management of eclampsia 47% stated that it would be the consultant obstetrician and 50% stated that the responsibility for care would be collaborative.

All obstetricians and midwives were asked if their unit was a regional referral or advisory centre for severe hypertensive disorders and, if not, if referrals were made or advice was sought from other units. Forty-three per cent stated they were a regional referral centre and 32% said referrals were made to other units. Of the 16 consultants who stated that the units in which they practised were not regional referral centres, only two said they asked for advice from another unit. The remaining fourteen consultants said they managed these cases in house, that they would ask advice very rarely and could not state when they last had. In addition, they said that they only transferred women when a neonatal cot was required. These 16 units (52% of sample) conduct approximately 45,800 deliveries annually.

Discussion

Although nearly all units surveyed did have clinical guidelines the figure should have been 100% and units without guidelines need urgently to address this and also to ensure the guidelines are known to all staff involved in maternity care. The guidelines were clearly being kept up to date, with the interviewees revealing a universal change to the use of magnesium sulphate since the publication of the Collaborative Eclampsia Trial showing this to be the preferred treatment[10]. It was also of concern that the management of some severely ill women was still not considered to be a collaborative effort.

Recommendations

- *All units should review their clinical guidelines and ensure that they are developed by a multidisciplinary team, using current evidence from national guideldines.[11]*
- *It is of concern that the concept of regional advisory centres has still not been fully developed or where they are available they are not being fully utilised.*

Thromboembolic disorders

Previous Reports have emphasised the need for vigilance with regard to the risk factors for thrombo-embolic disorders, particularly in relation to caesarean section, with the use of prophylactic measures in vulnerable women. The last Report endorsed the recommendations from the 1995 RCOG working party on prophylaxis against thromboembolism[12], which was circulated to all members and fellows of the RCOG. The standards for this section of the audit are based on the RCOG report.

Postal survey

Sixty-six per cent (171/259) of consultant maternity units in the UK stated that they had clinical guidelines for the management of thromboembolic disorders. Table 18.4.

Interviews

All obstetricians and midwives were asked if there were guidelines available to identify women at risk of developing thromboembolic disorders, and, in addition, whether prophylactic measures were used for women who had had a previous thrombosis.

Ninety-seven per cent (29/30) of consultant obstetricians, 94% (17/18) of specialist registrar obstetricians, 48% (15/31) of senior midwives and 52% (11/21) of E/F grade midwives stated that they had guidelines for identifying women at risk. All consultant obstetricians, 78% (14/19) of specialist registrar obstetricians, 48% (15/31) of senior midwives, 52% (11/21) of E/F grade midwives, 97% (29/30) of consultant anaesthetists and 95% (18/19) of specialist registrars in anaesthetics stated that prophylactic measures were used for women at risk, the remaining 21% (32/149) of staff being unsure if prophylactic measures were used.

The RCOG working party report stated that "caesarean section is a major risk factor for pulmonary embolism and the risk appears greater after an emergency procedure"[12]. All the consultant obstetricians interviewed stated that they used the RCOG risk assessment profile for categorising risk to the individual woman.

All obstetricians, midwives and anaesthetists were asked if prophylactic measures were used for women undergoing an elective or emergency caesarean section and what form these took. Ninety-one per cent (136/149) stated that prophylactic measures were used for women who had a caesarean section. Those who stated that they used prophylactic measures ($n=136$) were asked what methods they utilised, whether anticoagulants, such as low molecular weight heparin, and/or mechanical methods, such as thromboembolic stockings or pneumatic leggings. In the case of elective caesarean sections, 16% (22/136) stated that anticoagulants were used in all cases, with 63% (86/136) saying that they were used for women who were classed as high-risk cases only. With the use of mechanical methods, 39% (53/136) stated they were used in all cases, with 46% (62/136) saying they were used in high-risk cases only. Similarly, following emergency caesarean sections, 25% (34/136) stated that all women were given anticoagulants, with 57% (77/136) stating they were only used for women considered to be at high risk. Forty-nine per cent (66/136) stated that mechanical methods were used in all cases and 37% (50/136) in high risk-cases only.

Despite caesarean section being a recognised risk factor and emergency procedures increasing this risk further, it appeared that not all staff were fully conversant with the need for thromboprophylaxis, with only 91% (136/149) stating that it was used after a caesarean section. The RCOG working party report states that women fulfilling the risk assessment profile for moderate and high risk should receive anticoagulants. An emergency caesarean section, without other risk factors, is considered to be a moderate risk factor. Although all consultant obstetricians stated that they followed the RCOG recommendations, only 20% (6/30) used anticoagulants for every woman undergoing an emergency caesarean section and only 67% (20/30) did so for women considered to be at high risk.

Discussion

Despite the RCOG recommendations being available to all Members and Fellows since 1995 it is of concern that only 66% of consultant maternity units have guidelines for the management and prophylaxis of thrombo-embolic disorders. Nevertheless, in the units which participated in the study, there appears to be a fair amount of consistency between the groups interviewed. In view of the lack of randomised controlled trials into thromboprophylaxis in pregnancy and childbirth the recommendations of the RCOG working party are based on authoritative consensus opinion. One particular area of concern has been in the use of anticoagulants following caesarean section. In order to address this, a randomised controlled trial on the use of low molecular weight heparin is proposed and the pilot study is underway[13].

Recommendations

- *This survey suggests that the recommendations are not being comprehensively practised and there is a need to re-emphasise these guidelines and evaluate whether these are being implemented.*
- *Until the results of further research are available, all maternity units should have guidelines based on the RCOG recommendations.*

Infection

Previous Reports have emphasised that infection must never be underestimated as it still remains a cause of maternal mortality. The RCOG recommends that guidelines are available for the management of women with suspected major sepsis[4] and that antibiotics are given in all cases of emergency caesarean section.

Postal survey

Twenty per cent (53/259) of consultant maternity units in the UK stated that they had clinical guidelines for the management of severe genital tract infection (Table 18.4).

Interviews

All obstetricians and midwives were asked if their unit had guidelines for the management of women with suspected severe infection. Thirty-one per cent (31/100) stated that they had management guidelines, 43% (43/100) did not and 26% (26/100) were unsure. In addition, all obstetricians, midwives and anaesthetists were asked if prophylactic antibiotics were given to women undergoing a caesarean section. Eighty-two per cent (122/149) stated that antibiotics were given. Of these, 97% (119/122) stated that they were always used in emergency caesarean sections and 88% (107/122) said they were also used in elective cases.

Several of those interviewed stated that they did not have guidelines for the management of infection because each case was dealt with separately. The 31 members of staff who said they had management guidelines for severe infection, represented 21 maternity units. The guidelines supplied by these 21 units were reviewed and only two of the units had specific guidelines detailing the management of women with severe infection. Of the remaining 19 units, 13 made reference to screening for infection following pre-labour spontaneous rupture of the membranes and the use of prophylactic antibiotics following caesarean section. The guidelines from the other six units made no reference to infection at all. The staff most likely to deal with the problem of infection in the first instance, particularly in the early postnatal period, are the specialist registrars and E/F grade midwives at ward level, but 39% (7/18) of specialist registrars and 57% (12/21) of midwives were unsure if any guidelines even existed.

Discussion

It would seem from the lack of guidelines that the problem of infection is not given the consideration that the RCOG recommends.

Recommendations

- *All units need to ensure that they have agreed guidelines for the management of suspected major sepsis.*
- *Guidelines should include an antibiotic schedule which has been agreed with the local microbiology department.*
- *There should be an agreed schedule for antibiotic prophylaxis at caesarean section.*
- *The implementation of these guidelines should be regularly audited.*

Overall conclusions

This study shows that there has been an encouraging improvement in the provision of facilities and services in the maternity services throughout the UK and that many of the recommendations from the Reports have been implemented. Nevertheless, there will always be improvements to be made and this study has highlighted some areas in which these should be made as soon as practicable. Recommendations have been made at the end of each section and all maternity units, not just consultant units, are encouraged to implement these. The two main issues are concerned with the communication between all those responsible for the care of women during childbirth, particularly in relation to the development, dissemination and implementation of clinical guidelines, and the care of ill women during pregnancy and childbirth, particularly the education, training and maintenance of skills of all those responsible for their care.

The key message is that there is a commitment to the continuous improvement in the quality of care within the maternity services. The advent of clinical governance, with its assurance that quality will resume its rightful place at the heart of the NHS, will assist all those involved in maternity care to continue this process.

References

1. Department of Health. *A First Class Service: Quality in the new NHS*. London: Department of Health; 1998.

2. Hibbard, B. & Milner, D. Reports on Confidential Enquiries into Maternal Deaths: an audit of previous recommendations. *Health Trends* 1994; **26**:26-8.

3. Patel, N. (ed.) *Maternal Mortality - The Way Forward*. London: Royal College of Obstetricians & Gynaecologists; 1992.

4. Royal College of Obstetricians & Gynaecologists. *Deriving Standards from the Maternal Mortality Reports*. London; Royal College of Obstetricians & Gynaecologists; 1994.

5. The Report of the National Confidential Enquiry into Perioperative Deaths 1991-1992. *The National Confidential Enquiry into Perioperative Deaths*. London; 1993.

6. Cordingley, J. J. & Rubin, A. P. A survey of facilities for high risk women in consultant obstetric units. *International Journal of Obstetric Anesthesia* 1997; **3**:156-60.

7. Royal College of Obstetricians & Gynaecologists, Clinical Audit Unit. *Effective Procedures in Maternity Care Suitable for Audit*. London: Royal College of Obstetricians & Gynaecologists; 1997.

8. NHS Executive. *Clinical Guidelines: Using clinical guidelines to improve patient care within the NHS*. NHS Executive; 1996.

9. Royal College of Obstetricians & Gynaecologists, Clinical Audit Unit Guideline Appraisal Tool: criteria for evaluating maternity unit guidelines. Derived from Instrument as: Cluzeau F, Littlejohn J, Grimshaw J, Fader G. Draft Appraisal Instrument for Clinical Guidelines, in RCGP The Development and Implementation of Clinical Guidelines 1995, Report 26. London: Royal College of Obstetricians & Gynaecologists; 1997.

10. The Eclampsia Trial Group. Which anticonvulsant for women with eclampsia? Evidence from the Collaborative Eclampsia Trial. *Lancet* 1995; **345**: 1455-63.

11. Management of Eclampsia, Green Top Guideline No 10. London: The Royal College of Obstetricians & Gynaecologists; November 1996.

12. Royal College of Obstetricians & Gynaecologists *Report of the RCOG Working Party on Prophylaxis Against Thromboembolism in Gynaecology and Obstetrics*. London: Royal College of Obstetricians & Gynaecologists; 1995.

13. Prevention of Pulmonary Emboli and Deep Venous Thromboses After Casearean Section with Low Molecular Weight Heparin - The PEACH Pilot study 1998. Contact: Peter Brocklehurst, Perinatal Trials Service, National Perinatal Epidemiology Unit, Radcliffe Infirmary, Oxford.

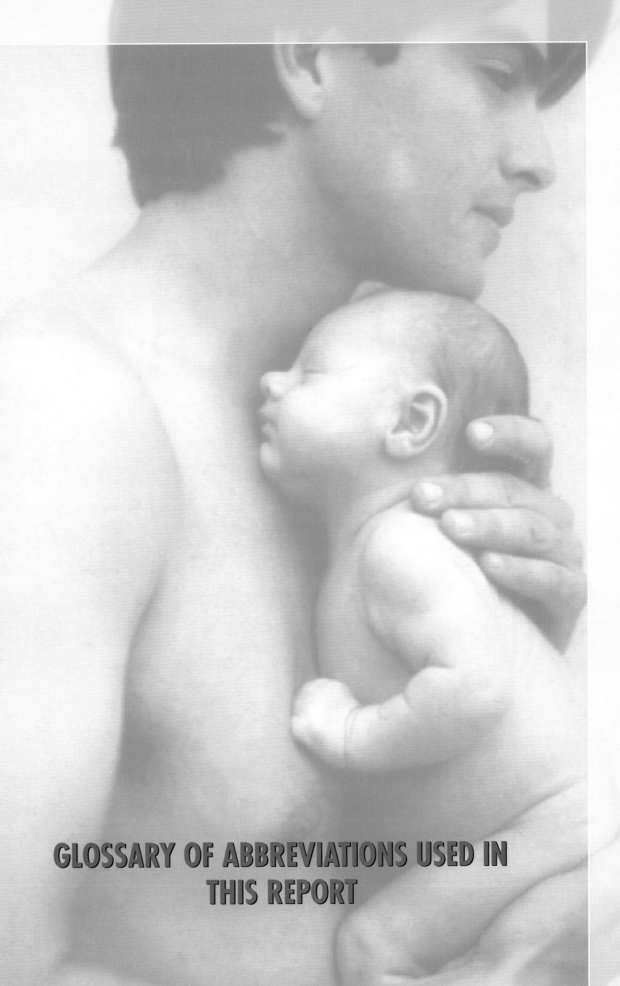

GLOSSARY OF ABBREVIATIONS USED IN
THIS REPORT

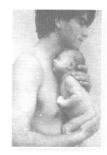

GLOSSARY OF ABBREVIATIONS USED IN THIS REPORT

A&E	-	Accident and Emergency
AFE	-	Amniotic Fluid Embolism
AIDS	-	Aquired Immune Deficiency Syndrome
APH	-	Antepartum Haemorrhage
ARDS	-	Acute Respiratory Distress Syndrome
ARM	-	Artificial Rupture of Membranes
BEST	-	British Eclampsia Survey Team
BMI	-	Body Mass Index
BP	-	Blood Pressure
CAMO	-	Chief Administrative Medical Officer
CPN	-	Community Psychiatric Nurse
CPR	-	Cardiopulmonary Resuscitation
CEMD	-	Confidential Enquiries into Maternal Deaths
CS	-	Caesarean Section
CTG	-	Cardiotocograph
CT (CAT)	-	Computerised Axial Tomography
CVP	-	Central Venous Pressure
D&C	-	Dilatation and Curettage
DGH	-	District General Hospital
DIC	-	Disseminated Intravascular Coagulation
DOA	-	Dead on Arrival
DPH	-	Director of Public Health
DVT	-	Deep Vein Thrombosis
ECG	-	Electrocardiogram
ECM	-	External Cardiac Massage
EMD	-	Electromechanical Dissociation
FFP	-	Fresh Frozen Plasma
FH	-	Fetal Heart
GP	-	General Practitioner
Hb	-	Haemoglobin Concentration
HDU	-	High Dependency Unit

HELLP	-	Haemolysis, Elevated Liver Enzymes and Low Platelets
HES	-	Hospital Episode Statistics
HIV	-	Human Immunodeficiency Virus
ICD	-	International Classification of Diseases
ICU	-	Intensive Care Unit
IUCD	-	Intrauterine Contraceptive Device
IUD	-	Intrauterine Death
IV	-	Intravenous
IVF	-	In Vitro Fertilisation
LSA	-	Local Supervising Authority
MDR UK(1)	-	Maternal Death Report Form for the United Kingdom (from October 1995)
MRI	-	Magnetic Resonance Imaging
NCEPOD	-	National Confidential Enquiry into Peri-Operative Deaths
OC	-	Oral Contraceptive
ONS	-	Office of National Statistics
PA	-	Pulmonary Artery
PE	-	Pulmonary Embolism
PET	-	Pre-eclamptic Toxaemia
PG	-	Prostaglandin
PIN	-	Pregnancy Induced Hypertension
PPH	-	Postpartum Haemorrhage
PROM	-	Premature Rupture of Membranes
PTE	-	Pulmonary Thromboembolism
RCOG	-	Royal College of Obstetricians & Gynaecologists
RHA	-	Regional Health Authority
RMA	-	Regional Midwifery Assessor
SB	-	Stillbirth
SHO	-	Senior House Officer
SpR	-	Specialist Registrar
SLE	-	Systematic Lupus Erythematosus
SSRI	-	Serotonin Selective Reuptake
SVD	-	Spontaneous Vaginal delivery
TED	-	Thromboembolic Disease
URTI	-	Upper Respiratory Tract Infection
VSD	-	Ventricular Septal Defect
VTE	-	Venous Thromboembolism
WBC	-	White Blood Count

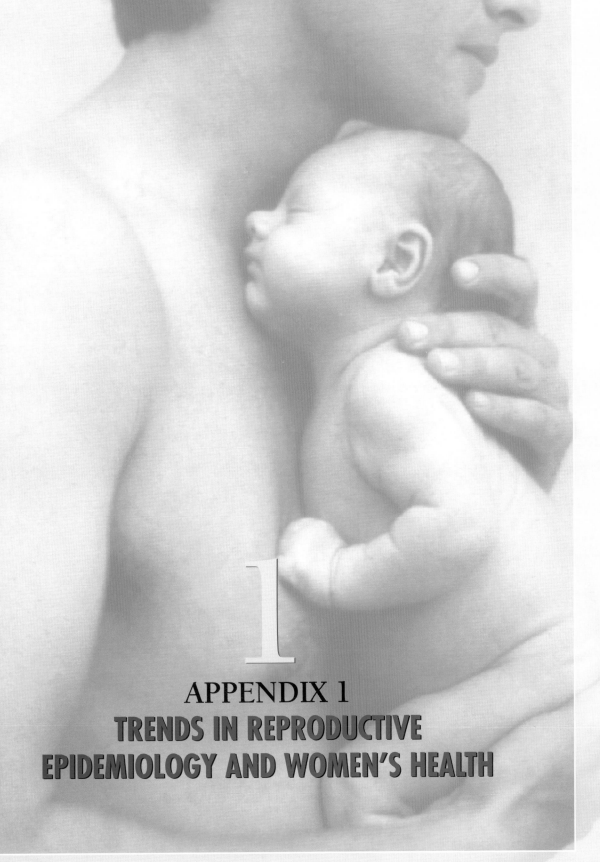

1

APPENDIX 1
TRENDS IN REPRODUCTIVE
EPIDEMIOLOGY AND WOMEN'S HEALTH

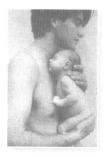

APPENDIX 1
TRENDS IN REPRODUCTIVE EPIDEMIOLOGY AND WOMEN'S HEALTH

Introduction

The purpose of this Appendix is to provide statistics which place in context the data on maternal deaths given earlier. Changes in the population at risk could change the number of deaths expected if rates remain at the same level. This Appendix will provide an overview of trends in reproductive epidemiology by discussing conceptions, abortions and births. It will discuss the fertility of women in different age groups and at different parities, and also present relevant information about problems around the time of delivery. The Appendix will also discuss other aspects of women's health highlighted in this Report. In particular, a section is devoted to statistics on obesity and on smoking in pregnancy.

Overall trends in reproductive epidemiology

Maternities and estimated pregnancies

Maternities are pregnancies that result in a live birth at any gestation or a stillbirth occurring at 24 completed weeks' gestation or later. Statistics on these outcomes can be given with great confidence since they are required by law to be registered. It is impossible, however, to know the exact number of pregnancies which occurred during this, or any preceding, triennium, since not all pregnancies result in a registrable live or stillbirth. Other outcomes of a pregnancy can be a legal termination (which is also registrable by law), a miscarriage, or an ectopic pregnancy.

Estimated pregnancies

The combination of the number of maternities, together with legal terminations, hospital admissions for spontaneous abortions (at less than 24 weeks' gestation) and ectopic pregnancies, with an adjustment to allow for the period of gestation and maternal ages at conception, provide an estimate of the number of pregnancies as shown in Table A.1. The resulting total, however, is still clearly an underestimate of the actual number of pregnancies since these figures do not include other pregnancies which miscarry early, those where the woman is not admitted to hospital, or indeed those where the woman herself may not even know she is pregnant. Data in previous Reports were given for England and Wales only, and these are included for comparison.

Table A.1

Triennia	Maternities	Legal abortions	Spontaneous abortions	Ectopic pregnancies	Total estimated pregnancies
Estimated number of pregnancies (in thousands); England & Wales 1976-93 and United Kingdom; 1991-96.					
England and Wales					
1976-1978	1781.3	324.6	158.3+	11.6	2275.8
1979-1981	1910.9	380.5	134.3*	12.1	2437.8
1982-1984	1905.8	393.1	113.6*	14.4	2426.9
1985-1987	1987.9	451.1	N/A	N/A	2439.0
1988-1990	2073.0	512.7	277.2*	24.0	2886.9
1991-1993	2045.3	485.7	233.8*	27.0	2791.8
United Kingdom					
1991-1993	2315.2	525.7	266.4*	30.2	3137.4
1994-1996	2197.6	518.8	164.7*	33.5	2914.6

+ ICD (8th revision) 640-645
* ICD (9th revision) 634-638
N/A: Not available
Source: ONS Birth statistics Series FM1
 ONS Abortion statistics Series AB
 Dept of Health: Hospital Episodes Statistics
 Welsh Office: Hospital Activity Analysis
 Scottish Morbidity Records (SMR) 1 Inpatients and Daycases Acute
 Scottish Morbidity Records (SMR) 2 Inpatients and Daycases Maternity
 DHSS Northern Ireland

Using these sources of data, ONS estimated that 75 % of pregnancies in the UK between 1994 and 1996 led to a maternity which resulted in one or more registrable live or stillbirths. A further 18% of pregnancies were legally terminated under the 1967 Abortion Act. The remaining 7% of known pregnancies were admitted to hospital because of a spontaneous abortion or an ectopic pregnancy. Spontaneous abortions which resulted in a day stay or where the woman was not admitted to hospital are not included in these data. The striking changes in the estimated number of spontaneous abortions and ectopic pregnancies between 1982-84 and 1988-90 are most likely to be due to the different ways the data were collected during these triennia and the different sampling and grossing-up procedures used. There appears to be no obvious change in clinical patterns over this period which could have contributed to this increase in number.

Trends in legal abortion

Some women die following legal (and in the past, illegal) abortion. Legal abortion was introduced in 1968, following the Abortion Act 1967, in England, Wales and Scotland. By the end of 1996, over 3.9 million legal terminations of pregnancy had been carried out on residents of Great Britain. The Abortion Act 1967 does not apply to Northern Ireland, where only a small number of legal terminations are performed each year on medical grounds under the case law that applied in England and Wales before the Abortion Act 1967. However, some women having legal terminations in Great Britain, of which there were 4,808 in 1994-96, gave a usual address in Northern Ireland.

Table A.2

Legal abortions in Great Britain to women resident in United Kingdom; 1988-96.		
Triennia	Number of abortions	Rate per 1,000 women aged 15-44
1988-90	545618	15.0
1991-93	520451	14.5
1994-96	518764	14.1

Source: England and Wales - ONS Abortion statistics Series AB
           Scotland - Information & Statistics Division

Figure A.1

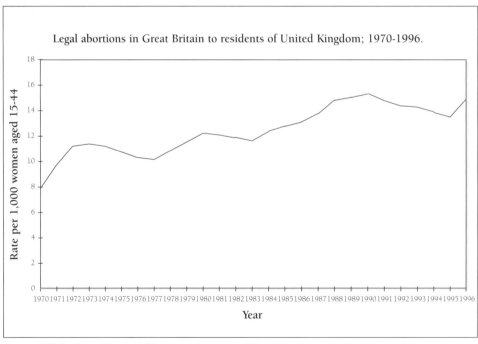

Legal abortions in Great Britain to residents of United Kingdom; 1970-1996.

Source: ONS Abortion statistics Series AB
            Scotland - Information & Statistics Division

Table A.2 shows the number of legal abortions in Great Britain and the rate per 1,000 women aged 15-44, for each of the most recent three triennia. Figure A.1 shows the legal abortion rate for each individual year over the period 1970 to 1996. From 1970 to 1995 the rate of abortion to women aged 15-44 decreased continually. This trend reversed in 1996, however, when the rate increased. This was due, at least in part, to a pill scare in September 1995[1]. In this current Report, one woman died after legal abortion.

Following the introduction of legal abortion the number of maternal deaths following illegal abortions fell sharply. In 1970-72 (the first full triennium during which legal abortion was available) there were 37 reported deaths from illegal abortion, falling to one in 1979-81. No maternal deaths from illegal abortion have been reported since, including this triennium.

Birth rates and general fertility trends

Birth rates and fertility trends are important in the context of this Enquiry as changes in patterns of childbearing may affect the number of maternal deaths. Since the England and Wales Enquiry started in 1952, joined by Scotland and Northern Ireland in 1985, almost 36 million births have been registered in the United Kingdom. The total number of births and the fertility rate for each triennium since 1976-78 are given in Table A.3. Figure A.2 shows the general fertility rate (births per 1,000 women aged 15-44) over the period 1952-96.

Table A.3

Total number of births (live and still) and fertility rate, United Kingdom; 1976-96.		
Triennia	Total births (in 1,000's)	Fertility rate per 1,000 women aged 15-44
1976-78	2083.3	60.9
1979-81	2235.4	64.2
1982-84	2183.2	60.7
1985-87	2293.7	61.9
1988-90	2374.8	62.5
1991-93	2346.8	63.4
1994-96	2228.6	60.9

Source: England and Wales - ONS Birth statistics Series FM1
        Scotland - Registrar General's Annual Report series
        Northern Ireland - Registrar General's Annual Report series

As can be seen in Figure A.2, fertility increased from 1952 until it peaked in 1964 at 94 births per 1,000 women. This was followed by a steady decrease in the general fertility rate until 1977, when it reached a minimum of 59 births per 1,000 women. The rate then fluctuated, but between 1982 and 1990 there was a small but sustained increase, reaching 64 per 1,000 in 1990. The rate for the three years covered by this Report fell to 61 per 1,000.

Figure A.2

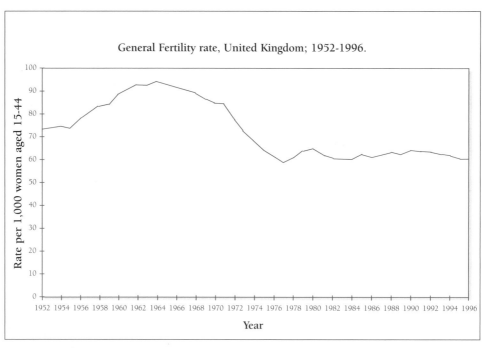

General Fertility rate, United Kingdom; 1952-1996.

Source: ONS Birth statistics Series FM1

The small fluctuations in fertility rates since 1977 conceal wider medical and social changes affecting reproductive epidemiology. Reduced perinatal and infant mortality mean that more babies are surviving into childhood. An increasing proportion of births are outside marriage, and there are changing patterns in the age at which women have children.

Maternities by age and parity

The pattern of fertility in terms of maternal age and age at first birth has changed over recent years. Women are, on average, older at childbirth, in part due to older age at marriage. On the other hand, figures for parity remain constant. These changes can make an important contribution to maternal mortality because the risk of maternal mortality becomes higher with increasing age and parity.

Between 1986 and 1996 fertility rates among women in their thirties and forties increased considerably. In contrast, rates among women in their twenties fell. Nevertheless, the late twenties remain the peak child-bearing years, with fertility rates substantially above those for all other age groups.

As a result of a special exercise undertaken in England and Wales, shown in Table A.4, it is possible to estimate separately, using survey data, the changes in the age and parity distribution of live births in England and Wales for each triennium between 1988-90 and 1994-96. More women are delaying childbearing. In 1988-90, 49% of women having their first child were aged under 25 whereas by 1994-96 only 39% were aged under 25. Similar data are not routinely available for Scotland and Northern Ireland.

Table A.4

Percentage distribution of all live births by parity and age at first birth 1988-96; England and Wales only.			
	1988-90	1991-93	1994-96
Parity			
0	41	40	40
1	34	34	34
2	16	17	18
3	6	6	6
4	3	3	3
Total	100	100	100
Age (years)			
<20	8	7	7
20-24	27	24	20
25-29	35	35	34
30-34	21	24	28
35-39	7	8	10
40+	1	1	2
Total	100	100	100
Age (years) at first birth			
<20	16	15	14
20-24	33	29	25
25-29	33	34	33
30-34	14	17	21
35+	4	5	7
Total	100	100	100

Source: ONS
Source: Unpublished ONS fertility tables
Note - Figures may not exactly total due to rounding
Note - Exact parity figures are only available for births inside marriage
The data in this table are based on estimates of "true" parity order estimated by using information from the General Household Survey

Maternities by marital status

One of the most striking trends in recent years has been the dramatic increase in both the number and proportion of births occurring outside marriage. By 1996, 35% of births in the UK were outside marriage. Nevertheless, this increase has been concentrated in births outside marriage registered by both parents, usually giving the same address. During the period 1980 to 1996 the proportion of all births that occurred outside marriage and were registered by the mother alone remained at 6-8%. The proportions of births outside marriage in England and Scotland were the same (36%). In Wales the proportion of births outside marriage has been increasing faster than for the other countries, reaching 41% in 1996. The proportion of births outside marriage in Northern Ireland (26%), was smaller than in Great Britain, although the rate of increase over the previous decade was similar, as shown in Figure A.3.

Figure A.3

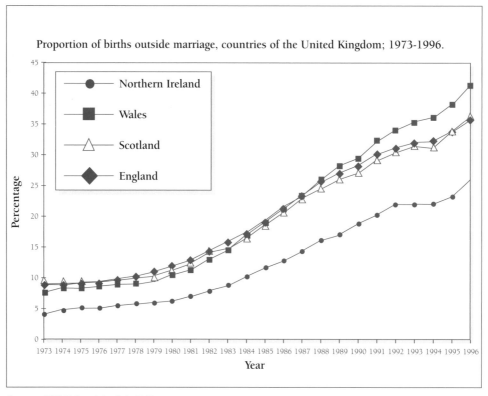

Proportion of births outside marriage, countries of the United Kingdom; 1973-1996.

Source: ONS Birth statistics Series FM1
          Registrar General for Scotland Annual Report
          Registrar General Northern Ireland Report

Fertility rates in the four constituent countries of the UK follow the same pattern but those for Northern Ireland always remain higher than for the other countries. In 1994-96, 34% of births within marriage in Northern Ireland were the woman's third or higher order birth, compared with 24% of births in England and Wales.

Maternities by ethnic origin

Since 1994 ethnic origin has been collected on the Enquiry notification forms. To place these data in context it would be ideal to compare them with the proportion of maternities by the mother's ethnic origin. Unfortunately, however, ethnic origin is not recorded at birth registration. Instead, the parents' countries of birth are recorded. This is becoming a less reliable proxy for ethnic origin as increasing proportions of women from different ethnic groups were born in the United Kingdom. For comparisons with the data recorded for this Enquiry, therefore, we analyse the population of all women aged 15-44 by their ethnic group. Ethnic origin was asked for the first time in the 1991 Census of Great Britain and can be estimated from the Labour Force Survey. Table A.5 shows the female population of Great Britain in 1996 in the childbearing ages by ethnic group. In 1996, 3% of all women aged 15-44 considered themselves of Black ethnic origin (including mixed), 2% Indian, and 1% Pakistani. In total 7% of women in these age groups considered themselves to belong to an ethnic minority group.

Table A.5

Female population of Great Britain by Ethnic group and age; 1996 (in thousands).						
Ethnic group	Total 15-44	15-19	20-24	25-29	30-34	35-44
Black - Caribbean	143	17	13	23	37	53
Black - African	93	8	13	20	27	25
Black - Other (non-mixed)	34	5	5	8	10	6
Black - Mixed	32	7	7	6	6	6
Indian	225	37	25	40	43	80
Pakistani	142	31	28	31	18	34
Bangladeshi	44	9	11	10	5	9
Chinese	38	5	8	6	6	13
Other - Asian (non-mixed)	45	6	5	6	10	18
Other - Other (non-mixed)	30	3	4	6	9	8
Other - Mixed	41	11	7	7	7	9
All ethnic minority groups	**867**	**139**	**126**	**163**	**178**	**261**
White	10834	1510	1618	1970	2102	3634
Not stated	4	1	1	0	1	1
Total females	**11705**	**1650**	**1745**	**2133**	**2281**	**3896**

Source: Labour Force Survey (average of 1996 Spring Summer Autumn and Winter quarters)

Mode of delivery

The proportion of deliveries by caesarean section, whether elective or emergency, has been increasing steadily. The level was 3% in the 1950s and rose to about 10% in the early 1980s. It then rose from 11% in 1989-90 to about 15% in 1994-95[2]. This trend is important in the context of this Enquiry since complications of a caesarean section may lead to a maternal death. An increase in the proportion of deliveries by caesarean section means that more women are at risk of these complications. This is discussed in Chapter 1.

The mode of delivery is highly related to both parity and age. In 1994-95 in England 5% of deliveries to women aged under 25 were elective caesareans, compared with 8% of those aged 25-34 and 13% of those aged 35 or over. Within these age groups, however, primiparous women were less likely than other women to have an elective caesarean (Table A.6). The same pattern of increasing proportions with age was also seen in the proportion of women whose delivery was by emergency caesarean. In contrast, however, emergency caesarean rates were higher for primiparous women in each age group.

Table A.6

Percentage of singleton deliveries by caesarean section by parity and age, 1994-1995; England.		elective caesarean	emergency caesarean
All ages	Total	7	9
	0	5	12
	1+	9	6
Under 25	Total	5	7
	0	4	9
	1+	6	5
25-34	Total	8	9
	0	5	14
	1+	9	5
35 and over	Total	13	12
	0	11	21
	1+	13	8

Source: HES

Complications during delivery

Hypertension was mentioned as an antenatal complication in 7% of deliveries in England in 1994-95[2]. Labour was induced in about half of all cases where hypertension was recorded as having complicated pregnancy. Over 80% of deliveries reported the use of anaesthetics or analgesics before or during delivery. General anaesthetic was administered in 6% of deliveries, an epidural in 20%, and spinal anaesthetic in 5%. Postpartum haemorrhage was reported in 4% of spontaneous deliveries, 11% of instrumental deliveries and 8% of deliveries by caesarean section.

Other aspects of women's health

Obesity

The Body Mass Index (BMI) is the most widely used measure of obesity. It is defined as weight (kg) divided by the square of height (m^2). Adults with a BMI between 25 and 30 inclusive are described as overweight, and those with a BMI over 30 as obese. In 1996 in England the mean BMI for women aged 16-64 was 25.8 kg/m^2. Seventeen per cent of women aged 16-64 were obese[3]. Between 1993 and 1996 the mean BMI increased, and the prevalence of obesity increased by 1.6% for women in this age group (Figure A.4). The increase was greater in women aged 25-34 and 55 and over than in the other age groups.

Figure A.4

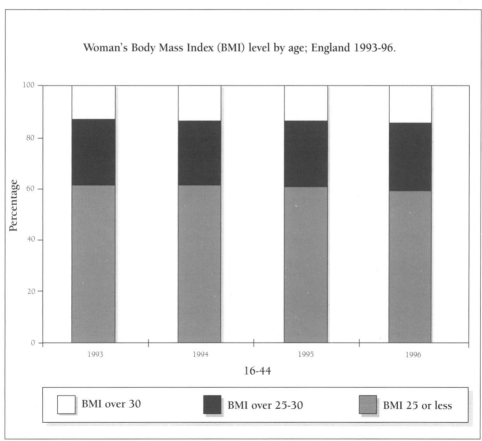

Source: Health Survey for England 1996

REPORT ON CONFIDENTIAL ENQUIRIES INTO MATERNAL DEATHS IN THE UNITED KINGDOM

Blood pressure

Raised blood pressure is a risk factor for both coronary heart disease and stroke. Various initiatives have been suggested to reduce the mean systolic blood pressure, including promoting healthy eating, sensible drinking and the reduction of obesity. Table A.7 shows that in 1996, 4% of obese women were hypertensive compared to 1% of women with a BMI below 30. A further 4 % of obese women were not hypertensive but were taking medication affecting blood pressure, compared with 1% of other women.

Table A.7

Blood pressure level of females aged 16-44 by body mass index and age, England; 1996.					
Blood pressure level*	BMI level				Total
	20 or under %	Over 20-25 %	Over 25-30 %	Over 30 %	%
Normotensive untreated	98	99	98	92	97
Normotensive treated	0	1	1	4	1
Hypertensive treated	0	0	0	1	0
Hypertensive untreated	1	1	1	3	1

* Informants were considered hypertensive if their systolic blood pressure was 160 mmHg or over or their diastolic blood pressure was 95 mmHg or over or they were taking medicine affecting blood pressure. 'Treated' means taking medication affecting blood pressure.
Source: Health Survey for England 1996

Smoking

Women's cigarette smoking in England was about half a percentage point higher in 1996 than in the previous 3 years. This suggests that the long-term downward trend in cigarette smoking amongst women has halted. There is evidence, however, that women do reduce their levels of smoking when they are pregnant. In England in 1995 a survey of women who had recently given birth showed that although 35% of these women smoked before pregnancy, only 23% continued to smoke during pregnancy. Figure A.5 shows that this reduction in the prevalence of smoking during pregnancy was seen in all age-groups, although the overall prevalence of smoking was highest for the youngest mothers and reduced at higher ages[4].

Figure A.5

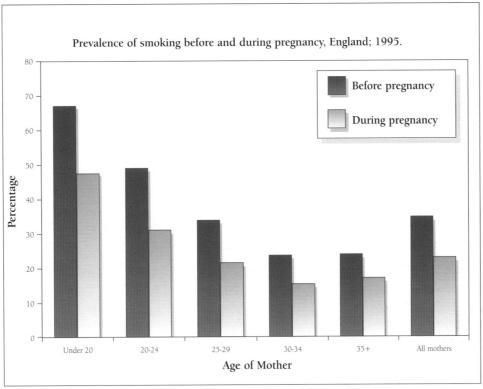

Prevalence of smoking before and during pregnancy, England; 1995.

Source: Infant feeding survey 1995

Contraceptive pill usage

In Great Britain during the period covered by this enquiry, it is estimated that one-quarter of all women aged 16-49 used the contraceptive pill. This proportion varied for different age groups as seen in Table A.8, from just under half of women aged 16-24 to around 10% of women in the oldest group. In the past there have been suggestions that the contraceptive pill carried a relatively higher risk of thrombosis. The most recent warning about possible risks of this form of contraception was during the period covered by this Enquiry. On 18 October 1995 the Committee on Safety of Medicines issued a warning that seven brands of the contraceptive pill carried such a risk. There were concerns that this scare would result in an increase in unplanned pregnancies. There was a rise in conception rates which coincided with the timing of the announcement about the safety of contraceptive pills, and so it seems likely that the pill scare had an upward effect on conceptions[1].

Table A.8 gives data from the contraception module of the Omnibus Survey. Whilst the data show a dip in the proportion of women using the pill in November 1995, around the time of the pill scare, the changes are not statistically significant. Analysis of prescription data in the Northern and Yorkshire region suggests that up to 5% of oral contraception users may have stopped using effective contraception in the October 18 to December period of 1995. Many women changed brands[5].

Table A.8

Proportion of women aged 16-49 reporting pill usage, Great Britain; 1993-97.				
Date of interview	Age of woman at interview			
	all ages	age 16-24	age 25-34	age 35 and over
November 1993	24	42	37	7
January 1994	25	50	34	7
March 1994	24	39	37	10
November 1994	26	43	37	11
January 1995	26	47	30	13
November 1995	23	36	31	10
March 1996	26	49	38	9
June 1996	26	46	36	9
September 1996	23	45	30	7
January 1997	25	37	37	10

Source: Department of Health (ONS Omnibus Survey modules)

References

1.   Wood, R., Botting, B. & Dunnell K. Trends in conceptions before and after the 1995 pill scare. *Population Trends* 89.London: TSO; 1997.

2.   NHS Maternity Statistics, England:1989-90 to 1994-95, Department of Health Statistical Bulletin, December 1997.

3.   Prescott-Clarke, P. & Primatesta P.(eds) *Health Survey for England 1996*. London: TSO;. 1998.

4.   Foster, K., Lader, D. & Cheeseborough, S. *Infant Feeding Survey 1995*. London: TSO; 1997.

5.   Roberts, S.J. The immediate effects of the pill safety scare on usage of combined oral contraceptives in North East England. *Journal of Epidemiology and Community Health*, 1997; **51**: 332-3.

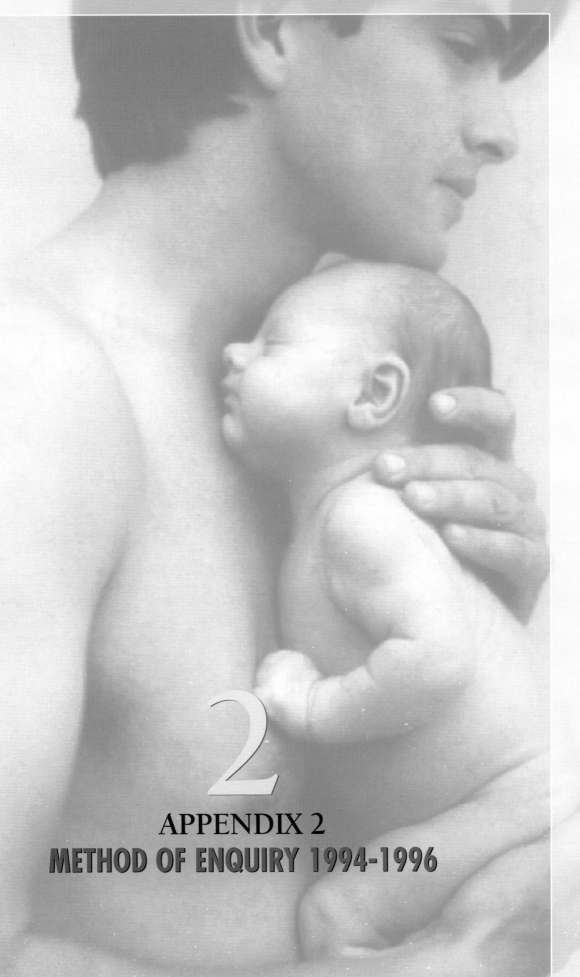

2

APPENDIX 2
METHOD OF ENQUIRY 1994-1996

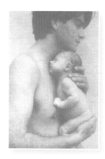

APPENDIX 2
METHOD OF ENQUIRY 1994-1996

Historical background

This is the fourth Report to cover the whole of the United Kingdom, replacing the three separate Reports for England and Wales, Scotland and Northern Ireland. The England and Wales reports were published at three-yearly intervals from 1952 to 1984. The Reports for Scotland were published at different intervals from 1965 to 1985, the last covering both maternal and perinatal deaths. Northern Ireland Reports were started in 1956 and were published four-yearly until 1967; because of the small number of maternal deaths the next Report covered 10 years from 1968 to 1977, and the last Report covered the seven year period 1978 - 1984. The relatively small number of deaths in Scotland and Northern Ireland led to the decision of the four Chief Medical Officers to change to a combined UK Report after 1984. This decision also ensured maintenance of confidentiality.

England and Wales

The responsibility for initiating an enquiry into a maternal death rests with the Director of Public Health (DPH) in England, or in Wales with the Director of Public Health Medicine/Chief Administrative Medical Officer (CAMO) of the District in which the woman was usually resident. An enquiry form MDR(UK)1 is sent to obstetricians, anaesthetists, pathologists, general practitioners, midwives and any other professionals who were concerned with the care of the woman.

When all available information about the death has been collected the DPH forwards the form to the appropriate Regional obstetric assessor in England, or the DPHM/CAMO to the Welsh obstetric assessor. The relevant anaesthetic assessors review all cases where there had been involvement of an anaesthetist, and midwifery assessors where the involvement of a midwife may have affected the outcome. In addition every possible attempt is made to obtain full details of any autopsy or pathological investigations, which are then reviewed by the appropriate pathology assessors. The assessors add their comments and opinions regarding the cause or causes of death.

Statistical data are supplied by the Office for National Statistics (ONS).

The completed form is returned to the Medical Co-ordinators, acting on behalf of the Chief Medical Officers of the Department of Health or for Wales, as appropriate. The central Assessors in obstetrics and gynaecology, anaesthetics, pathology, psychiatry, general medicine or midwifery as required then review all available recorded facts about each case and assess the factors that may have led to death.

Scotland

In Scotland, the system of enquiry is broadly similar except that a single panel of assessors considers all cases. Each obstetric assessor is responsible for a geographical area which includes more than one Health Board. Two anaesthetic assessors cover one half of the country each and all cases are seen by a single pathology assessor. The allocation of cases to diagnostic category is undertaken by the full panel of assessors each year.

On receipt in the Scottish Office Department of Health (SODH) of a certificate of maternal death from the General Registrar's Office (Scotland) an enquiry form is sent to the Chief Administrative Medical Officer (CAMO) of the Health Board of residence of the woman concerned. Since August 1995 the enquiry form used is MDR(UK)1; prior to this it was a specific form for Scotland, the MD1. As in England and Wales, the CAMO takes responsibility for organising completion of the form by all professional staff involved in caring for the woman. When this is achieved it is passed to the appropriate obstetric assessor, who determines whether further data are required before the case is submitted for discussion and classification to the full panel of assessors. In cases where an anaesthetic had been given or an autopsy or pathological investigation undertaken he passes the form to the appropriate assessors for their further comments. The form is then returned to the Medical Co-ordinator at SODH, who retains it from that time until it has been fully considered, classified and used for preparation of the Report. As for the other countries at all times each form is held under conditions of strict confidentiality and is anonymised before being provided to assessors compiling the Report.

Additional information is obtained from statistics collected and analysed by the Information and Statistics Division of the Scottish Health Service Common Services Agency. This is available from routine hospital discharge data collected by general and maternity hospitals. The coverage by Form SMR2, the maternal discharge summary, is now almost universal at 98% of registered births. General practitioners and hospital and community medical and midwifery staff assist in ensuring that deaths occurring at home are included in the Enquiry.

Northern Ireland

Maternal deaths are reported to the Director of Public Health (DPH) of the appropriate Health and Social Services Board, who initiates completion of the maternal death form, by those involved in the care of the patient. On completion, forms are sent to the Department of Health and Social Services. As in Scotland, one panel of assessors deals with all cases. The assessors are asked to consider the report, to give their views on classification and indicate whether avoidable factors were present.

Central Assessment

The Assessors review each case thoroughly, taking into account the case history, the results of pathological investigations and findings at autopsy, before allotting the case to be counted in a specific Chapter in the Report. Their assessment occasionally varies with the underlying cause of death as given on the death certificate and classified by the Registrars General using the International Classification of Diseases, Injuries and Causes of Death - tenth revision (ICD10). This is because, although the death may have been coded for multiple organ failure as the terminal event, it could have been precipitated by an obstetric cause such as septicaemia from an infected caesarean section. Although maternal deaths reported to this Enquiry are assigned and counted only in one Chapter, they may also be referred to in other Chapters; thus a death assigned to hypertensive disorder of pregnancy, in which haemorrhage and anaesthesia also played a part, may be discussed in all three Chapters.

Authors

Chapters are drafted by Central Assessors. Strict confidentiality is observed at all stages of the Enquiry, and identifying features are erased from all forms. After preparation of the Report, and before publication, all the maternal death report forms and related documents are destroyed.

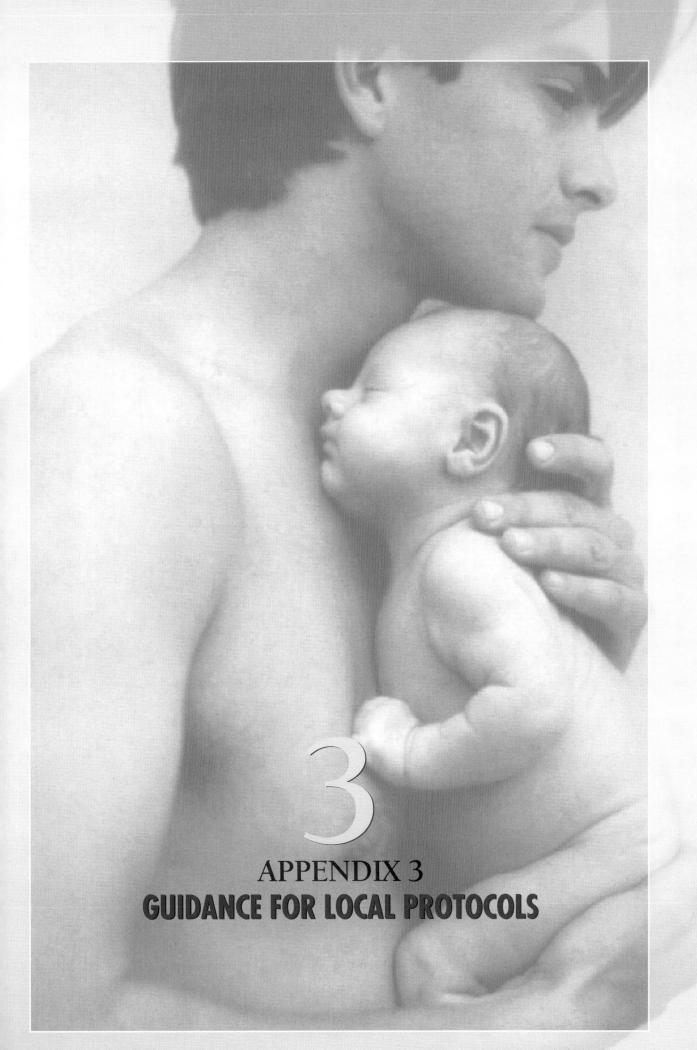

3
APPENDIX 3
GUIDANCE FOR LOCAL PROTOCOLS

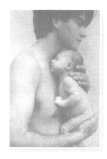

APPENDIX 3
GUIDANCE FOR LOCAL PROTOCOLS

With thanks to Kathie Bell and Dr Jean Chapple of Kensington & Chelsea and Westminster Health Authority for allowing this adaptation of a local protocol developed for North Thames Regional Health Authority to be given as an example which can be modified to suit local circumstances.

1   Introduction

1.1   The Confidential Enquiry into Maternal Deaths is a triennial Report which gives an overview of the numbers and causes of maternal deaths in the United Kingdom. The collated and anonymised information shows where improvements in clinical practice or service provision may help to prevent future deaths. It is therefore important that all cases are notified promptly so that full information on each case is readily available.

1.2   The purpose of these guidelines is to assist professionals working in both primary and secondary care in developing local policies which ensure effective management in the rare event of a maternal death.

1.3   Professionals who are involved in providing both primary and secondary care play an important role in participating in the on-going Confidential Enquiry into Maternal Deaths firstly by recognising that a maternal death has occurred and secondly by ensuring that the appropriate people have been notified.

2   Definition of a maternal death (International Classification of Diseases (ICD code 9))

2.1   A maternal death is defined as **any** death which occurs **during or within one year of pregnancy, ectopic pregnancy or abortion** which is **directly** or **indirectly** related to these conditions.

2.2   A **Direct** maternal death is defined as a death resulting from obstetric complications of the pregnancy state (pregnancy, labour and puerperium), from interventions, omissions, incorrect treatment, or from a chain of events resulting from any of the above.

2.3   An **Indirect** maternal death is defined as a death that resulted from previously existing disease, or disease that developed during pregnancy and which was not due to direct obstetric causes, but which was aggravated by the physiological affects of pregnancy. These include cases of self harm as a consequence of postnatal depression

2.4   A **Fortuitous** death is defined as a death that occurs from unrelated causes which happen to occur in the pregnancy or puerperium, i.e. some malignancies, domestic violence, road traffic accidents, etc. They are also important causes of death from the aspect of wider public health.

2.5   A **Late** death is defined as a death that occurs between 42 days and one year after abortion, miscarriage or delivery that is due to **direct or indirect** maternal causes. *Late Fortuitous* deaths can sometimes also be important.

3   Recognising a maternal death

3.1   The International Classification of Diseases (ICD) definition of a **Direct**, **Indirect** or **Fortuitous** maternal death is one which occurs during or up to 42 days after a termination of pregnancy, miscarriage, ectopic pregnancy or delivery. In addition, the ICD recognises **Late** maternal deaths which occur between 42 days and one year after delivery and are also subject to Enquiry and therefore require reporting. Thus it is apparent that a maternal death may occur in a multitude of both clinical and non-clinical settings.

3.2   A maternal death may include those women who die following a miscarriage, termination of pregnancy, suicide from postnatal depression, death from cardiac disease or any medical disorder, ectopic pregnancy, following a surgical procedure and even following a road traffic accident. It often includes women who die in ICUs from conditions such as ARDS or HELLP which develop as result of the predisposing cause.

3.3   When developing local policies it is therefore important both to involve and disseminate information on the notification of and management of the subsequent enquiry into a maternal death to the following professionals who may have cared for the woman:

Obstetricians and Gynaecologists
Midwives, (both hospital and community)
General Practitioners
Health Visitors
Community Nurses
Practice Nurses
Psychiatrists and community psychiatric nurses
Physicians
Surgeons
Managers of maternity or obstetric trusts
Mortuary Department
Hospital Nurses
Accident & Emergency Staff
Registrars and Senior House Officers
Intensive Care Unit Staff
Pathology Consultants

4 Responsibility for reporting a maternal death

4.1 A maternal death may occur in the community or in the hospital. The Enquiry is started by the Director of Public Health of the district in which the woman lived. The responsibility for notifying the Director of Public Health that a maternal death has occurred should rest with either the consultant, or midwife, or general practitioner who had overall responsibility for the pregnancy or with the consultant or general practitioner treating the woman during her final illness if the death occurs within one year following the end of her pregnancy. It does not matter if more than one professional notifies the Director of Public Health as case ascertainment is more important than duplication of notifications.

5 Managing a maternal death: provider unit guidelines

5.1 For maternal deaths occurring in hospital it is advisable for the director of the relevant department to appoint one person who has overall responsibility for ensuring that the local policies are followed. The policy should detail who, for the particular department, will act as co-ordinator. Because a maternal death may occur in a variety of clinical areas within the hospital setting (for example, in Intensive Care units or Accidents & Emergency departments) it may be advisable always to nominate a senior midwife or supervisor of midwives to undertake the role of co-ordinator.

5.2 The role of the co-ordinator may be both complex and demanding. He/she must ensure that a confidential accurate record of each part of the procedure that has been followed is maintained. The development of a quick check list containing dates and times may be useful. The co-ordinator for the duration of this process should be released from their normal duties.

5.3 The co-ordinator should then ensure a check list of the following is drawn up and completed:

- An experienced member of staff is nominated to act as the relatives' main point of contact to prevent conflicting information being given.

- The consultant on call, if not already present, should be contacted and must meet the relatives as soon as possible. If the woman already has a named consultant he or she should be informed when next on duty.

- If a supervisor of midwives has not been nominated to act as co-ordinator then, in accordance with The Midwives Code of Practice (UKCC 1994) Code 59, a supervisor must be notified that a maternal death has occurred.

- The mortuary department should be informed that a maternal death has occurred and to expect the patient. The mortuary attendant may inform the pathologist on-call; if not it will be the responsibility of the woman's consultant to do so. Guidelines for the procedures to be followed in a maternal autopsy are available from the Royal College of Pathologists. If at all possible, a post-mortem should be undertaken in order to confirm the cause of death. The consultant present should seek permission for a post-mortem from the woman's next of kin. If the cause of death is unknown, the coroner is informed and he/she will be responsible for ordering a post-mortem.

- The case notes and all documentation should be completed, photocopied and secured at the first opportunity. It should be noted that the coroner may decide to hold a hearing on the case. If this happens the case notes and documentation will be sent to the Coroners office.

- If appropriate, the local untoward incident policy should be activated and an internal investigation initiated.

- Staff involved in the case may require support. Local policies may already be in place to address this issue; if policies do not exist then support may be sought from personnel such as the hospital chaplain or the provider unit staff counsellor.

5.3   In the event of the baby dying in the uterus the following should be taken into consideration:

The definition of a stillbirth does not include the removal of a dead baby from its dead mother at post-mortem for the purpose of ascertaining the cause of death. This is because the post-mortem is being carried out on the mother rather than the baby. Therefore, registration of a baby in these circumstances over 24 weeks gestation as a death is not **legally** required. This advice has been given by Registrar General (Office for National Statistics). However, consideration must be shown to the wishes of the family. A medical practitioner may issue a death certificate for the dead baby as stillborn. Most Registrars of Births, Deaths and Marriages will comply but local policies in this respect should be checked in order to prevent confusion and further distress for the family.

As the majority of pathologists will tend to remove the baby from the mother's body at post-mortem it is sensible for the local stillbirth/neonatal death procedure to be followed whether the baby is to be registered as a death or not. It would also be helpful for the normal CESDI procedure to be followed.

5.4   The relative may wish for their local priest, vicar, rabbi, or whoever is applicable to their religious denomination, to be notified. They may also wish for this person to be with them at the hospital. If they are uncertain or would like someone of faith to be with them, the hospital chaplain should be contacted.

5.5   The Trust Chief Executive Officer, the Director Clinical Director, the Consumer Affairs, Complaints, and Risk Manager should be notified when next on duty.

5.6   If applicable, the community midwife (midwives) and general practitioner who were involved in the patient's care should be notified.

5.7   Clinical managers within the Department should be notified when next on duty particularly in case they receive a query in relation to the case.

5.8   Arrangements should be made for the woman's family to meet as soon as possible with her consultant. At least one further meeting should be arranged for when the results of investigations are available, in order for the findings to be comprehensively discussed with the woman's close relatives.

6 Those whom the provider unit must inform in the event of a maternal death

6.1 A death certificate must be promptly and accurately completed by the consultant. It is appropriate for the relatives to deliver the certificate to the registrar of births and deaths.

6.2 The Coroner should be notified if the cause of death is unknown.

6.3 The "Coroner's officer" (who is often a policeman) usually works with the coroner but may not necessarily be based in the same area. It is worth having the local telephone numbers and addresses of both the coroner and his officer detailed in the local policy.

6.4 In some areas the Coroner's officer may insist on being present when the relatives visit the body (bodies) in the mortuary. Sensitive handling and co-ordination will be required if this situation occurs.

6.5 The consultant responsible for the case **must** inform their Director of Public Health at the Health Authority that a maternal death has occurred. It is appropriate for this to be done during office hours.

6.6 Once notified, the Director of Public Health will liaise with the consultant and request further information which may be required for the official report.

6.7 If the death of the baby has also occurred the local Confidential Enquiry into Stillbirths, Deaths and Infancy office must be notified.

6.8 The woman's general practitioner and health visitor must be informed as soon as possible on the next working day.

6.9 The Local Supervising Authority Officer must be informed as soon as possible on the next working day.

6.10 If the woman has been admitted having been treated or booked in another area, the senior midwife and consultant at the hospital must be informed.

6.11 If the woman was not resident in the hospital's local district, the local Director of Public Health will ensure that the Director of Public Health in the area of residence is notified.

6.12 If the death has occurred outside the maternity department, the consultant, general practitioner or midwife in charge of the pregnancy should be informed.

6.13 Social services should also be notified if the family social circumstances are applicable or if a live baby requires care and the family requires support.

7   Managing a maternal death in primary care

7.1   The woman's general practitioner will be responsible for ensuring that the Director of Public Health at the Health Authority has been notified.

7.2   The general practitioner should also notify the hospital on the next working day if the woman had delivered or received care there.

7.3   Each general practice should ensure that all staff in the primary care team have access to and understand the procedures to be followed if a maternal death occurs.

7.4   The recommendations outlined above should reflect this.

8   Completing the enquiry form

8.1   When the local Director of Public Health in the woman's district of residence is informed of a maternal death he/she must request a confidential enquiry form from the Department of Health Dr Gwyneth Lewis (Principal Medical Officer; 0171 972 4345) and have as many details as possible to hand (i.e. Name, DoB, DoD, address).After completing initial details of the case the form will be passed back to the clinicians involved for local completion of the form for each death, and to ensure that forms are not lost within the hospital.

8.2   **In order to preserve anonymity no photocopies of the confidential enquiry form should be made at any time.**

9   Where to go for further advice

9.1   Further advice in reporting a maternal death may be sought from Director of Public Health at the Health Authority [append local list of DPHs to this protocol or directly from the CEMD Secretariat (see 8.1)]. Dr Lewis, at the Department of Health (see 8.1 above) is also available to give advice.

9.2   Advice may also be sought from the Regional Obstetric Assessor (append list to this protocol). It should be noted that the Director of Public Health must be informed of any written information that has been passed directly to a Regional Assessor.

9.3   The Local Supervising Authority Midwife will also be able to provide support and advice.

9.4   The local CESDI co-ordinator will advise on information that is required if the baby has also died.

Appendix

Append lists of local DPHs, CEMD Assessors, CESDI Co-ordinators and Local Supervising Authority Midwives.

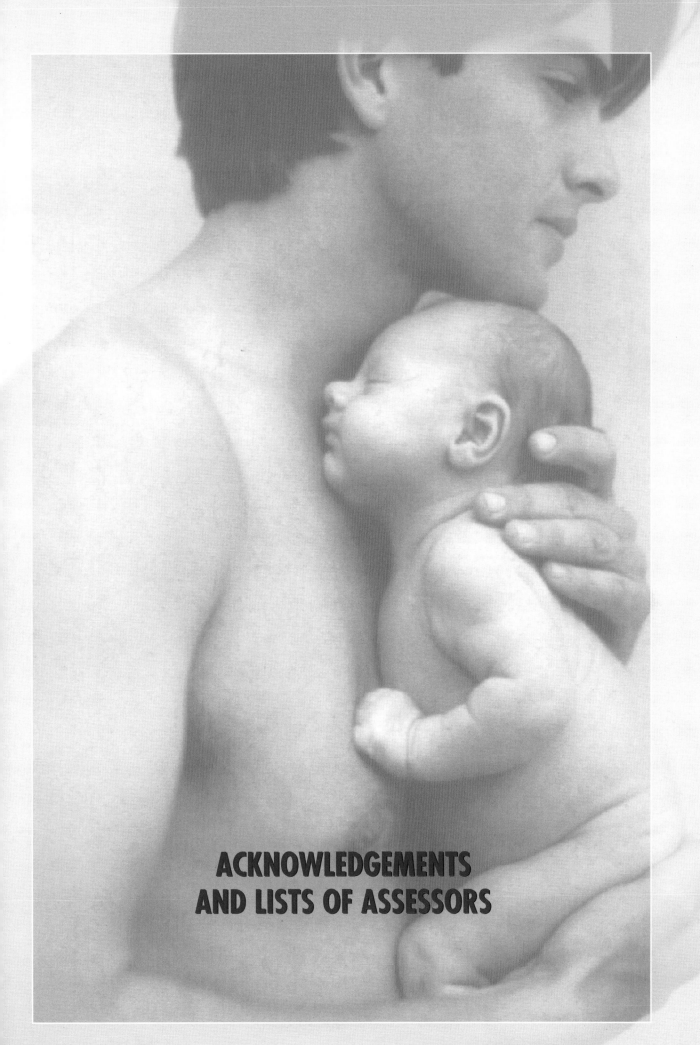

**ACKNOWLEDGEMENTS
AND LISTS OF ASSESSORS**

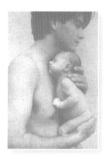

ACKNOWLEDGEMENTS AND LISTS OF ASSESSORS

Acknowledgements

This Report would not have been possible without significant help by the District Directors of Public Health in England and Northern Ireland and the Chief Administrative Medical Officers in Wales and Scotland, who initiated case reports and collected the information, and all those consultant obstetricians, anaesthetists and pathologists, general practitioners and midwives who have supplied the detailed case records and autopsy reports.

Considerable assistance has also been given by procurators fiscal who have supplied copies of reports of autopsies, and by coroners who have supplied autopsy reports and occasionally inquest proceedings to the assessors.

The staff of the Child Health Branch of the Office of National Statistics in England have worked with the Information and Statistics Division of the Common Services Agency in Scotland and Departmental statisticians in Wales and Northern Ireland to collate the statistical data and helped prepare some tables and figures.

ENGLAND
Central Assessors

Obstetrics	Professor J Drife	MD FRCOG FRCPEd FRCSEd
	Professor J Neilson	MD FRCOG
Anaesthetics	Dr S Willatts	MD FRCA FRCP
Pathology	Dr G H Millward-Sadler	BSc MB ChB FRCPath
Psychiatry	Professor R C Kumar	MD PhD FRCPsych
Medicine	Dr Michael de Swiet	MD FRCP
Midwifery	Mrs N Shaw	SRN SCM MTD BA(Hons)
	Mrs K Sallah	RN RM ADM DipPH

Local Assessors in Obstetrics

Northern Region	Professor J M Davidson MD FRCOG
Yorkshire	Mr P S Vinall FRCOG (until September 1996)
	Mr D M Hay FRCOG (from September 1996)
Trent	Miss H J Mellows FRCOG
East Anglia	Mr P J Milton MA MD FRCOG
North West Thames	Mr H G Wagman FRCSE FRCOG
North East Thames	Mr M E Setchell FRCS FRCOG
South East Thames	Professor L D Cardozo MD FRCOG (until Sept 1996)
	Mr J A Elias FRCOG (from September 1996)
South West Thames	Professor G V P Chamberlain MD FRCS FRCOG (until September 1996)
	Mr P M Coats MRCP FRCS FRCOG DCH (from September 1996)
Oxford	Mr M Gillmer MD FRCOG (until September 1996)
	Miss S Sellers (from September 1996)
South Western	Professor G M Stirrat MA MD FRCOG
West Midlands	Mr H Oliphant Nicholson FRCSE FRCOG (until September 1996)
	Professor M Whittle MD FRCOG (from September 1996)
North West	Mr P Donnai MA FRCOG
Mersey	Miss A Garden FRCOG
Wessex	Mr C P Jardine Brown FRCS FRCOG

Local Assessors in Anaesthetics

Northern	Dr M R Bryson FRCA
Yorkshire	Professor F Richard Ellis PhD FRCA (until September 1996)
	Dr I F Russell FRCA (from September 1996)
Trent	Dr A Caunt FRCA (until September 1996)
	Dr D Bogod FRCA (from September 1996)
East Anglia	Dr B R Wilkey FRCA (until September 1996)
	Dr A Nicholl FRCA FFARCSI (from September 1996)
North West Thames	Dr M Morgan FRCA (until September 1996)
	Dr A P Rubin FRCA (from September 1996)
North East Thames	Dr Miriam Frank FRCA (until September 1996)
	Dr W Aveling FRCA DRCOG (from September 1996)
South East Thames	Dr P B Hewitt FRCA
South West Thames	Dr H F Seeley MSc FRCA (until September 1996)
	Dr I Findley (from September 1996)
Oxford	Dr L E S Carrie FRCA (until September 1996)
	Dr M B Dobson MRCP FRCA (from September 1996)
South West	Dr T A Thomas FRCA
West Midlands	Dr A M Veness FRCA (until September 1996)
	Dr M Lewis FRCA (from September 1996)
North West	Dr E L Horsman MB ChB FRCA (from September 1996)

Mersey	Dr T H L Bryson FRCA (until September 1996)
	Dr R G Wilkes FRCA (from September 1996)
Wessex	Professor John Norman PhD FRCA (until September 1996)
	Dr D Brighouse BM MA FRCA (from September 1996)

Local Assessors in Pathology

Northern	Dr A R Morley MD FRCPath (until September 1996)
	Dr J N Bulmer MBChB PhD FRCPath (from September 1996)
Yorkshire	Professor M Wells MD FRCPath (until September 1996)
	Dr A Andrew MRCPath (from September 1996)
Trent	Dr L J R Brown FRCPath
East Anglia	Dr P F Roberts FRCP FRCPath (from September 1996)
North West Thames	Dr I A Lampert FRCPath
North East Thames	Dr J Crow MB BS FRCPath
South East Thames	Dr N Kirkham MD FRCPath
South West Thames	Dr M Hall FRCPath
Oxford	Dr W Gray FRCPath
South West	Professor P P Anthony FRCPath (until July 1998)
West Midlands	Dr D I Rushton MB ChB FRCPath
North West	Dr C H Buckley MD FRCPath
Mersey	Dr I W McDicken MD FRCPath
Wessex	Dr G H Millward-Sadler BSc MB ChB FRCPath (until May 1996)
	Dr A Hitchcock FRCPath (from May 1996)

Local Assessors in Midwifery

Northern	Miss L Robson MA RN RM ADM PGCAE
Yorkshire	Miss W Robinson RN RM QIDNS (until March 1998)
	Mrs E Sheppard RN RM
Trent	Miss I Cooper RN RM
East Anglia	Miss E Fern RGN RM MTD
North West Thames	Miss C Nightingale BA RN RM RSCN DipN
North East Thames	Mrs M Grant RN RM (until September 1996)
	Ms M McKenna RM RN DPSM (from September 1996)
South East Thames	Mrs I Bryan RN RM DMS
South West Thames	Mrs M Wheeler RN RM ADM BSc (Hons)
Oxford	Mrs C Osselton RN RM
South West	Mrs V Beale RN RM Dip Man MSc
West Midlands	Mrs J Goulding (until September 1996)
	Ms C McCalmont RN RM
North West	Miss J Bracken RGN RM MTD
Mersey	Miss C Whewell RN RM ADM MTD
Wessex	Mrs J Duncan RGN RM

Department of Health

| Dr Gwyneth Lewis | MSc MRCGP MFPHM |

SCOTLAND

Chairman
Dr G Gordon FRCS FRCOG

Obstetric Assessors
Dr J G Donald FRCOG (until March 1996)
Professor I Greer. MD MRCP MRCOG
Dr M Hall FRCOG
Dr W A Liston FRCOG
Dr K S Stewart MD FRCS FRCOG
Dr H P McEwan MD FRCS FRCOG

Anaesthetic Assessors
Dr J H McClure FRCA
Dr J Thorburn FRCA

Pathology Assessor
Dr E S Gray MRCPath

Midwifery Assessors
Mrs C S Docherty RN RMN RM ADM
Miss M Stewart   SRN SCM ADM

Scottish Office Department of Health
Dr Sheila Lawson degree (until September 1998)
Dr Ian Bashford MSc MRCOG (from September 1998)

NORTHERN IRELAND

Obstetric Assessor
Professor W Thompson MD FRCOG

Anaesthetic Assessor
Dr I M Bali Phd FFARCS

Pathology Assessor
Professor P G Toner DSc FRCPG. FRCPath

Midwifery Assessor
Mrs E Millar RGN RGM CHSM

Department of Health and Social Services: Northern Ireland
Dr Patrick Woods degree (to August 1997)
Dr Margaret Boyle MSc FFARCSI MFPMH (from August 1997)

REPORT ON CONFIDENTIAL ENQUIRIES INTO MATERNAL DEATHS IN THE UNITED KINGDOM

WALES

Obstetric Assessor
Professor R W Shaw MD FRCOG FRCSEd

Anaesthetic Assessor
Professor M Harmer MD FRCA

Pathology Assessor
Dr R J Kellett FRCPath

Midwifery Assessor
Ms K Isherwood RGN RM DAM

Welsh Office
Dr Joan Andrews MD FRCOG (until June 1997)
Dr Jane Ludlow FFPHM (from June 1997)

Printed in the United Kingdom for The Stationery Office
J64976, 11/98, 5673